Forensic Anthropology

Published and forthcoming titles in the Forensic Science in Focus series

Published

The Global Practice of Forensic Science
Douglas H. Ubelaker (Editor)

Forensic Chemistry: Fundamentals and Applications
Jay A. Siegel

Forensic Microbiology
David O. Carter, Jeffrey K. Tomberlin, M. Eric Benbow and Jessica L. Metcalf

Forensic Anthropology: Theoretical Framework and Scientific Basis
C. Clifford Boyd Jr and Donna C. Boyd

Forthcoming

The Future of Forensic Science
Daniel A. Martell

Humanitarian Forensics and Human Identification
Paul Emanovsky and Shuala M. Drawdy

Forensic Anthropology

Theoretical Framework and Scientific Basis

EDITED BY

C. Clifford Boyd Jr

Department of Anthropological Sciences, Radford University Forensic Science Institute
Radford University, USA

Donna C. Boyd

Department of Anthropological Sciences, Radford University Forensic Science Institute, Radford University, USA
Department of Biomedical Science, Virginia Tech Carilion School of Medicine, Roanoke, USA

WILEY

This edition first published 2018

Registered Office(s)
John Wiley & Sons, Inc., 111 River Street, Hoboken, NJ 07030, USA
John Wiley & Sons Ltd, The Atrium, Southern Gate, Chichester, West Sussex, PO19 8SQ, UK

Editorial Office
The Atrium, Southern Gate, Chichester, West Sussex, PO19 8SQ, UK

For details of our global editorial offices, customer services, and more information about Wiley products visit us at www.wiley.com.

Wiley also publishes its books in a variety of electronic formats and by print-on-demand. Some content that appears in standard print versions of this book may not be available in other formats.

Library of Congress Cataloging-in-Publication Data

Names: Boyd, C. Clifford, Jr, 1952– editor. | C. Boyd, Donna, 1960– editor.
Title: Forensic anthropology : theoretical framework and scientific basis /
edited by C. Clifford Boyd Jr, Donna C. Boyd.
Other titles: Forensic anthropology (Boyd)
Description: First edition. | Hoboken, NJ : Wiley, 2018. | Includes bibliographical
references and index.
Identifiers: LCCN 2017044528 (print) | LCCN 2017041632 (ebook) | ISBN 9781119226383 (hardback) |
ISBN 9781119226406 (pdf) | ISBN 9781119226420 (epub)
Subjects: | MESH: Forensic Anthropology–methods
Classification: LCC RA1055 (ebook) | LCC RA1055 (print) | NLM W 750 | DDC 614/.17–dc23
LC record available at https://lccn.loc.gov/2017044528

Cover Design: Wiley
Cover Images: Microscopic images courtesy of Donna C. Boyd

Set in 10.5/13.5pt Meridien by SPi Global, Pondicherry, India

10 9 8 7 6 5 4 3 2 1

We dedicate this book to our children, Merritt, Emily, and Forrest,
because butterflies taste with their feet.

Contents

About the Editors

C. Clifford Boyd Jr, PhD, RPA, received his PhD in Anthropology from the University of Tennessee–Knoxville in 1986, with a specialty in archaeology. Since 1986, he has taught at Radford University, Virginia, and is currently professor of anthropological sciences, codirector of the RU Forensic Science Institute, and consultant for the Virginia Office of the Chief Medical Examiner. He has conducted archaeological and skeletal analyses of remains from prehistoric, historic, and forensic sites in Tennessee and Virginia for 38 years. In 1998, he was named Professional Archeologist of the Year by the Archeological Society of Virginia. In 2008, he received an Outstanding Faculty Award from the State Council of Higher Education in Virginia. In 2016, he was awarded the Ellis R. Kerley Foundation Research Award for excellence in forensic anthropology research. His research interests include prehistoric and historic archaeology of the southeastern United States, human osteology, forensic archaeology, and anthropological theory.

Donna C. Boyd, PhD, D-ABFA, is eminent professor of anthropological sciences at Radford University, codirector of the Radford University Forensic Science Institute, professor of biomedical science at Virginia Tech Carilion School of Medicine, and consultant for the Virginia Office of the Chief Medical Examiner (VOCME). Dr. Boyd received her PhD in Anthropology in 1988 from the University of Tennessee–Knoxville and has taught at Radford University since 1989. She is the recipient of numerous awards honoring her teaching and research, including the Donald N. Dedmon Professorial Excellence Award for outstanding teaching at Radford University (1998), the Outstanding Faculty Award from the State Council of Higher Education in Virginia (2006), and the United States CASE/Carnegie Outstanding Professor of the Year Award (2006). She is a fellow of the American Academy of Forensic Sciences (AAFS), secretary for the AAFS Standards Board (Anthropology Consensus Group), and secretary and public information officer for the American Board of Forensic Anthropology Board of Directors. She is also a member of the US Department of Health and Human Service's National Disaster Medical System's Disaster Mortuary Operational Response Team (DMORT), through which she was deployed to Haiti in February 2010, to recover, analyze, and identify American and Haitian–American earthquake victims. Her current research is on the macroscopic and microscopic skeletal signatures of antemortem and perimortem pediatric and elderly trauma, the estimation of time since injury in pediatric death investigations, and microevolutionary change in the human mandible.

Notes on contributors

Janna M. Andronowski, PhD, is an assistant professor in the Department of Biology, University of Akron, Akron, Ohio. She was formerly a research intern with the Forensic Anthropology Unit at the Office of Chief Medical Examiner in New York City, a research assistant at Simon Fraser University's Center for Forensic Research, and a postdoctoral fellow in the Department of Anatomy and Cell Biology at the University of Saskatchewan.

William W. Baden, PhD (retired), worked in the Information Technology and Institutional Research Units of Indiana University–Purdue University Fort Wayne. His research focuses on the application of quantitative approaches to anthropological questions, specifically developing nonlinear models of cultural phenomena and, in particular, prehistoric maize agriculture in the Southeastern United States and Mexico.

Eric J. Bartelink, PhD, D-ABFA, has taught for 11 years at California State University, Chico, where he is currently a full professor and director of the Human Identification Laboratory. His research interests focus on the bioarchaeology of Native California, dietary reconstruction using stable isotope analysis, and applications within forensic anthropology. He is a coauthor of *Essentials of Physical Anthropology* and *Forensic Anthropology: Current Methods and Practice* and has authored and coauthored numerous articles in scientific journals.

Hugh E. Berryman, PhD, D-ABFA, is a research professor with the Department of Sociology and Anthropology and director of the Forensic Institute for Research and Education at Middle Tennessee State University. Since 1997, Dr. Berryman has provided forensic anthropology consultation to the Defense POW/MIA Accounting Agency-Central Identification Laboratory in Hawaii and the Office of the Metropolitan and Davidson County Medical Examiner. He serves on the Crime Scene Subcommittee of the Organization of Scientific Area Committees (OSAC). His research interests include bone trauma, bone fracture interpretation, and skeletal crime scene processing. In 2012, he received the T. Dale Stewart Award for lifetime achievement.

John F. Berryman, MS, holds a BS degree in mechanical engineering from the University of Tennessee, Martin, and an MS in aerospace engineering from Virginia Tech, Blacksburg. His research interests have varied from the use of finite element analysis to examining bone fracture propagation to software development including coauthoring a book entitled *Relevant Search: With Applications for Solr and Elasticsearch*.

Soren Blau, PhD, is the senior forensic anthropologist at the Victorian Institute of Forensic Medicine (VIFM) where she has been employed since 2005. She is an adjunct associate professor in the Department of Forensic Medicine at Monash University, a founding fellow of the Faculty of Science of the Royal College of Pathologists of Australasia, and a recipient of a Churchill Fellowship (2013). She has undertaken consultancies for the International Criminal Court (ICC) and the International Committee of the Red Cross (ICRC) and participated in the recovery and analysis of human remains from archaeological and forensic contexts in numerous countries. She is the coeditor of the *Handbook of Forensic Anthropology and Archaeology* (2009, 2016).

Lesley A. Chesson, MS, is the president of IsoForensics, Inc., a private analytical services and research firm located in Salt Lake City, UT, that focuses on forensic applications of stable isotope techniques. She was approved as a forensic practitioner by the Forensic Isotope Ratio Mass Spectrometry Network (FIRMS) in 2013 and is a member of the FIRMS Steering Group. She has applied stable isotope analysis for more than 14 years to examine drugs, explosives, foods, and beverages. One of her current areas of focus is assisting law enforcement in investigations via the stable isotope analysis of unidentified human remains.

Christian M. Crowder, PhD, D-ABFA, is director of the Forensic Anthropology Division for the Harris County Institute of Forensic Sciences in Houston, Texas. Previously, he was the chief anthropologist for the Office of the Armed Forces Medical Examiner and deputy director of Forensic Anthropology Unit for the Office of Chief Medical Examiner in New York City. He has also worked as an anthropologist for the Defense POW/MIA Accounting Agency in Hawaii and the International Criminal Tribunal for the former Yugoslavia. In addition to his practitioner duties, he is adjunct faculty at Pace University in New York City and at the University of Toronto, Ontario.

Ronald W. Davis, PhD, is a former assistant professor of Geosciences and Natural Resources and National Resource Conservation and Management at Western Carolina University. His research interests include wildlife ecology and management, GIS, and remote sensing.

Victoria M. Dominguez, MA, spent 4 years with the Forensic Anthropology Unit of the Office of Chief Medical Examiner in New York City. Currently, she is a PhD candidate in the Division of Anatomy at the Ohio State University (OSU). She is also the laboratory manager for the Skeletal Biology Research Laboratory, a part of the Injury Biomechanics Research Center at OSU. Her principal research interest is in bone histology, particularly the use of histology for human versus nonhuman differentiation, age-at-death estimation, and the influence of microarchitecture on bone mechanics.

Beatrix Dudzik, PhD, is an assistant professor of anatomy at the DeBusk College of Osteopathic Medicine of Lincoln Memorial University. She received her PhD in biological anthropology at the University of Tennessee. Her research interests and publications focus on morphological variation of the skull in Asian populations, forensic age estimation methods, and forensic taphonomy.

James R. Ehleringer, PhD, is a distinguished professor at the University of Utah, where his research focuses on ecological, environmental, and forensic applications of naturally occurring stable isotopes (nature's natural recorders) in water, atmospheric gases, and biological materials. He is a member of the US National Academy of Sciences and a recipient of the Rosenblatt Prize for Excellence. He is also senior scientist at IsoForensics, Inc.

Amanda N. Friend, MA, is a PhD student in the Department of Anthropology at the University of Florida and is a forensic anthropology assistant in the C.A. Pound Human Identification Laboratory (CAPHIL) where she also currently serves as the senior analyst. Her research interests include undocumented border crosser deaths in Florida, ancestry assessment, and isotopic variation.

Joseph T. Hefner, PhD, RPA, D-ABFA, is currently an assistant professor of anthropology at Michigan State University. His research interests focus on morphological variation in cranial form within and between modern human populations. In particular, he works with morphoscopic traits, parametric and nonparametric classification statistics, and machine learning methods useful for the assessment of ancestry in forensic anthropology.

Richard L. Jantz, PhD (emeritus professor), has taught at the University of Tennessee since 1971, serving as director of the UT Forensic Anthropology Center from 2000 to 2011. His research interests mainly include quantitative human variation with an emphasis on American populations, both early and recent. In the mid-1980s, he established the forensic anthropology data bank and, along with Steve Ousley, developed ForDisc software that automates estimation of sex, ancestry, and height from skeletal measurements. His primary research in forensic anthropology deals with improving estimates of sex, ancestry, and height and documenting the changes occurring in the American population during the twentieth century. He is now an emeritus professor and is enjoying working on research that has been put off for decades.

Cheryl A. Johnston, PhD, D-ABFA, is a Lecturer at the Center for Life Sciences Education at the Ohio State University. She has worked as a consultant in forensic anthropology since 1991 for numerous agencies in North Carolina and Ohio, including the Ohio Attorney General's Office Consumer Protection Division, the Ohio Bureau of Criminal Identification and Investigation, and the US Fish and

Wildlife Service. Her interests in forensic anthropology include cultural modification of human bone, decomposition, and thermally altered bone.

Natalie R. Langley, PhD, D-ABFA, is a senior associate consultant in the Department of Anatomy at the Mayo Clinic School of Medicine in Scottsdale, AZ, and an adjunct faculty member in the University of Tennessee Anthropology Department and the DeBusk College of Osteopathic Medicine Anatomy Department. Her research interests include skeletal maturation in modern populations, age and sex estimation from the human skeleton, secular changes in skeletal biology, currency of forensic standards, skeletal trauma, and anatomy education. In 2007, the AAFS Forensic Sciences Foundation awarded her the Emerging Forensic Scientist Award for her research in skeletal maturation.

Jennifer C. Love, PhD, D-ABFA, is currently the forensic anthropologist and identification unit supervisor for the Office of Chief Medical Examiner (OCME) in Washington, DC. Prior to joining the OCME, she served as the forensic anthropology director at the Harris County Institute of Forensic Sciences in Houston, TX. She is a member of the Anthropology Subcommittee of the Organization for Scientific Area Committees (OSAC). Her research interests are bone trauma, bone pathology, and decedent identification. In 2011, she coauthored the textbook *Skeletal Atlas of Child Abuse*.

Miriam E. Soto Martinez, PhD, received her PhD in biological anthropology from the University of Tennessee in 2015. She has been working at the Harris County Institute of Forensic Sciences since 2013. Her research interests include child abuse, growth and development, and sexual dimorphism in subadults.

Stephen Ousley, PhD, has been a professor at Mercyhurst University in Erie, Pennsylvania, since 2007. From 1998 to 2007, he was the director of the Repatriation Osteology Laboratory in the Repatriation Office of the National Museum of Natural History at the Smithsonian Institution, where he developed multivariate statistical methods to estimate ancestry of human remains in the Smithsonian's collections. Most of his professional activities involve anthropological databases, computer programming, and statistical approaches to biological anthropology. His research interests include forensic anthropology, human growth and development, and human variation. With Richard Jantz, he coauthored ForDisc, discriminant function software for sex, ancestry, and height estimation.

Todd Park is a cold-case investigator for the Unified Police Department of Greater Salt Lake, Utah.

Deborrah C. Pinto, PhD, D-ABFA, is a forensic anthropologist with the Harris County Institute of Forensic Sciences in Houston, Texas, and has been with the agency since 2010. Her research and publications focus on adult and pediatric trauma as well as anthropological methods using bone histology.

Tiffany B. Saul, PhD, is currently a research assistant professor with the Forensic Institute for Research and Education at Middle Tennessee State University. Her research interests include the use of stable isotopes and trace elements for the identification of human remains, trauma analysis, and the role of anthropologists in humanitarian and human rights responses, including disaster response and human rights investigations.

John F. Schweikart, MA, RPA, is an archaeologist with Search Recovery Consultants, LLC, with over 20 years' field and laboratory experience working collaboratively with the Ohio Bureau of Criminal Investigation and Identification (BCII), North Carolina State Bureau of Investigation (SBI), the Franklin County (Ohio) Coroner, and various county law enforcement agencies in Ohio, North Carolina, and West Virginia. He has served as guest instructor for forensic anthropology training courses for the York Regional Police, Ontario, Canada.

Michala K. Stock, MA, is a PhD candidate in the Department of Anthropology at the University of Florida and a forensic anthropology analyst in the C.A. Pound Human Identification Laboratory (CAPHIL). Her research focuses on the growth and development of sexual dimorphism in the crania of humans and apes.

Brett J. Tipple, PhD, is a senior research scientist at IsoForensics, Inc. in Salt Lake City, Utah, and a research assistant professor within the Department of Biology at the University of Utah. His research interests are in the fields of isotope geochemistry, plant ecology, and social geochemistry. Some of his current areas of research are plant ecophysiology and applications of heavy isotopes from human tissues for provenancing.

Douglas H. Ubelaker, PhD, D-ABFA, is a curator and senior scientist at the Smithsonian Institution's National Museum of Natural History in Washington, DC, where he has been employed for nearly four decades. He is also a professorial lecturer with the Departments of Anatomy and Anthropology at the George Washington University, Washington, DC, and is an adjunct professor with the Department of Anthropology, Michigan State University. He has published extensively in the general field of human skeletal biology with an emphasis on forensic applications. He served as the 2011–2012 president of the AAFS and was named Distinguished Fellow in 2016. He has received numerous honors, including the Memorial Medal of Dr. Aleš Hrdlička, Humpolec, Czech Republic; the Anthropology Award of the Washington Academy of Sciences; the T. Dale Stewart Award of the Physical Anthropology Section of AAFS; the FBI Director's Award for Exceptional Public Service; and a special recognition award from the FBI.

Michael W. Warren, PhD, D-ABFA (retired), was director of the C.A. Pound Human Identification Laboratory at the University of Florida. His research areas of interest include forensic identification and trauma analysis, human variation, and forensic examination of cremated human remains. He is coeditor of *The Forensic Anthropology Laboratory.*

Daniel J. Wescott, PhD, is associate professor in the Department of Anthropology and the director of the Forensic Anthropology Center at Texas State University. His forensic anthropological research focuses on developing and testing methods for defining biological profiles, interpreting the postmortem interval, and reconstructing trauma from human skeletal remains. He is a recipient of the Ellis Kerley Award for excellence in forensic anthropology research.

John A. Williams, PhD, D-ABFA, is a professor of anthropology at Western Carolina University. His primary interests are in the interpretation of bone trauma, especially dismemberment. He has consulted with medical examiners, various law enforcement agencies, and the FBI.

Allysha Powanda Winburn, PhD, is an assistant professor of anthropology at the University of West Florida. She has worked previously as a forensic anthropologist at the Defense POW/MIA Accounting Agency and as quality assurance coordinator of the University of Florida's C.A. Pound Human Identification Laboratory. In addition to the study of ethics, error, and objectivity in forensic anthropology, her research interests include pelvic age estimation and medicolegal interpretations of ritual remains used in African diaspora religious practices.

Foreword

As the field of forensic anthropology has advanced and flourished, critics have emerged. During the formative years of the discipline, some anthropology colleagues, who were not engaged in forensic applications, contrasted forensic casework and research with more traditional endeavors, labeling the former as "police work" largely devoid of a theoretical foundation. Those of us active in forensic anthropology at that time simply shrugged these comments off, viewing them as reflective of ignorance of the reality of the field and also a bit of jealously regarding its visibility. With time, these critiques have waned. Fueled by surging student interest in forensic anthropology and administrative responses, some of these former critics now find themselves involved with teaching courses in forensic applications.

Today, forensic anthropology is recognized as an important subdiscipline of anthropology. Emerging forensic anthropologists can find jobs in university faculties, medical examiners' offices, human rights organizations, government facilities, and many other sites. Anthropologists are integrated into recovery teams. Anthropological analysis of recovered remains is sought after and highly valued. Data and interpretations offered by forensic anthropologists have contributed in critical ways to the solutions of many medicolegal problems.

In spite of this progress, some concern lingers, especially among the older generation of anthropologists, regarding the robusticity of method and theory within forensic anthropology. Today, much like before, such doubts remain rooted in ignorance of the complexity of the modern practice of forensic anthropology. Some concerns reflect criticism of the overall field of forensic science and its perceived needs of more robust methodology, error analysis, assessment of cognitive bias, and related issues.

This volume addresses such concerns in a comprehensive manner. Forensic anthropology, like other forensic science disciplines, is case-driven but also represents applied science. The quality of these applications reflects advances, as well as knowledge of the underlying science. To address issues presented by a particular case or set of evidence, the forensic anthropologist turns to the relevant science at hand. At the general level, the available science reflects method and theory in the studies of evolution, growth and development, anatomy, physics, engineering, chemistry, archaeology, and of course the broad fields of anthropology and physical anthropology. In addition, certain methods and theories derived from research and casework experience are specific to the unique forensic applications. This book presents detail on the many different levels of method and theory in forensic anthropology.

Nonlinear systems theory is included in this discussion. Throughout its history, progress in the field of forensic anthropology has been distinctly nonlinear.

Promising new methods have emerged from research on specific samples. However, in many cases, enthusiasm for these methods has waned when testing on different samples has revealed reduced accuracy. Although irregular, progress has been sustained by increasingly critical research and the growing availability of new documented collections. Research has become increasingly interdisciplinary and international. Simultaneously, anthropologists have eagerly taken on issues of error analysis, cognitive bias, and many of the concerns that ripple through forensic science today.

In my view, this volume represents a welcomed addition to the scientific literature in forensic anthropology and the more general field of forensic science. The book documents in a comprehensive and exhaustive manner what forensic anthropologists have known all along; method and theory are alive and well in the dynamic and rapidly growing field of forensic anthropology.

Douglas H. Ubelaker
Smithsonian Institution
Washington, DC, USA

Series preface

The forensic sciences represent diverse, dynamic fields that seek to utilize the very best techniques available to address legal issues. Fueled by advances in technology, research and methodology, as well as new case applications, the forensic sciences continue to evolve. Forensic scientists strive to improve their analyses and interpretations of evidence and to remain cognizant of the latest advancements. This series results from a collaborative effort between the American Academy of Forensic Sciences (AAFS) and Wiley to publish a select number of books that relate closely to the activities and Objectives of the AAFS. The book series reflects the goals of the AAFS to encourage quality scholarship and publication in the forensic sciences. Proposals for publication in the series are reviewed by a committee established for that purpose by the AAFS and also reviewed by Wiley.

The AAFS was founded in 1948 and represents a multidisciplinary professional organization that provides leadership to advance science and its application to the legal system. The 11 sections of the AAFS consist of Criminalistics, Digital and Multimedia Sciences, Engineering Sciences, General, Pathology/Biology, Questioned Documents, Jurisprudence, Anthropology, Toxicology, Odontology, and Psychiatry and Behavioral Science. There are over 7000 members of the AAFS, originating from all 50 States of the United States and many countries beyond. This series reflects global AAFS membership interest in new research, scholarship, and publication in the forensic sciences.

Douglas H. Ubelaker
Senior Scientist
Smithsonian Institution
Washington, DC, USA
Series Editor

Acknowledgments

The editors wish to thank the chapter contributors who accepted the challenge of exploring theoretical applications of their expertise in the discipline of forensic anthropology. They are particularly indebted to Dr. Douglas H. Ubelaker and the American Academy of Forensic Sciences for soliciting and supporting this project. Many thanks also to Jenny Cossham, Elsie Merlin, and P. Sathishwaran at Wiley Blackwell for their many helpful edits and suggestions.

CHAPTER 1

The theoretical and scientific foundations of forensic anthropology

C. Clifford Boyd Jr[1] and Donna C. Boyd[1,2]

[1] *Department of Anthropological Sciences, Radford University Forensic Science Institute, Radford University, Radford, VA, USA*

[2] *Department of Biomedical Science, Virginia Tech Carilion School of Medicine, Roanoke, VA, USA*

1.1 Introduction

Despite its acceptance as a section in the American Academy of Forensic Sciences over 45 years ago (Thompson, 1982; Ubelaker, 2009), forensic anthropology has continued to be plagued by questions of scientific validity and rigor (Nordby, 2002). The legitimacy of forensic anthropology as a science and as a stand-alone discipline has been challenged repeatedly due to its perceived lack of a "grounding body of theory" (Adovasio, 2012). Viewed as a laboratory-based applied subfield of biological anthropology, it has been characterized as emphasizing methodology over theory, with a narrow focus on reconstructing the biological profile and establishing human identification (Adovasio, 2012).

The authors of this volume aim to show that this view of forensic anthropology is not only antiquated but also inadequate and inaccurate. This volume is an outgrowth of a symposium entitled "Application of Theory to Forensic Anthropology," presented at the 67th annual meeting of the American Academy of Forensic Sciences in 2015, and all of the presenters in this symposium are also chapter authors. As will be seen in the following chapters, forensic anthropology, a discipline that examines various aspects of the physical environment and material remains contained in that environment that are of legal significance, is firmly grounded in well-established scientific, logical theory. The goal of this chapter (and volume) is to explicate the theoretical bases for various specialized fields of inquiry in forensic anthropology and, through this process, define the basic elements of forensic anthropology theories, their interrelationships, and their relation to the logical reasoning process of the legal system in which they interact. The ultimate focus of the volume is to illustrate how these theoretical

Forensic Anthropology: Theoretical Framework and Scientific Basis, First Edition.
Edited by C. Clifford Boyd Jr and Donna C. Boyd.

approaches form the scientific foundation for the discipline and shape the data collected and results obtained in forensic anthropological research.

1.2 A selective history of theory in forensic anthropology

Theories are explanations—answers to "why?" questions (Howard, 1993:7; Johnson, 1999:2; Hage, 2007:124–127; Boyd and Boyd, 2011). Scientific theories are explanations of observable, quantifiable phenomena (Salmon, 1982:158). They allow the construction of models to better understand dynamic events and their physical material consequences. As Johnson (1999:7) notes, "Facts are important, but without theory they remain utterly silent." Scientific theories are, importantly, amenable to testing by means of quantification and analysis of new observations.

Because of its strong applied nature, as noted earlier, it may be asked why scientific theories are important for forensic anthropology. As will be seen in the following chapters, theories provide a basis for generating and testing new hypotheses regarding forensic events and the evaluation of their likelihood and probability. They influence and direct every aspect of forensic anthropology, from field search and recovery to laboratory analysis to the courtroom. Clearly stating one's theoretical focus and methodology can reduce bias and mitigate unfounded, unsubstantiated statements in legal reports and testimony. Theory consequently strengthens arguments for plausibility, reliability, and relevance of data introduced in the courtroom—without it, forensic anthropologists risk having their credibility as expert witnesses dismissed and admissibility of their scientific evidence denied.

In order to fully understand the theoretical underpinnings of forensic anthropology, it is important to briefly review theoretical developments within its parent discipline, anthropology. Anthropologists have attempted to explain all aspects of what it means to be human; their theories have accommodated humans as biocultural creatures—dependent on behavior and social interactions as much as their biology for their ultimate adaptability and survivability. Any discussion of theory development in forensic anthropology must consider these broader historical influences.

Anthropology began as a recognized discipline in the mid-late nineteenth century, with the writings of Lewis Henry Morgan, Sir Edward Tylor, Herbert Spencer, and Karl Marx (McGee and Warms, 2012), who all expressed, in one form or another, an evolutionary view of human cultural development. These early writers felt that human cultures had evolved over time from primitive to more complex forms, adapting to their environments with new technologies and new forms of social organization.

This early cultural evolutionary view, although discredited due to its simplistic and inherently racist connotations, dovetailed nicely with the contemporaneous theoretical proposal of biological evolution by means of natural selection from Charles Darwin (1859). These evolutionary theories all considered adaptation, reproductive success and consequent population growth, and a progression of change over time as important elements in any explanation of humans' current social and biological condition.

As the subfield of cultural anthropology developed in the twentieth century, its focus on human social and behavioral characteristics fluctuated between the later evolutionists' (e.g., Julian Steward, Leslie White) materialist perspective and that of the idealists. Materialists emphasized the roles of technology, modes of production and trade, and adaptation to the environment, while idealists (mentalists) focused on psychological, linguistic, and mental developments and their resultant influence on perceptions of reality as major theories explaining human behavior.

This theoretical dichotomy was also expressed in archaeology in the second half of the twentieth century. Prior to this, archaeology was initially focused on recovering material remains from impressive ancient sites and civilizations. Theoretical orientation was largely inductive and was primarily focused on descriptive culture history—dating artifacts, sites, and civilizations and organizing them into a chronology. In America and Britain, this approach began to change in the 1960s and 1970s, with the advent of the "New Archaeology."

Theory was at the heart of this revolution. Lewis Binford (1977, 1983), Michael Schiffer (1976), and many others championed this "New Archaeology," which explicitly recognized the hidden theoretical basis of archaeology and the building of theory through actualistic (middle-range) studies. These researchers sought to establish a firmer foundation for archaeological theory, with the goal of developing scientifically-based broad foundational laws, models, and explanations of human behaviors.

An important publication within archaeology during this time with implications for forensic anthropological theory was Michael Schiffer's (1988) "The Structure of Archaeological Theory," which described "three great realms" (Schiffer, 1988:464) of archaeological theory applicable to the study of human behavior—social, reconstruction, and methodological. Within these categories, he also described the presence of three levels of theory—high, middle-range, and low. Schiffer's high-level theories were broad and comprehensive, while middle-range theories served to link these high-level theories to empirical generalizations (low-level theories). An example of high-level social theory would be diffusion theory, as espoused by many anthropologists in the early twentieth century. Independent inventions spread from their centers of origin over a period of time, and this explained culture change and adoption of new traits (Harris, 1968:380–383). Perhaps more obvious is the role of reconstruction theory (often considered "middle-range"), which attempts to link the static archaeological (or forensic) record to the dynamic forces that produced it. Here, theory is clearly more applied, focusing on the development of observation-based explanations and improved inferences about events of significance. Schiffer's (1988) discussion of lithic use-wear analysis and its application toward reconstructing stone tool use in the past serves as a good archaeological example. Microscopic use-wear analysis helps to identify the raw materials processed by lithic tools by comparing the edge wear on archaeological specimens to the wear on experimentally produced stone tools used on known, specific raw materials (Vaughan, 1985). Finally, Schiffer (1988) originally defined methodological theory as a separate "realm" in his hierarchical model. Within this category, he included what he called recovery theory (e.g., protocols for conducting an archaeological survey or excavating a burial) and analytic theory (methods of analysis); these were considered to be low-level because they are "... more empirical in content..." (Schiffer, 1988:462).

This acknowledgement of a theoretical foundation based on actualistic and experimental studies became a major aspect of archaeological research, leading to the recognition of archaeology as a science (at least as it was practiced by many archaeologists). The "positivist" science-oriented materialist view of the past became a hallmark of archaeology and related disciplines during this time. However, beginning in the late twentieth century, this positivist (Giddens, 1974; Comte, 1975; Mill, 2009) or (to use an archaeological term) processualist view of science as an objective, unbiased method of study that explains natural phenomena through the careful analysis of material physical objects began to be criticized (Robson, 2002; Wylie, 2002). Post-processualist archaeological theorists emphasized a focus on uncovering the mental attributes of past peoples and meanings they assigned to artifacts and features. It was also recognized by postpositive, post-processual critics that scientists' own biases and theoretical orientations can influence and color the results of their research. Although sometimes viewed as antiscience, it can be argued that this postpositive approach offers a sobering and perhaps more realistic perspective regarding research by consciously recognizing the biases that may influence scientists. By actively recognizing and controlling these biases, scientists may make more progress toward the positivist goal of objectivity (see Chapters 2, 3, and 5 of this volume for a more thorough discussion of how cognitive bias affects forensic anthropology research).

In the midst of twentieth-century theory development in other areas of anthropology, forensic anthropology was in its infancy. Although considered by many to be a "subdiscipline" of biological anthropology, it can trace its roots to the fields of medicine and anatomy in the nineteenth century, as some practitioners in these fields began to apply anatomical knowledge to the task of human identification (Ubelaker, 2009; Tersigni-Tarrant and Shirley, 2013). In this clinical context, the importance of theory was not recognized or emphasized. Although still predominantly housed within anthropology departments (at least in the United States), this close relationship of forensic anthropology with clinical medicine continues to the present, with many forensic anthropologists currently employed in university or medical school anatomy departments or medical examiner's offices (Bethard, 2017). Early twentieth-century practitioners of forensic anthropology were primarily anatomists or physical anthropologists who engaged only in "laboratory-based and episodic involvement in forensic cases" (Dirkmaat and Cabo, 2012:6). This also has, perhaps, contributed to the perception of a dearth of theory in forensic anthropology today, where its practice is often seen as providing a technical service to medical examiners, coroners, and law enforcement when decomposed or skeletal remains of a decedent are present.

A review of all research articles, case studies, and technical notes ($n=644$) with significant forensic anthropology content or relevance from the *Journal of Forensic Sciences* (*JFS*) from 1995 to 2014 recorded thematic content, theoretical foundation, methodological approach, and research focus across this 20-year period (Boyd and Boyd, 2015). A recent expansion of this study also includes *JFS* articles from 2015 to November, 2017 (n=182). Identification of decedents through their biological profile and antemortem conditions (e.g., facial reconstruction), relying on evolutionary principles of human variation, still comprises the majority of published research. However, papers on perimortem (trauma) and postmortem (taphonomic) processes have become more prominent since 2010, and, in the last 3 years (2015–2017), there has been a notable increase in articles relating to trauma, taphonomy, and recovery methods. The frequencies of these topics are greater than the frequency of articles on any specific aspect of the biological profile. The great majority of researchers employ the scientific method, relying on macro- or microevolutionary theory (including natural selection); however, the exact nature of their theoretical foundation is rarely discussed, and explicit statements regarding hypotheses being tested are inconsistent and often absent. Although often not explicitly discussed in the publications, interpretive theories linking theoretical concepts to observed phenomena (e.g., principles of physics to explanations of blunt force trauma fracture propagation) and methodological theory discussions on archaeological search and recovery or new laboratory analysis techniques are primarily correlated with the previously noted research on perimortem and postmortem processes.

In sum, although it is clear that a firm theoretical (and, scientific) foundation underlies the majority of forensic anthropology research, this theoretical basis has not been explicitly recognized, developed, or communicated. Evolutionary theory (as per Darwin) and its explanatory power for interpreting human skeletal variation are still at the heart of much of what forensic anthropologists study, but modern forensic anthropology research has significantly expanded this foundation, particularly through its interdisciplinary engagement with aspects of physics, engineering, biology, chemistry, geology, anatomy, and other sciences. Eclectic borrowing of theoretical ideas from these and other disciplines serves to strengthen our theoretical base and scientific framework.

1.3 A modern perspective on forensic anthropology theory

It is apparent from the aforementioned discussion that forensic anthropology has not historically had a distinctive, unifying theory of its own and when theoretical approaches are borrowed from other disciplines, they are not overtly recognized.

In response to this conundrum, in 2011, Boyd and Boyd incorporated many elements of the Schiffer (1988) model into an exploration of forensic anthropology theory, and they applied his hierarchy of high-level, middle-range, and low-level theoretical concepts to forensic anthropological research. They also illustrated the relevance of several theoretical models derived from archaeology (e.g., agency theory, nonlinear systems theory) to interpretation of the more recent (forensic) past and emphasized the importance of the case study in initial theory building and hypothesis testing.

Ultimately, these aspects of hierarchical theory building have as their goal improving our inferences about the past—whether recent or distant. Forensic anthropology is, therefore, analogous to other historical sciences that rely on current observations to build theoretical interpretations of prior events. This is one reason Schiffer's (1988) model of archaeological theory was considered a good starting point for building forensic anthropological theory.

While a general application of the Schiffer model in forensic anthropology has been instructive as a heuristic device for clarifying and organizing theoretical approaches (Boyd and Boyd, 2011), as with all models, particularly hierarchical ones, it can be overly simplistic and obfuscate the actual process of theory building, particularly in developing sciences (see Salmon, 1982:178). We therefore recommend a more modern and realistic interpretation of forensic anthropological theory—one that, as we will see, is not hierarchical or static but based on three dynamic interacting *forms* of theory: foundational, interpretive, and methodological.

Foundational theories are those that are general, broad, and overarching and ground the discipline in a solid scientific framework. Since, ultimately, forensic anthropology focuses on once-living, sexually reproducing biological organisms, the most basic theory that grounds the discipline, as noted earlier, is Darwinian biological evolution by means of natural selection (Darwin, 1859; Mayr, 2001; Quammen, 2006). This theoretical base allows us to address several issues of relevance to forensic anthropologists, including human and nonhuman anatomical similarities and differences, human variation, sexual dimorphism, and ontogeny. These are all important concepts enabling the estimation of the biological profile and establishing personal identification from the remains of a decedent—traditionally the major goals of forensic anthropological practice. Although foundational theories like these are well established, they can be strengthened or modified with new interpretations or methods—the traditional phyletic gradualism model of evolution by means of natural selection was modified by the concept of punctuated equilibrium, for example (Elderidge and Gould, 1972). In forensic anthropology, evolutionary theory has been reflected in recent studies of secular trends and intergroup variation in aspects of the biological profile—notably stature—that stress the need for population-specific standards and the revision of standards based on nineteenth- to early twentieth-century skeletal collections (Meadows and Jantz, 1995; Jantz *et al.*, 2008; Spradley *et al.*, 2008; Wilson *et al.*, 2010; Gocha *et al.*, 2013). An understanding of biological evolutionary theory, therefore, forms the ultimate grounding for forensic anthropological analysis and interpretation.

Interpretive theories build research-generated and validated explanations that can be used to interpret specific events and underlie the forensic anthropological analyses of antemortem, perimortem, and postmortem processes. The classic application of interpretive theory is found in taphonomic research, which has long been recognized as a major area of interest in forensic anthropology because of its importance in determining the postmortem interval (PMI) (Lyman, 1994; Haglund and Sorg, 1997, 2002; Pokines and Symes, 2014). This form of interpretive theory defines how recovered remains may have been altered by natural forces or human behavior and permits the more accurate differentiation of peri- and postmortem events. A focus in taphonomic research is on the behavioral effects of various agents on the body and the forensic scene and their interpretation. These agents can range in scale and influence, from the blowflies initially infesting a corpse and the animals dismembering it, to the activities of field investigators documenting the forensic scene, to the medical examiners and forensic anthropologists conducting their laboratory analysis and interpretation (Boyd and Boyd, 2011). Schiffer and Skibo's (1997) concept of a "behavioral chain," with interactions between various agents and material remains all along the trajectory of transformation and recovery, is quite an applicable model for the creation of a forensic scene. All of the agents involved and their activities affect the final interpretation of the scene and its structure. Awareness of the potential biases introduced by these agents (including forensic anthropologists) in all contexts is a very important product of interpretive taphonomic research and theory building.

The empirical basis for interpretive theory is also important in the study of the effects of trauma on the human skeleton. For example, research documenting the process and timing of bone fracture repair for different age groups through macroscopic, microscopic, and radiographic observations is important in identifying prior injuries and can also be used to investigate claims of abuse, especially in children or the elderly. Theoretical models defining violent behavior, its timeline, and its consequences can then be developed (Walker *et al.*, 1997; Love *et al.*, 2011; D. Boyd, Chapter 9, this volume). Experimental and case studies involving perimortem blunt force, sharp force, and gunshot trauma (Symes *et al.*, 2002; Passalacqua and Fenton, 2012; Berryman *et al.*, 2013; Powell *et al.*, 2013; Love *et al.*, 2015) also exemplify interpretive research by providing a rigorous database for the recognition and interpretation of these events in actual cases.

Methodological theory includes recovery theory, analytical theory, and statistical theory. Methodological theory is just that—it provides the reasons behind *why* we use a certain protocol for the collection and analysis of relevant data. Methodological theory tests and develops valid methods and procedures for conducting both field recovery and laboratory research (see Chapters 8, 11, 12, and 14 for examples). Detailed procedures have been developed for the accurate recovery of both surface and buried human remains (Rhine, 1998; Dupras *et al.*, 2012; Hunter *et al.*, 2013; Groen *et al.*, 2015) to ensure that maximum contextual integrity is preserved and documented. The rationale for following certain procedures is based on robust inductive experiential and experimental data derived from thousands of prior case studies in a variety of environments. Without robust methodological theory and its application, a forensic scene and the data recovered from it can be permanently compromised.

Once the material items and human remains from a forensic scene are removed to the laboratory, analytical and statistical methodological theory become prominent. Why are certain procedures used for processing human remains? What statistical methods and measurements are most appropriate for the analysis of human remains? The answer to the "why?" theory question is, therefore, that certain procedures work best and are standards that other forensic anthropologists are following (or should follow). Methodological theory forms the basis for many forensic anthropology articles published in the *JFS*, in that these studies are often testing prior analytical methods or proposing new ones. Of course, following the optimum analytical protocols strengthens our inferences about prior events. Appropriate methodology guides the observation and collection of data and influences the interpretation (explanation) of *any* past event. As such, methodological theory should be considered the basic tool from which *all* theories are built.

These three forms of theory are critical for the process of theory building in forensic anthropology and serve to strengthen the scientific framework of the discipline. However, their relationship with each other is not necessarily linear or hierarchical. They come together in a flexible, interactive process that is dependent upon logical reasoning, described as follows.

1.3.1 Three forms of logical reasoning

In the late nineteenth century, the American philosopher and logician Charles Sanders Peirce defined three categories of reasoning—deduction, induction, and abduction (1965:99). He briefly defined their distinctiveness: "Deduction proves that something must be; Induction shows that something is actually operative; Abduction merely suggests that something may be" (Peirce, 1965:106; Walton, 2004, emphasis in original).

Deduction can be more specifically envisioned as an inference for which if the premises are true, then the conclusion must also be true (Walton, 2001). Deductive statements are non-defeasible (irrefutable) facts. For example, humans, as bipedal creatures, have a uniquely shaped innominate (relatively compact, with a wide, curved ilium) compared with terrestrial quadrupeds. *If* an innominate with the attributes described earlier is recovered from a forensic scene, *then* deductively it *must* be from a bipedal animal (i.e., a human).

Inductive inferences are based on probability. These are the statements produced as a result of experimentation on and statistical analysis of a data set. So, for example, adult stature estimates can be obtained (for a specific sex) by calculation using linear regression. The result is a statistical forensic mean *estimate* of the living stature of the person, with an associated range, indicating that the *true* biological stature is within that range (probably). Discriminant functions for sex and ancestry estimation in ForDisc will produce estimates with probabilities assessing the accuracy of their determination (Ousley and Jantz, 2005).

In both deductive and inductive reasoning, the logical process proceeds from premises to conclusions (if the innominate has these characteristics, then it must be human; if we use the long bone measurements of individuals of known stature, we can then derive a formula for predicting stature of unknown individuals). Both forms of logic are, of course, components of the classic hypothetico-deductive method of reasoning and investigation in science (Leblanc, 1973; Gibbon, 1984:12–13; Komar and Buikstra, 2008), wherein a hypothetical if-then (deductive) statement is tested by experimentation with new evidence (induction) and either supported or rejected as a result.

But how are those hypotheses created in the first place? Peirce (1965), Magnani (2001), Walton (2001, 2004), and many other logicians (e.g., Shelley, 1996; Gabbay and Woods, 2005) see the source of these hypotheses as abduction. Unlike deduction and induction, abductive reasoning "starts from the known facts and probes *backward* into the reasons or explanations for those facts" (Walton, 2001:145; emphasis ours). Peirce (1965:325) describes abduction in this way: "when we find some very curious circumstance, which would be explained by the supposition that it was a case of a certain rule, and thereupon adopt that supposition." This statement illustrates the *first* meaning or form of abduction: discovery and the creative process of generating a plausible hypothesis. The *second* meaning of abduction is evaluative and is referred to as inference to the best explanation (Lipton, 1991; Magnani, 2001:19; Taroni *et al.*, 2006:27). This second meaning is the one most commonly applied to abduction (Walton, 2001). However, both meanings can be considered part of a logical process: a "surprising" or "curious" object or event is discovered, and initial hypotheses are generated to explain it. Then, based on available evidence and the knowledge base of the observer, the best of these hypotheses is selected as the most likely explanation. This can be envisioned as the initiating stage of the hypothetico-deductive analytical process described earlier.

Abductively-selected best explanations or arguments are both presumptive and plausible, compared with their rejected competitors. Presumptive arguments are based on the specific context that one is trying to understand. Using contextual data (e.g., the location and position of a body at a forensic scene), several presumptive hypothetical explanations can be made and evaluated, leading to the recognition of the most plausible (or reasonable, based on available information). Then "...we infer that the best *potential* [plausible] explanation is an *actual* explanation" (Lipton, 1991:60). For example, at our hypothetical forensic scene in a somewhat isolated rural area, there is the body of an individual with severe blunt force trauma to the chest and face lying 20 m from a car that has left the road and crashed into a tree. The car door on the driver's side is open and there are blood stains leading from the car along the ground surface to the body. The most plausible explanation, given the contextual evidence, is that the body and the crashed car are related and that the injured driver of the car expired after leaving the vehicle to seek help. The lack of any contradictory evidence (gunshot trauma, evidence for another occupant of the car) for intentional injury of the deceased by another party strengthens this abductive explanation.

As shown in the aforementioned example, the evaluation and determination of the best explanation is a dialectical process—each abductive hypothesis needs to be evaluated in a dialogue with other competing hypotheses (Walton, 2001). The hypothesis that best explains the available evidence or facts is, as Lipton (1991) noted earlier, selected as the actual explanation. It should be emphasized, however, that abductive explanations *are* defeasible (falsifiable), unlike deductive explanations. They are *tentative* assessments of the truth. New evidence or facts can lead to the rejection of a prior "best" explanation. As an example, note the several cases of exoneration of individuals by DNA evidence who were previously judged "guilty" (Berger, 2006). So, one might think of abductive reasoning as a somewhat open-ended process, contingent on current knowledge.

1.3.2 Theory building in forensic anthropology: Linking logic and theory

Science is a process that utilizes these three forms of reasoning to develop and test hypotheses and to consequently build theory. The relationship between these three types of logical reasoning and theory building is reiterative and dynamic—logical reasoning and theory building are clearly nonlinear processes. Figure 1.1 illustrates the interactive nature of these three forms of theory and reasoning that are linked together and provide necessary feedback for each other in the process of theory building. As shown in the figure, foundational theory provides the basis for abductively developing a hypothesis (a tentative interpretation) to explain initial observed data. Deductive if-then statements, which delineate expectations that may be confirmed by testing, are generated, and the observed data, along with new information, are inductively collected and tested using methodological theory. This testing may support the hypothesis, thus establishing an interpretive theory for the observations in question, or the hypothesis may be rejected, leading to a new cycle of hypothesis generation, deduction, and inductive data collection and testing. While deduction and induction are applied to address specific research problems in forensic anthropology, much of the reasoning process used—especially regarding specific cases and their interpretation—is abductive in nature, postulating and deriving prior causes for currently perceived effects, based on the best available evidence. Successful hypothesis testing may eventually enhance or strengthen foundational theory.

In a comparable example, Magnani (2001:23) describes the theory building process as it relates to medical diagnoses: "...*selective abduction* is the making of a preliminary guess that introduces a set of plausible diagnostic hypotheses, followed by deduction to explore their consequences, and by induction to test them...."He therefore feels that the inference to the best explanation model actually describes the whole scientific "abduction—deduction—induction cycle" (Magnani, 2001:25; also see Gabbay and Woods, 2005:79) at all levels. Abductive reasoning is clearly a predominant form of reasoning in all historical sciences (Fogelin, 2007). By definition, geologists, paleontologists, archaeologists, and forensic anthropologists observe present-day objects or contexts of interest and seek to develop plausible explanations about the past historical processes (premises) that led to their present form.

As shown in Figure 1.1, methodological theory generates the empirical data that ultimately form the basis for broader, more general foundational theory. How did Darwin *see* natural selection? By following the traditional scientific method (i.e., using inductive methodological theory) and carefully collecting specimens and recording observations on his *Beagle* voyage and, afterward, documenting the results of selective animal breeding around his rural Down House home in England (Quammen, 2006). From these data, he deduced the theory of natural selection.

In taphonomic research, how do we build interpretive theory regarding the postmortem effects of carnivore (Haglund, 1997a; Colard, *et al.*, 2015), rodent (Haglund, 1997b), and vulture (Reeves, 2009) activity on human remains? We abductively infer explanations based on initial observations, develop testable hypotheses, and then inductively through our established research design (methodology) collect empirical data to evaluate those hypotheses.

It is clear then that abductive, deductive, and inductive logic are all operative within and provide an important link between methodological, interpretive, and

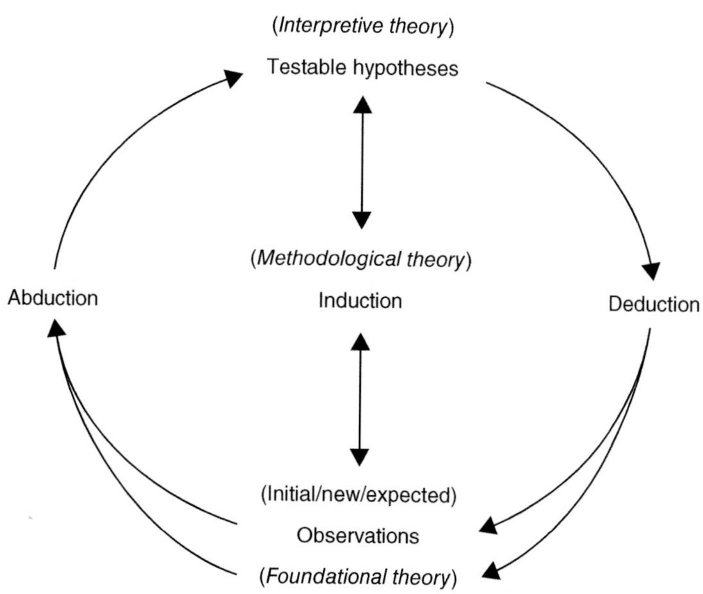

Figure 1.1 The interrelationships between forms of theory and logic in scientific research and theory building. Source: adapted from Magnani, 2001.

foundational theory. However, the interaction of all these forms of theory and logical reasoning is not reflected in a simple, linear model, but involves a great deal of feedback and information from a variety of sources. Thus, theoretical development is a "messy" and complex process, even in the sciences, and involves subjective insights gained through experience and observation, as well as rigorous, structured experimental testing. As Salmon (1982:173) states:

> Theories are usually developed in a very unsystematic manner. Scientists employ a variety of "methods," approaches, and techniques. Comparative studies, observations of "dynamics," extrapolation from other theories in related areas, pursuit of hunches—these and a host of other means not easily fitted within any rigorous "logic of discovery" are used.

In sum, theories should be envisioned as dynamic, vibrant explanatory statements, subject to expansion and revision at *all* levels and types, given new data.

1.4 Forensic anthropology theory and modern practice

Although not often recognized, aspects of logical reasoning and theory building that form the scientific basis of our discipline are prominent in forensic anthropology. The chapters in this volume exemplify this.

Contributions from positivism, processualism, and post-processual theoretical approaches are explored, as they are related to forensic anthropology, in Chapters 2–4 of this volume. Chapters 2 and 3 by Winburn and Warren *et al.* consider problems of bias and objectivity in forensic anthropological research and practice—something that affects all scientific endeavors. Allysha Winburn (Chapter 2) discusses the influence of both subjectivity and objectivity in the practice of forensic anthropology, noting the importance of recognizing sources of error. Purely objective, unbiased interpretations are not possible. Instead, she emphasizes the need for a more "mitigated objectivity" that realistically and critically evaluates the limitations and capabilities of forensic anthropology research.

Mike Warren, Amanda Friend, and Michala Stock (Chapter 3) address the problem of cognitive bias in forensic anthropological practice and the need to recognize the contextual and interpretive factors that create this bias. They suggest methods (such as established laboratory policies and procedures) that can help alleviate this problem or, at least, recognize its effects on forensic interpretation.

Soren Blau (Chapter 4) provides an international perspective on theory development in forensic anthropology and stresses the need for better communication between forensic practitioners and academics in this endeavor. She emphasizes the importance of ethical considerations when working internationally and sensitivity to other cultures' views regarding their dead. She focuses on the applied aspects of forensic anthropology and the important development of a sound "theory of practice."

As discussed earlier, a traditional focus in forensic anthropology has been estimating biological profile and establishing personal identification. Chapters 5 and 6 address the theoretical basis for the analysis and interpretation of major aspects of the biological profile—ancestry and age. Chapter 5, by Stephen Ousley, Richard Jantz, and Joseph Hefner, notes the biases in both past and current anthropological conceptions of ancestry (or "race"). They show that many current genetic analyses, which address covariation among multiple traits, do "indicate strong geographical patterning" and regional variation between populations. Designations of social race are indeed corroborated by multivariate morphological and genetic analyses.

Natalie Langley and Beatrix Dudzik (Chapter 6) delve into the history and theory behind the estimation of age from the skeleton, emphasizing the importance of the environment as well as genes in phenotypic development. They therefore stress the need to develop "population-specific standards" for age estimation using modern samples rather than ignoring secular change and continuing to rely on nineteenth- and early twentieth-century skeletal collections.

Additional methodological applications to forensic anthropological identification questions are exemplified by Chapters 7 and 8. Christian Crowder, Deborrah Pinto, Janna Andronowski, and Victoria Dominguez discuss the historical development of theories regarding bone biology in Chapter 7, specifically focusing on the process of bone growth and remodeling in response to mechanical loading. Histological analyses used to estimate age at death and differentiate human from nonhuman bone are described as examples of the application of all levels of theory to the understanding of bone development and its reaction to stress.

In Chapter 8, Lesley Chesson, Brett Tipple, James Ehleringer, Todd Park, and Eric Bartelink describe the use of stable isotope analysis to create "isoscapes," which can delineate the geographical/environmental source of human remains and the movements of decedents over time and across space. This method can play a useful role in the identification of unknown individuals by placing them in their antemortem contexts.

The scientific foundation for interpretations of antemortem, perimortem, and postmortem processes is explored in Chapters 9–13. Trauma analysis and interpretation is an increasingly important aspect of forensic anthropology and includes both antemortem and perimortem processes. In Chapter 9, Donna Boyd reviews the anatomical basis for fracture repair and its applications for evaluating forensic non-accidental pediatric and elderly deaths. She documents the significant variation in bone healing processes and rates, which are dependent on a number of intrinsic and extrinsic factors, and stresses the need for anatomically-informed, microscopically-based documentation of time since injury (TSI) estimates. A new model for TSI estimation, based on an archival bone fracture database, is presented.

Following along the child abuse theme, Chapter 10 by Jennifer Love and Miriam Soto Martinez describes the theoretical basis for differentiating between accidental and non-accidental trauma in children. They emphasize the importance of using the pediatric skeletal examination (PSE) methodology to more accurately analyze remains from suspected child abuse decedents. Knowledge of bone biomechanics, an understanding of the stages of motor skill development in growing children, and the identification of specific fracture types and their frequencies all are important sources of information for building an inductive model to evaluate possible child abuse cases.

Chapter 11, by Hugh Berryman, John Berryman, and Tiffany Saul, addresses bone trauma analysis through the perspective of material science and engineering. They propose a fracture assessment triad model for the analysis of bone fractures, consisting of documentation of fracture behavior (resulting from tension and stress), an understanding of the intrinsic characteristics of bone, and an evaluation of extrinsic factors (such as the direction and duration of the force causing the fracture). When two of these factors are known, the third can be logically inferred, given the known mechanical and physical properties affecting fracture.

John Williams and Ronald Davis (Chapter 12) apply Locard's theory regarding the transfer of evidence to GIS mapping of the different striation patterns on the cut surfaces of sawed bones. They show that GIS can assist in the interpretations of fine scale cuts on individual bones and that this method can be used to identify different classes of saws from kerf wall striations.

Daniel Wescott defines the interpretive theory behind taphonomic research and its use in PMI estimation in Chapter 13. Identifying taphonomic causes and their effects is a complex process, and he makes a strong case for the importance of cross-disciplinary collaboration in research and methodology to enhance this analysis. Because we are anthropologists with an ability to interact with different cultures, people, and settings, forensic anthropology should lead this collaborative effort.

The last section of the volume addresses connections between forensic anthropology and other disciplines and addresses the importance of theory in a legal context. In Chapter 14, Clifford Boyd and William Baden address the relationship between theoretical development and organization in archaeology and forensic anthropology with specific applications to the postmortem process of decay. Agency and nonlinear systems theory provide the basis for computer modeling of decay rates from 30 forensic cases to develop a model for PMI estimation. Nonlinear modeling is shown to accurately and realistically depict the decay process.

John Schweikart and Cheryl Johnston in Chapter 15 discuss influences of methodological theory derived from archaeology and also geophysics on forensic anthropology. They note that "backflow" from these influences has led to the development of forensic archaeology and forensic anthropologists well versed in the archaeological methods of search, recovery, and documentation. In addition, many forensic anthropologists are now trained and experienced in the use of geophysical remote sensing methods and their interpretation in forensic contexts.

Forensic anthropology, as an applied science, operates within a legal setting, and in Chapter 16, Donna and Clifford Boyd address the importance of theory in this context. Law and science differ in their views of truth, proof, and timeline. However, some commonalities between the two include their use of abductive logic and dialogue as well as statistically-based assessments of probability in the evaluation of data (evidence). It is shown that acceptance of forensic anthropologists as expert witnesses and admissibility of their evidence and testimony ultimately depends upon a sound theoretical and scientific basis for everything (methods and analyses) that they do. Mechanisms to develop an understanding between law and science through education and discourse between these entities are proposed.

Chapter 17 (Epilogue) summarizes some of the most important points of the volume, particularly as they relate to the identification of past and current theoretical approaches and their applications in forensic anthropology casework and research. Suggestions for meaningful future research and theory development, particularly in interpretive and methodological areas, are also discussed.

1.5 Final comments

As a largely applied enterprise, forensic anthropology has had its theoretical and scientific basis unrecognized for decades. However, whether implicit or explicit, theory guides all data collection and interpretation in the sciences. As section members within the American Academy of Forensic Sciences and as participants in legal proceedings, the need for forensic anthropologists to address the scientific *why* questions about the methods and analyses they use in their research and practice is clearly fundamental.

The chapters in this volume document the varied theoretical bases for specialized areas of study in forensic anthropology and the multiple forms of theory that they represent. However, the editors stress that this volume should not be considered the end point in any discussion of theory and its application to the field. Instead, it is hoped that the authors' presentations will engender future richer theoretical discussions and critical evaluations of theory and science in forensic anthropology—discussions that will only strengthen the discipline as a whole.

References

Adovasio, J. M. (2012) An "outsider" look at forensic anthropology. In: *A Companion to Forensic Anthropology* (ed. D. C. Dirkmaat). Wiley-Blackwell, Chichester, UK, pp. 683–689.

Berger, M. A. (2006) The impact of DNA exonerations on the criminal justice system. *The Journal of Law, Medicine & Ethics*, **34**, 320–327.

Berryman, H. E., Shirley, N. R., and Lanfear, A. K. (2013) Basic gunshot trauma and interpretation in forensic anthropology. In: *Forensic Anthropology: An Introduction* (eds. M. A. Tersigni-Tarrant and N. R. Shirley). CRC Press, Boca Raton, FL, pp. 291–306.

Bethard, J. D. (2017) Historical trends in graduate research and training of diplomates of the American Board of Forensic Anthropology. *Journal of Forensic Sciences*, **62**, 5–11.

Binford, L. R. (ed.) (1977) *For Theory Building in Archaeology*. Academic Press, New York.

Binford, L. R. (1983) *Working at Archaeology*. Academic Press, New York.

Boyd, C. C. and Boyd, D. C. (2011) Theory and the scientific basis for forensic anthropology. *Journal of Forensic Sciences,* **58**, 1407–1415.

Boyd, C. C. and Boyd, D. C. (2015) Theory in Forensic Anthropology: A Retrospective and Look Forward. *Proceedings of the 67th Annual Meeting of the American Academy of Forensic Sciences,* Orlando, FL, February 21, 2015, **XXI**, 193–194.

Colard, T., Delannoy, Y., Naji, S., *et al.* (2015) Specific patterns of canine scavenging in indoor settings. *Journal of Forensic Sciences,* **60**, 495–500.

Comte, A. (1975) (orig. 1922) Plan of the scientific operations necessary for reorganizing society. In: *Auguste Comte and Positivism: The Essential Writings* (ed. G. Lenzer). Harper Torchbooks, New York, pp. 9–69.

Darwin, C. (1859) *The Origin of Species* (reprinted 1998). The Modern Library, New York.

Dirkmaat, D. C. and Cabo, L. L. (2012) Forensic anthropology: Embracing the new paradigm. In: *A Companion to Forensic Anthropology* (ed. D. C. Dirkmaat). Wiley-Blackwell, Chichester, UK, pp. 3–40.

Dupras, T. L., Schultz, J. J., Wheeler, S. M., and Williams, L. J. (2012) *Forensic Recovery of Human Remains: Archaeological Approaches* (2nd edn.). CRC Press, Boca Raton, FL.

Elderidge, N. and Gould, S. J. (1972) Punctuated equilibrium: An alternative to phyletic gradualism. In: *Models in Paleobiology* (ed. T. J. M. Schopf). Freeman, Cooper & Company, San Francisco, CA, pp. 82–115.

Fogelin, L. (2007) Inference to the best explanation: A common and effective form of archaeological reasoning. *American Antiquity,* **72**, 603–625.

Gabbay, D. M. and Woods, J. (2005) *The Reach of Abduction: Insight and Trial, a Practical Logic of Cognitive Systems,* vol. 2. Elsevier, Amsterdam.

Gibbon, G. (1984) *Anthropological Archaeology.* Columbia University Press, New York.

Giddens, A. (1974) *Positivism and Sociology.* Heinemann, London.

Gocha, T. P., Vercellotti, G., McCormick, L. E., and Van Deest, T. L. (2013) Formulae for estimating skeletal height in modern South East Asians. *Journal of Forensic Sciences,* **58**, 1279–1283.

Groen, W. J. M., Marquez-Grant, N., and Janaway, R. C. (2015) *Forensic Archaeology: A Global Perspective.* Wiley-Blackwell, Chichester, UK.

Hage, J. (2007) The intersection of philosophy and theory construction: The problem of the origin of elements in a theory. In: *Philosophy of Anthropology and Sociology* (eds. S. P. Turner and M. W. Risjord). Elsevier, Amsterdam, pp. 121–156.

Haglund, W. D. (1997a) Dogs and coyotes: Postmortem involvement with human remains. In: *Forensic Taphonomy: The Postmortem Fate of Human Remains* (eds. W. D. Haglund and M. H. Sorg). CRC Press, Boca Raton, FL, pp. 367–381.

Haglund, W. D. (1997b) Rodents and human remains. In: *Forensic Taphonomy: The Postmortem Fate of Human Remains* (eds. W. D. Haglund and M. H. Sorg). CRC Press, Boca Raton, FL, pp. 405–414.

Haglund, W. D. and Sorg, M. H. (eds.) (1997) *Forensic Taphonomy: The Postmortem Fate of Human Remains.* CRC Press, Boca Raton, FL.

Haglund, W. D. and Sorg, M. H. (eds.) (2002) *Advances in Forensic Taphonomy: Method, Theory, and Archaeological Perspectives.* CRC Press, Boca Raton, FL.

Harris, M. (1968) *The Rise of Anthropological Theory: A History of Theories of Culture.* Harper and Row, New York.

Howard, M. C. (1993) *Contemporary Cultural Anthropology* (4th edn.). HarperCollins College Publishers, New York.

Hunter, J., Simpson, B., and Sturdy Colls, C. (2013) *Forensic Approaches to Buried Remains.* Wiley-Blackwell, Chichester, UK.

Jantz, R. L., Kimmerle, E. H., and Baraybar, J. P. (2008) Sexing and stature estimation criteria for Balkan populations. *Journal of Forensic Sciences*, **53**, 601–605.

Johnson, M. (1999) *Archaeological Theory: An Introduction*. Blackwell Publishers, Oxford, UK.

Komar, D. A. and Buikstra, J. E. (2008) *Forensic Anthropology: Contemporary Theory and Practice*. Oxford University Press, New York.

Leblanc, S. (1973) Two points of logic concerning data, hypotheses, general laws, and systems. In: *Research and Theory in Current Archeology* (ed. C. Redman). John Wiley & Sons, Inc., New York, pp. 199–214.

Lipton, P. (1991) *Inference to the Best Explanation*. Routledge, New York.

Love, J. C., Derrick, S. M., and Weirsema, J. M. (2011) *Skeletal Atlas of Child Abuse*. Humana Press/Springer, New York.

Love, J. C., Derrick, S. M., Weirsema, J. M., *et al.* (2015) Microscopic saw mark analysis: An empirical approach. *Journal of Forensic Sciences*, **60**, S21–S26.

Lyman, R. L. (1994) *Vertebrate Taphonomy*. Cambridge University Press, Cambridge, UK.

Magnani, L. (2001) *Abduction, Reason and Science: Processes of Discovery and Explanation*. Kluwer Academic/Plenum, New York.

Mayr, E. (2001) *What Evolution Is*. Basic Books, New York.

McGee, R. J. and Warms, R. L. (2012) *Anthropological Theory* (5th edn.). McGraw-Hill, New York.

Meadows, L. and Jantz, R. L. (1995) Allometric secular change in the long bones from the 1800s to the present. *Journal of Forensic Sciences*, **40**, 762–767.

Mill, J. S. (2009) (orig. 1865) *Auguste Comte and Positivism*. Cosimo Classics, New York.

Nordby, J. J. (2002) Is forensic taphonomy scientific? In: *Advances in Forensic Taphonomy: Method, Theory and Archaeological Perspectives* (eds. W. D. Haglund and M. H. Sorg). CRC Press, Boca Raton, FL, pp. 31–42.

Ousley, S. and Jantz, R. L. (2005) FORDISC 3.0 Personal computer forensic discriminant functions. The University of Tennessee, Knoxville.

Passalacqua, N. V. and Fenton, T. W. (2012) Developments in skeletal trauma: Blunt force trauma. In: *A Companion to Forensic Anthropology* (ed. D. C. Dirkmaat). Wiley-Blackwell, Chichester, UK, pp. 400–411.

Peirce, C. S. (1965) *Collected Papers of Charles Sanders Peirce* (reprinted) (eds. C. Hartshorne and P. Weiss), vols. 5 and 6. Harvard University Press, Cambridge, MA.

Pokines, J. T. and Symes, S. A. (2014) *Manual of Forensic Taphonomy*. CRC Press, Boca Raton, FL.

Powell, B. J., Passalacqua, N. V., Baumer, T. G., *et al.* (2013) Fracture characteristics of entrapped head impacts versus controlled head drops in infant porcine specimens. *Journal of Forensic Sciences*, **58**, 678–683.

Quammen, D. (2006) *The Reluctant Mr. Darwin*. Atlas Books/WW Norton, New York.

Reeves, N. M. (2009) Taphonomic effects of vulture scavenging. *Journal of Forensic Sciences*, **54**, 523–528.

Rhine, S. (1998) *Bone Voyage: A Journey in Forensic Anthropology*. University of New Mexico Press, Albuquerque.

Robson, C. (2002) *Real World Research: A Resource for Social Scientists and Practitioner-Researchers* (2nd edn.). Blackwell, Malden, MA.

Salmon, M. H. (1982) *Philosophy and Archaeology*. Academic Press, New York.

Schiffer, M. B. (1976) *Behavioral Archeology*. Academic Press, New York.

Schiffer, M. B. (1988) The structure of archaeological theory. *American Antiquity*, **53**, 461–485.

Schiffer, M. B. and Skibo, J. M. (1997) The explanation of artifact variability. *American Antiquity*, **62**, 27–50.

Shelley, C. (1996) Visual abductive reasoning in archaeology. *Philosophy of Science*, **63**, 278–301.

Spradley, M. K., Jantz, R. L., Robinson, A., and Peccerelli, F. (2008) Demographic change and forensic identification: Problems in metric identification of Hispanic skeletons. *Journal of Forensic Sciences*, **53**, 21–28.

Symes, S. A., Williams, J., Murray, E., *et al.* (2002) Taphonomic context of sharp-force trauma in suspected cases of human mutilation and dismemberment. In: *Advances in Forensic Taphonomy: Method, Theory, and Archaeological Perspectives* (eds. W. Haglund and M. Sorg). Charles C. Thomas, Springfield, IL, pp. 403–434.

Taroni, F., Aitken, C., Garbolino, P., and Biedermann, A. (2006) *Bayesian Networks and Probabilistic Inference in Forensic Science*. John Wiley & Sons, Ltd, Chichester, UK.

Tersigni-Tarrant, M. T. A. and Shirley, N. R. (eds.) (2013) *Forensic Anthropology: An Introduction*. CRC Press, Boca Raton, FL.

Thompson, D. D. (1982) Forensic anthropology. In: *A History of American Physical Anthropology: 1930–1980* (ed., F. Spencer). Academic Press, New York, pp. 357–369.

Ubelaker, D. H. (2009) Historical development of forensic anthropology: Perspective from the United States. In: *Handbook of Forensic Anthropology and Archaeology* (eds., S. Blau and D. H. Ubelaker). Left Coast Press, Walnut Creek, CA, pp. 76–86.

Vaughan, P. C. (1985) *Use-Wear Analysis of Flaked Stone Tools*. University of Arizona Press, Tucson.

Walker, P. L., Cook, D. C., and Lambert, P. M. (1997) Skeletal evidence for child abuse: A physical anthropological perspective. *Journal of Forensic Sciences*, **42**, 196–207.

Walton, D. N. (2001) Abductive, presumptive, and plausible arguments. *Informal Logic*, **21**, 141–169.

Walton, D. N. (2004) *Abductive Reasoning*. The University of Alabama Press, Tuscaloosa.

Wilson, R. J., Herrmann, N. P., and Meadows Jantz, L. (2010) Evaluation of stature estimation from the database for forensic anthropology. *Journal of Forensic Sciences*, **55**, 684–689.

Wylie, A. (2002) *Thinking from Things: Essays in the Philosophy of Archaeology*. University of California Press, Berkeley.

PART 1
Bias and objectivity in forensic anthropology theory and practice

CHAPTER 2

Subjective with a capital S? Issues of objectivity in forensic anthropology

Allysha Powanda Winburn
Department of Anthropology, University of West Florida, Pensacola, FL, USA

2.1 Introduction

In 1973, in the wake of the pro-science processualist turn in archaeological theory and several decades before the "science wars" pitted the allegedly dichotomous natural and social sciences against each other, Kent Flannery published *Archeology with a Capital "S."* In it, he summarized (and satirized) attempts by the archaeological community to elevate its practice from "imprecise pseudoscience" to "science with a capital S"—to make archaeology explicitly scientific (Flannery, 1973:53). Today, over 40 years later, forensic anthropologists struggle with the same issue faced by archaeologists during the processualist and ensuing post-processualist years: the goal of elevating their field to rigorous objectivity in the face of the subjectivity inherent in scientific knowledge production. This chapter critiques the pursuit of pure objectivity by forensic anthropologists by highlighting the presence of subjectivity in their methods and discussing the ramifications of ignoring it. The chapter then suggests ways to constrain that subjectivity, enabling forensic anthropologists to achieve not a pure but a mitigated objectivity, along with a more realistic view of their capabilities. Ultimately, this chapter poses the question of whether forensic anthropology can be "*subjective* with a capital S," and it answers in the affirmative.

Forensic Anthropology: Theoretical Framework and Scientific Basis, First Edition.
Edited by C. Clifford Boyd Jr and Donna C. Boyd.

2.2 Objectivity, subjectivity, and forensic anthropological theory

In discussing practitioners' attitudes toward science, this chapter contributes to the current volume's dialogue on the theoretical foundation for the science of forensic anthropology. However, this chapter does not deal with theory in the hypothetico-deductive sense, wherein a theory is an idea proposed to explain an empirical phenomenon that is supported or rejected through hypothesis testing (*sensu* Komar and Buikstra, 2008; Boyd and Boyd, 2011). The chapter does not address evolution, inheritance, growth and development, or any of the other theories explicitly underlying forensic anthropological analyses. Rather, it is concerned with *implicit* theories—the biases with which analyses, data, and even basic observations are infused. It argues that scientific data, and the ways in which scientists collect them, are theory-laden, whether they realize it or not.[1] In its argument for a rejection of the rhetoric of pure objectivity, the chapter also addresses the different "ways of thinking" that orient anthropologists' approaches to data collection and give their data meaning (Moore and Sanders, 2006:xi; McGee and Warms, 2008). These *are* theories in the broadest and most overarching sense of the term: positivism, anti-positivism, and post-positivism are the theoretical stances with which practitioners of forensic anthropology engage in order to create meaning from the evidence they analyze; objectivity, subjectivity, and mitigated objectivity are the epistemological perspectives that guide their methodological choices and shape their interpretations (Box 2.1).

As *objectivity, subjectivity,* and *bias* can be defined in different ways, it is appropriate to begin with a brief discussion of definitions (Box 2.2). In their introductory forensic anthropology text, Komar and Buikstra (2008) define objectivity as scientific disinterest. Subjectivity, its opposite, is tantamount to advocacy (Komar and Buikstra, 2008). By their definition, bias is the "loss of objectivity," or inclination or prejudice on the part of the researcher (Komar and Buikstra, 2008:48). These are likely the prevailing definitions used by forensic anthropologists; certainly, these or similar definitions are the ones that tend to put practitioners on the defensive, causing them to view subjectivity and bias as negatives to be avoided at all cost. Although these are valid definitions, they are not the ones employed in the current chapter. For the purposes of this chapter, a definition of bias includes no assumption of intentional inclination or unintentional prejudice, but simply refers to the implicit ideas that color scientists' observations and interpretations. This chapter's definitions of objectivity and subjectivity are less akin to the oft-cited, value-laden dichotomy of scientific distance versus *un*scientific advocacy and more akin to the Cartesian definitions of theoretical objectivism and subjectivism (Jones, 2002). In this view, while

[1]It should also be noted that although it discusses bias, this chapter does not address the issues of dishonesty or deliberate falsification in forensic science. This chapter holds (*sensu* Risinger *et al.*, 2002) that unwitting subjectivities play an even more important role than overt prejudices or deliberate falsehoods because their presence is often unnoticed or unacknowledged.

Box 2.1 Relevant anthropological theories (informed by Binford, 1968; Watson *et al.*, 1971; Wylie, 1982; Guba, 1990; Shanks and Tilley, 1992; Wylie, 1992; Bhaskar, 1994, 2005, 2008; Wallace, 2011)

Theory	Epistemology	Methodological approaches and ontologies
Positivism	Objectivity	Explicitly scientific; uses experiments and hypothesis testing to search for natural laws/generalizations explaining an external and universal reality
Anti-positivism	Subjectivity	Uses dialectic approach and subject–object interaction to create any of an almost infinite set of realities, each of which is a relativist construction (specific, contingent, and socially based)
Post-positivism	Mitigated objectivity	Uses scientific approach (qualitative and quantitative) to access a pluralistic, theory-laden reality that exists but can never be fully understood (often employs critical realism to critique the modernist thinking underlying positivism)

Box 2.2 Definitions (informed by Guba, 1990; Wylie, 1992; Jones, 2002)

Objectivity	Scientific distance and disinterest, non-interaction between scientist and object of study; reality exists outside the observer, and data on this reality are collected completely without bias, with no introduction of the scientist's theories or values
Subjectivity	Scientific embeddedness, interaction between scientist and object of study; reality exists, but perceptions of it are context-dependent, and data are culturally situated, necessarily infused with the scientist's theories and values
Mitigated objectivity	An approximation of objectivity: pursues the goal of scientific rigor but acknowledges interaction between scientist and object of study, possibility of bias, and social, theory-laden nature of data; constrains these with strong scientific methods and theories
Bias	Implicit theories, beliefs, and/or expectations that color scientific observations and interpretations

both objectivity and subjectivity are valid scientific stances, the former is employed to study *objects* that exist separate from the human cultural sphere, and the latter is employed to study active social *subjects* like humans (Guba, 1990; Wylie, 1992; Jones, 2002). This nature-versus-culture, subject–object dichotomy may be a false one (Latour, 1993, 1999; Marks, 2009; Wallace, 2011), but it adequately captures the divide between the epistemological stances of objectivity and subjectivity, as discussed in the following text (see Boxes 2.1 and 2.2).

2.3 Subjectivity in science

It is not a radical statement to note that true objectivity (see Box 2.2) is difficult, if not impossible, to achieve. As early as the seventeenth century, Sir Francis Bacon acknowledged that factors like emotion, expectation, and suggestion compromise scientific objectivity; further, Bacon identified what cognitive scientists now call selective attention and confirmation bias (Risinger *et al.*, 2002). Even in the fields traditionally considered to be natural science—chemistry, physics, molecular anthropology, and other "science with a capital S"—analysis can be subjective when there is an element of human interpretation (Risinger *et al.*, 2002). This is particularly true in cases where data are ambiguous (Dror and Hampikian, 2011).

All human knowledge is, necessarily, constructed by humans; and science is itself a social process (Bhaskar, 2005, 2008). The process of scientific knowledge production is culturally embedded and in a constant state of transformation (Latour, 1999). The *social studies of science* movement introduced this idea to anthropology, highlighting that scientific facts do not come into existence independently of social factors, but are lodged within historical processes (Latour and Woolgar, 1979a, b). The work of Bruno Latour and others has shown that the production of scientific knowledge is context-specific and that the context matters just as much as the particulars of the discovery (Marks, 2009). Scientific models necessarily reduce heterogeneity to homogeneity, creating docile, theory-laden representations (Law and Whittaker, 1988). These scientific products (representations, *sensu* Latour, 1988) become actors that can take on lives of their own (Gillespie, 2011). The explicit and implicit values of scientists affect the representations they create and influence their interpretations of them (Gould, 1981; Moser, 1992; van Reybrouck, 1998; Sommer, 2006). Thus, all data are theory laden; essentially, scientists' ideas and beliefs infuse the data they observe, collect, and interpret.

2.3.1 Subjectivity in forensic anthropology

In light of this increasing evidence that human subjectivities and biases preclude true scientific objectivity, many anthropologists have rejected their earlier attempts for purely objective analyses. In the fields of cultural anthropology and archaeology, for example, anthropologists are turning from positivism to embrace theoretical leanings that acknowledge the subjectivity of human scientific analysis (see Box 2.1). However, much of the field of forensic anthropology still maintains the positivist ideal of value-free, objective science. This may be due to the frequent status of forensic anthropologists as expert witnesses and their desire to portray results as accurate, precise, replicable, and statistically (and legally) defensible. Forensic anthropologists are more than just scientists: they are *forensic* scientists. In the post-*Daubert* era, the forensic sciences have been increasingly scrutinized for their standardization and objectivity (*Daubert v. Merrell Dow Pharmaceuticals, Inc.*, 1993; NRC, 2009). While the rest of anthropology rejects the idea of purely objective science, it seems that forensic anthropologists are increasingly pursuing it, asking "Is forensic anthropology *scientific* enough? Can it be 'science with a capital S'?"

Concurrent with this push for objectivity in forensic anthropology, however, the reality of the discipline's subjectivity has become increasingly difficult to ignore. A recent series of cognitive bias studies by Itiel Dror and his colleagues has brought home to forensic anthropologists the message of subjectivity in science—and in *forensic* science in particular (e.g., Dror *et al.*, 2005; Dror and Charlton, 2006; Dror *et al.*, 2006; Dror and Hampikian, 2011; Nakhaeizadeh *et al.*, 2014a, b). Cognitive bias studies show that the emotions and expectations of even expert forensic scientists can affect the conclusions they draw. These potentially biasing factors—also termed *observer effects*—are particularly influential when a scientist's methods rely on subjective human judgment (Risinger *et al.*, 2002). Human observation and subjective interpretation remain the major methods of reaching conclusions for scientists in most forensic disciplines; principal among them, forensic anthropologists frequently utilize qualitative, opinion-based methods (Grivas and Komar, 2008; Christensen and Crowder, 2009). Even forensic anthropology's more quantitative methods cannot truly be considered objective, as they are limited by the samples on which they were developed and by the experience of the analyst applying them (Grivas and Komar, 2008). Moreover, there is evidence that the field's faith in the reliability of so-called standard measurements is misplaced (Adams and Byrd, 2002; Smith and Boaks, 2014; Jantz *et al.*, 2015; Ousley *et al.*, 2015). Due to the vagaries of preservation, anthropological specimens are frequently of poor quality; due to the complexities of human variation, the data forensic anthropologists collect are frequently ambiguous. The intersection of human interpretation and ambiguous data produces conditions under which bias can thrive (Risinger *et al.*, 2002; Dror *et al.*, 2005; Dror and Hampikian, 2011; Nakhaeizadeh *et al.*, 2014b).

2.3.2 Effects of bias on forensic anthropology

Despite its often negative connotation, the term "bias" might bring to mind the sort of prejudice, impartiality, or emotional investment that could potentially be identified and overcome. In reality, however, cognitive studies show that humans are often unable to determine what factors are biasing them or to what extent they are being influenced (Wilson and Brekke, 1994; Pronin *et al.*, 2004; Pronin, 2006). Overt prejudices surely influence those forensic anthropologists who harbor them, but obvious, explicit influences are not the only factors that compromise their objectivity. Theories acquired from mentors and colleagues may influence them in ways they do not recognize; subconscious mental "controlling models" can infuse their analyses and conclusions with implicit ideas and beliefs (Clarke, 1972:5). As the differing theoretical perspectives, research foci, and casework practices of forensic anthropologists originating from disparate academic backgrounds illustrate, *forensic anthropology data are theory-laden.*

Even the basic act of scientific observation is affected by expectation. Observation is not the same as seeing: seeing is physical; it is a photochemical and neurological process. Observation, although implicit and instantaneous, is organized (in a *Gestalt* sense) by human experiences, beliefs, and expectations (Rock and Palmer,

1990; Nordby, 1992). In an example provided by Jon Nordby (1992), a pathologist and a kindergarten student may *see* the same histology slide, but where the former *observes* evidence of a pathological condition, the latter merely observes colors and patterns. The experiences and expectations of the pathologist differ from those of the kindergartener, and those experiences and expectations shape what each observer perceives. This is somewhat of a paradox: the human brain organizes what we perceive in order to make meaning, but then that organization limits the meaning we can make (Risinger *et al.*, 2002). In other words, "if we see what we believe, we may not be warranted in believing what we see" (Nordby, 1992:1123).

Thus, if scientific data are theory-laden, scientific observations are *expectation-laden* (Nordby, 1992). These layers of implicit theory and expectation bias the decisions forensic anthropologists make throughout their analyses. Forensic anthropologists *choose* how to process a scene based on their level of experience and on what they expect to find (Haglund and Sorg, 1997). They *choose* what is collected and processed as evidence based on their expectations for the type of scene being processed (Nordby, 1989). During analysis, they *choose* which variables to emphasize and which to background based on their subjective experiences. In the courtroom, they instruct jurors how to interpret the evidence *they have created*, molding their theory-laden data into what jurors perceive as self-evident scientific facts (Daemmrich, 1998). In all of these contexts, forensic anthropologists *decide* what counts as data—they are the active agents who *make* evidence (Daemmrich, 1998; Marks, 2009).

2.3.3 Subjective science is not bad science

Subjectivity is an inextricable part of the human observation and interpretation experience. Forensic anthropology, like all science, is colored by it. Yet, this chapter does not contain a message of despair. Rejecting the rhetoric of pure scientific objectivity does not necessarily entail a regression into a morass of "anything goes" relativism (Wylie, 1992:172; see Box 2.1). On the contrary, this chapter's message is a positive one: subjective science does not have to be bad science. *Science works*—in spite of scientific subjectivity, the socially embedded nature of science, and the fact that scientific models reduce complexity to simplicity. Through sound scientific practice, scientists accumulate knowledge that constrains their biases and enhances their observations and interpretations. Forensic anthropology, like archaeology, paleontology, and other studies of the past, is a historical, not an experimental, science. It depends not on conducting replicable experiments in controlled laboratory settings, but on interpreting past events based on the traces they leave in the present. Historical scientists may not always engage in the explicit hypothesis testing that forms the allegedly objective basis of experimental science, but this does not mean that their conclusions are any less valid. By thoroughly investigating the traces left by past processes and connecting them with strong theoretical frameworks, historical scientists too can draw definite and defensible conclusions about past events (Cleland, 2002).

Forensic anthropologists may not be capable of achieving pure objectivity, but if they attempt to understand how bias works, take measures to reduce it, and constrain subjectivity with sound methods, theories, and technologies, they can approximate objectivity in some form. This is the epistemological perspective of *mitigated objectivity* (*sensu* Wylie, 1992; see Box 2.2), and this chapter represents an argument for its application. Mitigated objectivity is not a pure but a "guarded" (Hodder, 1992:33) or "relative objectivity" (Binford, 1989:230)—a "particular and contingent objectivity" (Shanks and Tilley, 1992:43). Within the epistemology of mitigated objectivity, pluralism is possible, and the theory-laden nature of data is acknowledged, but interpretations are constrained by the existence of reality, strong theory, and sound scientific practice (Wylie, 1992; Bhaskar, 1994; Latour, 1999; Lewis *et al.*, 2011).

2.4 Mitigated objectivity: A path forward...

The first step toward achieving mitigated objectivity in forensic anthropology is simply acknowledging the subjectivities inherent in forensic anthropological practice. If the field denies that these subjectivities exist, practitioners will never be able to manage them appropriately (Dror *et al.*, 2005). The next step is attempting to understand those subjectivities. "Subjectivity does not necessarily equal unreliability" (Christensen and Crowder, 2009:1214), but forensic anthropologists must be honest and direct about the error it introduces. They must establish where error exists and communicate it responsibly to each other and in the courtroom (Dror, 2013). This means that in addition to critiquing and revising methods, forensic anthropologists can focus on validation studies and ascertaining error rates for their most frequently used methods (*sensu* Christensen and Crowder, 2009), looking at error in both the samples on which they were based and the different populations to which they are applied (Komar and Buikstra, 2008). Risinger and colleagues (2002:9) call this a "science of science"—studying what causes error, how to recognize it, and how to minimize it. The discipline of forensic anthropology has begun to engage in earnest with the quantification of error and uncertainty due to method inadequacies; now it must extend this "science of science" to the error introduced by human subjectivity.

As forensic anthropologists begin to understand their biases and subjectivities, they can take steps to constrain them. As experienced and educated as forensic experts may be, they cannot eliminate implicit biases and subjectivities through sheer force of will. Cognitive studies show that no humans have this capacity—forensic scientists included (Thompson *et al.*, 2011). Many other scientific fields take measures to minimize extraneous, biasing information (e.g., the double-blind and placebo trials used in medical research; Risinger *et al.*, 2002; Thompson *et al.*, 2011), and the field of forensic anthropology must engage in these practices as well. If practitioners know where subjectivities exist and how they contribute to error, they can mitigate that error and constrain subjectivity. In lieu of pure objectivity, they can pursue the goal of mitigated objectivity.

There are great benefits to striving for this approximation of objectivity: forensic anthropologists will improve their methods, develop quality-assurance protocols, learn more powerful statistical tools, and engage with new equipment and technologies—all of which will improve the state of their science. The current push within the field for increased method quantification represents an important step toward mitigated objectivity. Quantitative data collection and analysis constrain observer subjectivity, and the resulting probabilistic statements represent a vast improvement from the overly conclusive, statistically indefensible individualization claims for which the forensic sciences have been criticized (Steadman *et al.*, 2006; NRC, 2009; Kaye, 2010; Koehler, 2011). However, while forensic anthropologists pursue increasingly quantitative methods, they cannot neglect the importance of their qualitative techniques, which rely on the experience of the observer and are strengthened by that experience (Grivas and Komar, 2008). Moreover, they must acknowledge that there are many occasions on which subjective expert opinions (rather than objective facts) can be both valid and valuable—as long as the accompanying error can be identified and constrained (Dror, 2013). In their quest for mitigated objectivity, forensic anthropologists cannot ignore their own subjectivities.

2.4.1 Constraining subjectivity and bias

As long as humans are practicing science, there will always be a human filter on scientific methods. Yet, the epistemology of mitigated objectivity holds that forensic anthropologists can strive to constrain that human element of subjectivity (Box 2.3).

Box 2.3 Mitigated objectivity in forensic anthropology: potential constraints for subjectivity and bias

Minimum standards	Establish and enforce standards for education, training, testing, and qualifications
Quality control	Accredit laboratories; designate quality-control personnel; practice competency testing, peer review, external review, blind analysis, sequential unmasking
Foregrounding bias	Make biases explicit; test identifiable biases
Method and theory	Strengthen methods with anthropological and other theory; establish method error and realistic method performance
Publication and discussion	Exchange ideas and technologies with other members of the anthropological and forensic science community
Education and outreach	Convey mitigated objectivity (i.e., realistic view of method performance and field capabilities) to each other and the public

By applying multiple layers of constraint, scientists can mitigate the subjectivity of their interpretations and reduce bias in their conclusions.

An important first layer of constraint is standardization: establishing minimum standards of practice for the discipline of forensic anthropology and setting standards for education and qualifications to constrain the subjectivities of untrained analysts. The former Scientific Working Group for Forensic Anthropology began this standardization process by establishing consensus best-practice guidelines for forensic anthropologists. The current National Institute of Standards and Technology Organization of Scientific Area Committees and the American Standards Board Anthropology Consensus Body now continue the work, with the goal of setting and enforcing minimum standards for the field.

Quality control also mitigates subjectivity. Practices like laboratory accreditation, competency testing, peer review, external review, blind analysis, and the sequential unmasking of potentially biasing information reduce the potential for observer effects to bias analysts (Thompson *et al.*, 2011). Even an analyst's subjective opinion can be strengthened if an independent analyst comes to the same conclusion (Dror, 2013). Conclusions are further strengthened when the examiners themselves are constrained by competency testing and their laboratory's standard operating protocols are accredited. Funding and personnel limitations permitting, laboratories can appoint designated quality-control specialists to ensure transparency in case documentation and to act as gatekeepers at the beginning of analysis, providing analysts with necessary contextual data while filtering potentially biasing information (Risinger *et al.*, 2002). This increased quality control may translate to an increased workload for analysts, but extreme quality-control measures may not be necessary in every case. Laboratory management can ascertain when they are and craft case-specific analysis protocols accordingly (Risinger *et al.*, 2002; Dror, 2012; Nakhaeizadeh *et al.*, 2014b). Larger forensic anthropology laboratories across the country have already emplaced such quality-control measures (e.g., the New York City Office of Chief Medical Examiner, the Harris County Institute of Forensic Sciences, the Defense POW/MIA Accounting Agency), and the success of these laboratories demonstrates the utility and feasibility of applying such controls.

Even when analyses are compromised by biasing factors, forensic anthropologists can constrain this bias. If they identify the expectations that shape what they observe, they can examine and question these expectations, testing each one as they would a hypothesis (Nordby, 1992). Does reading the medical examiner report bias an analyst to expect a suicide? Does examining the associated material evidence cause the analyst to expect a female decedent? Those biases can be tested. Of course, not all of the "theories" behind the "theory-laden data" will be explicit or identifiable, but anthropologists can attempt to confront the biases they know they have. They can foreground and scrutinize these biases, evaluate the resulting data from an "ongoing critical perspective," and update these data as perspectives change, technologies advance, and theories and interpretations develop (Mnookin *et al.*, 2011:726).

Perhaps most importantly, forensic anthropologists must ensure that their methods have strong theoretical bases (Christensen and Crowder, 2009). The field has already begun to engage with quantifying and understanding method error. This pursuit is essential to a more realistic view of the accuracy that methods are capable of achieving. Yet, it is the theories underlying these methods that enable them to yield accurate biological determinations or doom them to inaccuracy and imprecision. Underpinning methods with strong theory will not only improve the methods—thus constraining subjectivity—but it will also help practitioners to understand *why* their methods work. As this volume attests, practitioners are only beginning to explore explicit applications of theory to the field. Still, the fact that they *are* beginning to do so is encouraging: the science of forensic anthropology is a developing one, and every science must start somewhere (Nordby, 2002). As the field develops, forensic anthropological practice is turning from a reliance on isolated observations to a focus on identifying and understanding underlying explanatory theories (Nordby, 2002). As it does so, its conclusions will be elevated from the level of subjective anecdote and observation to become more objective, rigorous, and reproducible (Haglund and Sorg, 1997).

The publication of this and other volumes in the *Forensic Science in Focus* series represents a further step toward developing these constraints, as does the continued, strong presence of forensic anthropological research in the *Journal of Forensic Sciences* and other peer-reviewed forensic journals. Continuous research, publication, and discussion form part of the robust research culture envisioned for the forensic sciences by Mnookin and colleagues (2011). As practitioners exchange ideas, learn new technologies and techniques, and engage with different theories and perspectives from the broader fields of anthropology and other disciplines, they contribute to the body of knowledge that constrains their interpretations. The field should be open to discussion of the sort broached by this chapter. Many forensic anthropologists are already aware of the possibility of subjectivity in their work. Many are aware of the ability of implicit theory to infuse their data and bias their conclusions. This awareness is good, but it is not good enough. Forensic anthropologists must be willing to state explicitly where subjectivities enter their work and enumerate the constraints applied to mitigate them (Box 2.4).

Finally, there is an education and public outreach component to this vision of mitigated objectivity. Forensic anthropologists must commit to conveying their realistic view of disciplinary capabilities and method performance not only to each other but also to the public. Forensic anthropology testimony must communicate mitigated objectivity. This may not be easy. Research indicates that the more forthcoming forensic experts are about the risks of human error in their methods, the less confident jurors are in the experts' conclusions—even though probabilistic evidence statements that incorporate error rates are inherently stronger than equivalent statistics that ignore risks of error (Koehler, 2011). However, forensic anthropologists have already begun to develop statistics that quantify the probability that their identifications are correct (Steadman *et al.*, 2006), and they must

Box 2.4 A case study in constraint: elucidating the process of constraining subjectivity and bias

Forensic anthropologists can apply theoretical and methodological constraints at multiple points during casework in order to reduce their inherent subjectivities. Through all stages of recovery, analysis, interpretation, and review, potential biases and constraining controls can be explicitly stated

Stage of casework	Potential biases	Constraints applied
Field recovery	Decisions about how deep to dig and how far to expand a search are subjective and experience-based	Use knowledge of archaeological principles (e.g., the laws of superposition and stratigraphic succession) to constrain subjectivity of recovery strategy
Field documentation	Scene maps are invaluable tools for depicting spatial relationships, but they are subjective, reductionist re-presentations of reality (i.e., anthropologists choose to present certain features and perspectives while backgrounding others)	Take comparative photographs showing the same views of the scene depicted in maps
Laboratory analysis and interpretation	Analyses of trauma, taphonomy, pathology, and the biological profile can be influenced by analysts' experiences and implicit biases	Constrain trauma determinations with biomechanical theories Strengthen taphonomic interpretations by conducting actualistic experiments Inform conclusions about pathology with theories from related fields (e.g., biology, paleodemography) Constrain age, sex, and ancestry assessments with an understanding of high-level theories (e.g., evolution, human growth and development) Follow standardized methods and quality-assurance protocols; ensure that both quantitative and qualitative methods have been validated and tested for error

(*Continued*)

Box 2.4 (Continued)

Stage of casework	Potential biases	Constraints applied
Reporting	Contextual case data and/or information gleaned during recovery of the remains can bias analysts' report conclusions	Sequentially unmask potentially biasing contextual information to ensure that analysts have the benefit of relevant contextual information only at key points during their analyses
Review	Peer reviewers may be influenced by primary analysts' conclusions, if these conclusions are available for review	Regularly test the proficiency of all analysts and remediate deficiencies Conduct blind peer review to test whether analysts reach similar conclusions with and without potentially biasing information

continue to rise to the challenge. This will potentially involve working with psychologists, legal scholars, statisticians, and other forensic scientists to devise ways to incorporate statements about subjectivity and bias into expert testimonies and to convey the meaning of such statistics to the lay public who serve as jurors (Koehler, 2011). Presenting "the logic of certainty"—implying that results are *facts* or portraying forensic science as rigorously objective—is dangerous (Hawley, 2005:108). The myth of pure objectivity can be as insidious as the "demon" of scientific certainty now rejected by both legal scholars and forensic scientists (Black, 1994:2129; Freudenburg *et al.*, 2008; DOJ and NIST NCFS, 2016). Espousing mitigated objectivity is more honest, more ethical, and more in keeping with the spirit of error and uncertainty analysis that has pervaded the post-*Daubert* era (*Daubert v. Merrell Dow Pharmaceuticals, Inc.*, 1993).

Indeed, applying the layers of constraint that allow forensic anthropologists to achieve mitigated objectivity represents progress toward the vision of objectivity called for by *Daubert*, the related *Kumho* decision, and the recent National Academy of Sciences (NAS) recommendations for advancing the state of the forensic sciences (*Daubert v. Merrell Dow Pharmaceuticals, Inc.*, 1993; *Kumho Tire Company, Ltd. v. Carmichael*, 1999; NRC, 2009). The method improvement, error quantification, and within-field communication discussed earlier are consistent with the *Daubert* call for forensic scientists to produce methods that are peer reviewed, rigorously tested, and widely accepted within the scientific community—with known error rates and standards for application (*Daubert v. Merrell Dow Pharmaceuticals, Inc.*, 1993). Working to advance the field's qualitative, opinion-based techniques, in addition to its more quantitative methods, guarantees improvement in the quality of both technical and scientific testimony (*Kumho Tire Company, Ltd. v. Carmichael*, 1999). Developing and enforcing standards for the field, emplacing quality-control measures, identifying and reducing bias, and validating and refining methods directly address NAS recommendations 3b, 5, 7, and 8 (NRC, 2009:190–191, 215). Finally, working to understand the theories underlying both quantitative and qualitative methods responds to the call by the NAS for studies establishing the scientific bases demonstrating the validity of forensic techniques (NRC, 2009: Recommendation 3a:190).

2.4.2 The continuing process of constraint

Possibilities abound for future research investigating the nature of subjectivity in forensic anthropological analysis and developing ways to constrain the bias that it entails. Recent research has highlighted the subjectivity of nonmetric forensic anthropological methods (e.g., Nakhaeizadeh *et al.*, 2014a, b). Metric methods must also be tested in order to ascertain whether these quantitative methods are truly as objective as forensic anthropologists would like to think they are. Ascertaining where interpretations of measurement definitions differ among observers will lead to the revision and clarification of these definitions (Ousley *et al.*, 2015; Langley *et al.*, 2016), increasing method reliability and forming part of the continuing process of constraint. Additional studies testing whether blind and context-dependent analysts come to the same analytical conclusions must be conducted—not only to highlight where subjectivities lie but also to identify gaps between what scientists think they know and what they only perceive based on the contextual biases that influence them. The theories assumed to underlie forensic anthropological methods must also be tested. In taphonomic analyses, for example, the principle of uniformitarianism presumably unites past observations with the results of current actualistic experiments (Haglund and Sorg, 1997), but instances where different processes can be identified in the past and present must be explored (e.g., patterns of animal scavenging observed today may differ from patterns described 50 years ago; Komar and Buikstra, 2008).

Another avenue for advancement toward the goal of mitigated objectivity involves the development of discipline-specific standards for the differentiation between relevant and irrelevant contextual information. Whether intentionally or unintentionally, analysts use context to give meaning to evidence and to organize what they observe (Rock and Palmer, 1990; Nordby, 1992). However, using contextual data to inform observations is not always a negative practice. Context can actually enhance inference if it is relevant to the analysis at hand (Haglund and Sorg, 1997; Warren, 2015). Not all context is irrelevant or biasing, and irrelevant must be differentiated from relevant context in ways that make sense for each discipline of forensic science (Risinger *et al.*, 2002). In the field of forensic anthropology, for example, while a confession from the suspect will always constitute irrelevant context, field-recovery data will always constitute *relevant* context (Haglund and Sorg, 1997; Risinger *et al.*, 2002; Dirkmaat *et al.*, 2008). If a forensic anthropologist does not participate in the recovery, she is one step removed from the recovery data—increasing the likelihood that detail will be lost (Haglund and Sorg, 1997). As forensic anthropology has transitioned from a predominantly laboratory-based discipline to one that increasingly incorporates archaeological recovery, analysts increasingly depend on recovery context to inform their laboratory analyses (Sorg and Haglund, 2002; Dirkmaat *et al.*, 2008). The scope of forensic anthropology has broadened over the past several decades, and that scope now includes not only human remains but also the context from which those remains were recovered (Dirkmaat *et al.*, 2008). Delineating relevant from irrelevant context in a way that is meaningful for the field of forensic anthropology will form an important part of developing standards for the field.

2.5 Conclusion

In this post-*Daubert* era of increasing method standardization, forensic anthropologists have demonstrated their commitment to understanding error so as not to overstate method performance (*Daubert v. Merrell Dow Pharmaceuticals, Inc.*, 1993). This chapter has argued that espousing the rhetoric of "true" or "pure" objectivity also overstates their capabilities. In the spirit of understanding error, forensic anthropologists must understand the limits of their own objectivity. They must evaluate their subjective biases, constraining interpretations with strong theory, methods, and quality control whenever possible and discussing the error those biases introduce whenever it is not. In lieu of pure objectivity, forensic anthropologists can strive for a mitigated objectivity that more accurately reflects the capabilities of their science.

If practitioners are willing to commit to approximating objectivity through this process of constraint, then the answer to this chapter's title question is *yes*. Yes, it is possible to practice subjective science that is also sound science. Yes, forensic anthropology can be subjective with a capital S.

References

Adams, B.J. and Byrd, J.E. (2002) Interobserver variation of selected postcranial skeletal measurements. *Journal of Forensic Sciences*, **46**, 1193–1202.

Bhaskar, R. (1994) *Plato Etc.: The Problems of Philosophy and Their Resolution*. Verso, London.

Bhaskar, R. (2005 [1979]) *The Possibility of Naturalism: A Philosophical Critique of the Contemporary Human Sciences*, 3rd edn. Routledge, New York.

Bhaskar, R. (2008 [1975]) Introduction. In: *A Realist Theory of Science*. Routledge, New York, pp. 12–20.

Binford, L.R. (1968) Some comments on historical versus processual archaeology. *Southwestern Journal of Anthropology*, **24**, 267–275.

Binford, L.R. (1989) *Debating Archaeology*. Academic Press, London.

Black, B. (1994) The Supreme Court's view of science: Has *Daubert* exorcised the certainty demon? *Cardozo Law Review*, **15**, 2129–2137.

Boyd, C. and Boyd, D.C. (2011) Theory and the scientific basis for forensic anthropology. *Journal of Forensic Sciences*, **56**, 1407–1415.

Christensen, A.M. and Crowder, C.M. (2009) Evidentiary standards for forensic anthropology. *Journal of Forensic Sciences*, **54**, 1211–1216.

Clarke, D.L. (1972) Chapter 1: Models and paradigms in contemporary archaeology. In: *Models in Archaeology* (ed. D.L. Clarke). Methuen, London, pp. 1–12.

Cleland, C.E. (2002) Methodological and epistemic differences between historical science and experimental science. *Philosophy of Science*, **69**, 447–451.

Daemmrich, A. (1998) The evidence does not speak for itself: Expert witnesses and the organization of DNA-typing companies. *Social Studies of Science*, **28**, 741–772.

Daubert v. Merrell Dow Pharmaceuticals, Inc. (1993) **509** U.S. 579.

Dirkmaat, D.C., Cabo, L.L., Ousley, S.D., and Symes, S.A. (2008) New perspectives in forensic anthropology. *Yearbook of Physical Anthropology*, **51**, 33–52.

DOJ (Department of Justice) and NIST (National Institute of Standards and Technology) NCFS (National Commission on Forensic Science) (2016) Testimony Using the Term "Reasonable Scientific Certainty." Views document by NCFS Subcommittee on Reporting and Testimony, adopted 22 March 2016. https://www.justice.gov/ncfs/file/839731/download (accessed August 29, 2017).

Dror, I.E. (2012) Letter to the editor—Combating bias: The next step in fighting cognitive and psychological contamination. *Journal of Forensic Sciences*, **57**, 276–277.

Dror, I.E. (2013) The ambition to be scientific: Human expert performance and objectivity. *Science and Justice*, **53**, 81–82.

Dror, I.E. and Charlton, D. (2006) Why experts make errors. *Journal of Forensic Identification*, **56**, 600–616.

Dror, I.E. and Hampikian, G. (2011) Subjectivity and bias in forensic DNA mixture interpretation. *Science and Justice*, **51**, 204–208.

Dror, I.E., Péron, A.E., Hind, S.-L., and Charlton, D. (2005) When emotions get the better of us: The effect of contextual top-down processing on matching fingerprints. *Applied Cognitive Psychology*, **19**, 799–809.

Dror, I.E., Charlton, D., and Péron, A.E. (2006) Contextual information renders experts vulnerable to making erroneous identifications. *Forensic Science International*, **156**, 74–78.

Flannery, K.V. (1973) Archeology with a capital "S." In: *Research and Theory in Current Archaeology* (ed. C.L. Redman). John Wiley, New York, pp. 47–53.

Freudenburg, W.R., Gramling, R., and Davidson, D. (2008) Scientific Certainty Argumentation Methods (SCAMs): Science and the politics of doubt. *Sociological Inquiry*, **78**, 2–38.

Gillespie, S.D. (2011) Archaeological drawings as re-presentations: The maps of Complex A, La Venta, Mexico. *Latin American Antiquity*, **22**, 3–36.

Gould, S.J. (1981) *The Mismeasure of Man*. W.W. Norton & Company, Inc., New York.

Grivas, C.R. and Komar, D.A. (2008) *Kumho, Daubert*, and the nature of scientific inquiry: Implications for forensic anthropology. *Journal of Forensic Sciences*, **53**, 771–776.

Guba, E.C. (1990) The alternative paradigm dialog. In: *The Paradigm Dialog* (ed. E.C. Guba). Sage Publications, Newberry Park, CA, pp. 17–27.

Haglund, W.D. and Sorg, M.H. (1997) Method and theory of forensic taphonomic research. In: *Forensic Taphonomy: The Postmortem Fate of Human Remains* (eds. W.D. Haglund and M.H. Sorg). CRC Press, Boca Raton, FL, pp. 13–26.

Hawley, T.M. (2005) *The Remains of War: Bodies, Politics, and the Search for American Soldiers Unaccounted for in Southeast Asia*. Duke University Press, Durham, NC.

Hodder, I. (1992) *Theory and Practice in Archaeology*. Routledge, London.

Jantz, L.M., Shirley, N.R., McNulty, S., *et al.* (2015) Evaluation and reformation of osteometric data in forensic anthropology: The foundations of DCP 2.0. *Proceedings of the 67th American Academy of Forensic Sciences*, Orlando, FL, February 19, 2015, **XXI**, 157–158.

Jones, A. (2002) The archaeology of "two cultures." In: *Archaeological Theory and Scientific Practice*. Cambridge University Press, Cambridge, U.K., pp. 1–22.

Kaye, D.H. (2010) Probability, individualization, and uniqueness in forensic science evidence: Listening to the academies. *Brooklyn Law Review*, **75**, 1163–1185.

Koehler, J.J. (2011) If the shoe fits they might acquit: The value of forensic science testimony. *Journal of Empirical Legal Studies*, **8**, 21–48.

Komar, D.A. and Buikstra, J.E. (2008) *Forensic Anthropology: Contemporary Theory and Practice*. Oxford University Press, New York.

Kumho Tire Company, Ltd. v. Carmichael (1999) 526 U.S. 137.

Langley, N.R., Jantz, L.M., Ousley, S.D., *et al.* (2016) *Data Collection Procedures for Forensic Skeletal Material 2.0*. The University of Tennessee Forensic Anthropology Center, Knoxville.

Latour, B. (1988) Visualisation and social reproduction: Opening one eye while closing the other...A note on some religious paintings. In: *Picturing Power: Visual Depiction and Social Relations* (eds. G. Fyfe and J. Law). Routledge, London, pp. 15–38.

Latour, B. (1993) *We Have Never Been Modern*. Harvard University Press, Cambridge, MA.

Latour, B. (1999) *Pandora's Hope: Essays on the Reality of Science Studies*. Harvard University Press, Cambridge, MA.

Latour, B. and Woolgar, S. (1979a) From order to disorder. In: *Laboratory Life: The Construction of Scientific Facts*. Sage Publications, Beverly Hills, CA, pp. 15–42.

Latour, B. and Woolgar, S. (1979b) The construction of a fact: The case of TRF(H). In: *Laboratory Life: The Construction of Scientific Facts*. Sage Publications, Beverly Hills, CA, pp. 105–149.

Law, J. and Whittaker, J. (1988) On the art of representation: Notes on the politics of visualisation. In: *Picturing Power: Visual Depiction and Social Relations* (eds. G. Fyfe and J. Law). Routledge, London, pp. 160–183.

Lewis, J.E., DeGusta, D., Meyer, M.R., *et al.* (2011) The mismeasure of science: Stephen Jay Gould versus Samuel George Morton on skulls and bias. *PLoS Biology*, **9**, e1001071.

Marks, J. (2009) *Why I am Not a Scientist: Anthropology and Modern Knowledge*. University of California Press, Berkeley.

McGee, R.J. and Warms, R.L. (2008) *Anthropological Theory: An Introductory History*, 4th edn. McGraw-Hill, Boston, MA.

Mnookin, J.L., Cole, S.A., Dror, I.E., *et al.* (2011) The need for a research culture in the forensic sciences. *UCLA Law Review*, **88**, 725–779.

Moore, H.L. and Sanders, T. (2006) *Anthropology in Theory: Issues in Epistemology*. Blackwell Publishing, Malden, MA.

Moser, S. (1992) The visual language of archaeology: A case study of the Neanderthals. *Antiquity*, **66**, 831–844.

Nakhaeizadeh, S., Hanson, I., and Dozzi, N. (2014a) The power of contextual effects in forensic anthropology: A study of biasability in the visual interpretations of trauma analysis on skeletal remains. *Journal of Forensic Sciences*, **59**, 1177–1183.

Nakhaeizadeh, S., Dror, I.E., and Morgan, R.M. (2014b) Cognitive bias in forensic anthropology: Visual assessment of skeletal remains is susceptible to confirmation bias. *Science and Justice*, **54**, 208–214.

Nordby, J.J. (1989) Bootstrapping while barefoot (crime models vs. theoretical models in the hunt for serial killers). *Synthese*, **81**, 373–389.

Nordby, J.J. (1992) Can we believe what we see, if we see what we believe?—Expert disagreement. *Journal of Forensic Sciences*, **37**, 1115–1124.

Nordby, J.J. (2002) Is forensic taphonomy scientific? In: *Advances in Forensic Taphonomy: Method, Theory, and Archaeological Perspectives* (eds. W.D. Haglund and M.H. Sorg). CRC Press, Boca Raton, FL, pp. 31–42.

NRC (National Research Council) Committee on Identifying the Needs of the Forensic Sciences Community (2009) Strengthening Forensic Science in the United States: A Path Forward. Document No. 228091. The National Academies Press, Washington, DC.

Ousley, S.D., Shirley, N.R., and Jantz, R. (2015) One hundred years since Martin's *lehrbuch*: Measurement confusion and DCP 2.0. *Proceedings of the 67th American Academy of Forensic Sciences*, Orlando, FL, February 19, 2015, **XXI**, 155–156.

Pronin, E. (2006) Perception and misperception of bias in human judgment. *Trends in Cognitive Science*, **11**, 37–43.

Pronin, E., Gilovich, T., and Ross, L. (2004) Objectivity in the eye of the beholder: Divergent perceptions of bias in self versus others. *Psychological Review*, **111**, 781–799.

Reybrouck, D. van (1998) Imaging and imagining the Neanderthal: The role of technical drawings in archaeology. *Antiquity*, **72**, 56–64.

Risinger, D.M., Saks, M.J., Thompson, W.C., and Rosenthal, R. (2002) The *Daubert/Kumho* implications of observer effects in forensic science: Hidden problems of expectation and suggestion. *California Law Review*, **90**, 1–56.

Rock, I. and Palmer, S. (1990) The legacy of Gestalt psychology. *Scientific American*, **263**, 84–90.

Shanks, M. and Tilley, C. (1992 [1987]) Positivism and the "New Archaeology." In: *Re-Constructing Archaeology: Theory and Practice*, 2nd edn. Routledge, London, pp. 29–45.

Smith, A.C. and Boaks, A. (2014) How "standardized" is standardized? A validation of postcranial landmark locations. *Journal of Forensic Sciences*, **59**, 1457–1465.

Sommer, M. (2006) Mirror, mirror on the wall: Neanderthal as image and "distortion" in early 20th-century French science and press. *Social Studies of Science*, **36**, 207–240.

Sorg, M.H. and Haglund, W.D. (2002) Advancing forensic taphonomy: Purpose, theory, and process. In: *Advances in Forensic Taphonomy: Method, Theory, and Archaeological Perspectives* (eds. W.D. Haglund and M.H. Sorg). CRC Press, Boca Raton, FL, pp. 3–29.

Steadman, D.W., Adams, B.J., and Konigsberg, L.W. (2006) Statistical basis for positive identification in forensic anthropology. *American Journal of Physical Anthropology*, **131**, 15–26.

Thompson, W.C., Ford, S., Gilder, J.R., *et al.* (2011) Commentary on: Thornton, J.I. Letter to the editor—A rejection of "working blind" as a cure for contextual bias. *Journal of Forensic Sciences*, **56**, 562–563.

Wallace, S. (2011) *Contradictions of Archaeological Theory: Engaging Critical Realism and Archaeological Theory*. Routledge, New York.

Warren, M.W. (2015) Context and cognitive bias: Informed applied science vs. working in the blind. *Proceedings of the 67th American Academy of Forensic Sciences*, Orlando, FL, February 20, 2015, **XXI**, 196.

Watson, P.J., LeBlanc, S.A., and Redman, C.L. (1971) *Explanation in Archaeology: An Explicitly Scientific Approach*. Columbia University Press, New York.

Wilson, T.D. and Brekke, N. (1994) Mental contamination and mental correction: Unwanted influences on judgments and evaluations. *Psychological Bulletin*, **116**, 117–142.

Wylie, A. (1982) Epistemological issues raised by a structuralist archaeology. In: *Symbolic and Structural Archaeology* (ed. I. Hodder). Cambridge University Press, Cambridge, UK, pp. 39–46.

Wylie, A. (1992) "Heavily decomposing red herrings": Middle ground in the anti-/postprocessualism wars. In: *Metaarchaeology* (ed. L. Embree). Kluwer Academic Publishers, New York, pp. 269–288.

CHAPTER 3

Navigating cognitive bias in forensic anthropology

Michael W. Warren, Amanda N. Friend and Michala K. Stock
Department of Anthropology, University of Florida, Gainesville, FL, USA

3.1 Introduction

Cognitive bias has long been recognized as part of the human condition. If one pays attention, it can be seen in our everyday lives during our interactions with others. A common form of cognitive bias, called belief perseverance, may be demonstrated by a stubborn neighbor who insists that the moon remains unconquered and that the Apollo missions were an elaborate hoax. Another form of cognitive bias arises when a family member *knows*, based on their loud music and clothing, that the kids across the street are "up to no good." These examples are relatively harmless, but within the domain of the forensic sciences and our legal system, these kinds of preconceived opinions and perceptions can have serious consequences.

Julius Caesar, recognizing the existence of observer effects, wrote "men generally believe quite freely that which they want to be true" (Risinger *et al.*, 2002). Later, this sentiment was reiterated by songwriter and poet Paul Simon, who wrote that "...a man hears what he wants to hear and disregards the rest" (Simon, 1970). Document examiner W. E. Hagan (1894) was perhaps the first forensic scientist to recognize that bias may affect interpretations and suggested that scientific examinations be carried out without the introduction of extraneous information. Since that period, social psychologists and cognitive behaviorists have corroborated Hagan's assessment. Errors associated with cognitive bias have been reported in numerous areas of the forensic sciences, including handwriting analysis (Found and Ganas, 2013), genetics (Dror and Hampikian, 2011), odontology (Page *et al.*, 2002), anthropology (Nakhaeizadeh *et al.*, 2014), firearms comparisons (Kerstholt *et al.*, 2012), and fire investigations (Bieber, 2012).

In recent years, cognitive bias has risen to the forefront among issues involving the forensic sciences, highlighted by the National Academy of Sciences (NAS) report (National Research Council, 2009), and was starkly demonstrated by the

Forensic Anthropology: Theoretical Framework and Scientific Basis, First Edition.
Edited by C. Clifford Boyd Jr and Donna C. Boyd.

erroneous fingerprint "identification" of Brandon Mayfield in the Madrid Bomber case (Kassin *et al.*, 2013). The NAS report not only recommended increased research on the effects of cognitive bias and error rates associated with bias but also suggested the development of "standard operating procedures" to control bias.

The forensic sciences have embraced the reality that confirmation bias exists and that it can negatively affect our conclusions and opinions. The standard procedures suggested in the NAS report are, or will be, written by the Organization of Scientific Area Committees, working groups, and other leaders within the disciplines as they establish best practices and minimum standards for each domain. Individual laboratories have already begun integrating policies and procedures for minimizing error due to bias. Some recommendations are obvious (e.g., limit access to biasing information), but even the most obvious solutions may be difficult to apply in some contexts. This chapter focuses on the complexity and special challenges we face in implementing strategies to reduce bias error within the field of forensic anthropology and proposes some open-ended questions for discussion of this subject.

3.2 Types of cognitive bias

Social psychologists and cognitive scientists identify several types of cognitive biases. The most relevant form pertaining to the forensic sciences is confirmation bias, in which people tend to favor information that confirms their theory over disconfirming information. This is applicable to science when a theory is based on information obtained prior to scientific testing. A subset within this category is prosecutory bias, which indirectly affects forensic scientists because it tends to dictate the types of evidence presented to forensic examiners and it channels existing *a priori* information toward a favored but potentially erroneous conclusion. In the US legal system, a prosecutor decides to pursue a case based on preliminary evidence that results in the belief that the defendant is guilty (Burke, 2005). At that point, the investigation tends to seek additional evidence confirming that belief and potentially filters out evidence that supports an alternate scenario. Forensic scientists should be buffered from this particular type of bias, since we should not harbor an opinion—and certainly do not assume—whether or not a particular defendant is guilty. The identity or existence of a defendant is often unknown to the forensic scientists performing analyses, and so at this basic level, they are not at risk.

Another type of cognitive bias is called selective information processing, which may be relevant when scientists cannot assign an appropriate level of probative value to evidence independent of their prior beliefs. This is especially true when the prior belief is based on extraneous information unrelated to the science being performed. An extension of this form of bias is called belief perseverance, in which individuals may hold on to a firmly held belief in the face of overwhelming evidence that discredits that belief. This is sometimes manifested by a prosecutor who has been confronted with exonerating evidence that the convicted person is innocent, but still insists that the defendant is guilty.

In science, errors related to bias are most commonly seen when scientists are exposed to extraneous information that shapes their opinion prior to scientific testing (Dror and Charlton, 2006). Dror and Hampikian (2011) call this domain irrelevant information. But bias can result from other factors. Those factors may include knowledge of the opinion of another scientist's conclusions, the influence of prior tests performed to reach a single conclusion, or preconceived theories or opinions based on experience or prior general observations. Additional sources may include practical matters related to employment or consulting relationships (e.g., a supervisor dictates policies about the information the analysts collect, or the pathologist only requests certain tests). Many of these factors are beyond the scope of this chapter, but all must be carefully considered if we are to find the most efficient and appropriate ways to reduce error caused by bias.

3.3 Research versus applied science

Research within the field of biological anthropology, or any scientific discipline, must be hypothesis-driven and performed in a way that does not influence our conclusions. Thus, scientific research, particularly in the "hard" sciences, is performed blind, and preferably double-blind, in which neither the subjects nor researchers have expectations based on prior knowledge that might affect the behavior or conclusions of either group. A common example is medical research in pharmaceutical clinical trials in which subjects are given either a test drug or a placebo. Neither the investigator nor the subject knows who is getting the placebo, which insures that both the test group and the control group are treated identically. Both groups are revealed at the end of the testing period and outcomes are recorded, interpreted, and compared against prestated hypotheses.

Should applied scientists always work in the blind, or should we integrate contextual clues into our analyses and conclusions? Do forensic anthropologists provide a better service to our consulting pathologists, law enforcement agencies, and attorneys when we are provided the context surrounding the case, or does that information unduly affect our interpretations? For example, when a pathologist provides us with the clinical radiographs of a putative decedent, are our results skewed because of some expectation that we will find a radiographic match? When we examine crime scene photographs of the area in which a body is found, does that alter our estimation of time since death, or facilitate it?

The practice of applied science is predicated upon the expectation that the research that generated the theories and methods being employed is (relatively) free from error produced by bias. Studies that do not control for bias are considered unsound and are therefore inappropriate to apply in practice. However, applied science often benefits from knowledge of the specific questions being asked by other parties. Especially in the fields of the forensic sciences, this knowledge can focus our efforts on aspects of a case that are most likely to yield results, thus avoiding dead-end paths that may waste the limited time and resources available to forensic practitioners.

The oft-cited analogy of clinical trials versus medical treatment considers the difference between research medicine and the practice of medicine. Medical practitioners are also applied scientists using medical research to guide their examination, diagnosis, and treatment of patients. The medical procedures, treatment modalities, and surgical/pharmacological interventions they use are based on sound research, which was conducted via hypothesis-driven testing and constrained *a priori* information. But in practice, physicians, nurses, and ancillary medical personnel do not limit *a priori* information, nor should they. When a middle-aged patient presents at the emergency department with severe chest pain, the physician does not prohibit the patient from relating this information because it may bias their diagnosis. Instead, she asks pertinent questions about the nature of the pain: *When did it start? Is it intermittent or steady? Have you had this type of pain before? What is your medical history?* This information is crucial in determining which diagnostic tests to perform, as well as guiding the physician in a preliminary diagnosis that will determine the appropriate treatment. Does the prior information provided by the patient affect the tests as they are being performed? No, the instrument that conducts the cardiac enzyme study and the electrocardiograph machine are blind to the patient's chest pain. However, the interview with the patient certainly plays a role in which tests are performed and may indicate which tests are nondiagnostic and unnecessary, or even harmful. The information given by the patient provides the context that guides the examination. In fact, much of the treatment in such a situation is most likely dictated by standing orders and protocols given the history, signs, and symptoms presented. Clinicians *want* to be biased by *a priori* information so they can begin to rule out alternate diagnoses and focus treatment on the primary diagnosis.

Similarly, forensic anthropologists may benefit from contextual information that will guide their approach to a specific case. Communication between the pathologist and anthropologist is vital in creating a thorough report of potential trauma that adequately addresses the needs of the pathologist. The skeletal exam must seek to address areas of interest noted by the pathologist during their initial exam and autopsy; however, the assessment of region of interest may be limited by the state of preservation of the remains.

A familiar example of these types of communication occurs when law enforcement requests that the anthropologist assist in a search for human remains. From a resource management perspective, it is a good idea to ask for basic information about why the agency is searching in a particular location. If the reason involves a witness to a clandestine burial, then it seems reasonable to assist if at all possible. However, if the reason for the search is a cell-phone call from the grave to a local psychic, then it seems prudent to carefully consider whether to provide personnel and valuable resources in that context. These decisions are made with the knowledge that the request for information about why the search is being conducted may, and often does, result in the agency revealing potentially biasing information (e.g., "We are missing a 20-year-old female and we have been informed that her body may be buried in her backyard"). Criminal investigations are closely bound to evidence and context, so law enforcement personnel see no reason to withhold information about the case. Unless the anthropologist has enough resources to dig up every area of interest to psychics in their geographic area, then managerial decisions must be made as to whether to risk receiving potentially biasing information prior to digging. This scenario may also impact how anthropologists deal with remains being examined in a laboratory setting if some lab personnel are intentionally excluded from a recovery in order to shield them from potentially biasing information prior to performing their analyses. This example highlights the balancing act that anthropologists and laboratory managers must perform in terms of resource allocation, as well as complications to the practicality of dealing with extraneous information.

3.4 Recommended solutions to mitigate confirmation bias

Several solutions have been proposed to isolate forensic analysts from irrelevant or potentially biasing information. The most obvious solution to control for the possible presence of biasing information is to have a second analyst conduct an independent examination, also called cross-laboratory verification. The second analyst, preferably from another laboratory, would be shielded from any communications or extraneous information the primary analyst received about the case and thus would be truly performing a blind examination. The second analyst would also be shielded from unavoidable information gleaned during the processing of remains in cases where the individual was fully fleshed upon arrival at the laboratory. The independent examination could also be performed in the same laboratory during a blind internal peer review in which the reviewer did not have access to the case file or the primary analytic notes. However, even quality assurance measures like peer review have the potential to introduce bias, especially when the reviewer knows the identity of the primary analyst. If the analyst is more experienced than the reviewer, it may be difficult for the reviewer to question the primary analyst's interpretations and conclusions.

A third method, called sequential unmasking, requires an appointed case manager who withholds potentially biasing information from the analyst(s) until such time as it can contribute to a forensic report without affecting testing. Sequential unmasking and internal peer review are both virtually impossible for the sole practitioner. However, in labs with multiple analysts (either employees or graduate students), the laboratory coordinator or director can serve as the case manager. The case manager is free to interact with crime scene investigators, detectives, and pathologists and collect case-related information. He/she can screen for potentially biasing information and coordinate the sequential unmasking of information as required by the analyst (Thornton, 2010; Thompson *et al.*, 2011). These solutions can also be used in various combinations depending on personnel, time, and/or resource constraints.

3.5 Challenges unique to forensic anthropology

3.5.1 Anthropologists work in a variety of professional contexts

Many of the solutions being developed to combat cognitive bias have been directed toward forensic scientists working within domains situated in accredited crime laboratories. These laboratories are staffed with multiple analysts in each discipline supported by a management structure utilizing surety-based quality controls. Within this idealized context, measures such as independent analysis, peer review, and sequential unmasking are relatively easy and cost-effective to implement and most likely increase laboratory efficiency.

Among the challenges facing forensic anthropologists is that we work in a wide variety of settings, most of which are far removed from the ideal laboratory environment referenced in the previous paragraph. Some forensic anthropologists work as sole practitioners, who may face the greatest obstacles to unbiased analyses. They serve as their own case managers and are hard pressed to use the aforementioned safeguards in their normal casework. However, these analysts can still acknowledge potentially biasing information by listing *a priori* information before beginning analysis. A large and still growing number of forensic anthropologists work within medical examiner offices under the direction of pathologists. If the pathologist does not favor specific quality assurance measures, such as accreditation, certification, or consensus best practices established by working groups, the anthropologist may be bound by policies that are less likely to address the influence of cognitive bias. Since the pathologist employs the anthropologists, they may be limited in their authority to write policies and procedures designed to address the cognitive biases that are specific to their field. Fortunately, the trend among most medical examiner offices—especially in larger jurisdictions—has been to hire many of our most talented colleagues, who are given the freedom and authority to write their own policies and procedures. Other anthropologists work in laboratories in university or college settings with the dual responsibilities of performing casework and training future forensic anthropologists. Some academic practitioners have codified standard operating procedures, while others do not. Differing laboratory management models are used for academic laboratories based on the number of faculty and available resources, not the least of which is the presence of highly trained graduate students who are qualified to serve as analysts.

All of these constraints are being discussed among our colleagues within the discipline and are being constantly addressed and updated through professional meetings, boards, working groups, and scientific area subcommittees. It has proven to be a Gordian knot of complexity in that the further one examines the theoretical solutions, the more apparent practical obstacles that make implementation difficult to apply in many real-world settings become.

3.5.2 The uniqueness of the forensic anthropology testing sample

Cross-laboratory verifications, as suggested by Koppl and colleagues (2008), are a valid and proven way of "checking on the propriety of the initial forensic work." In many forensic disciplines, it is possible that a small sample of blood, sputum, urine, or soft tissue may be retained and retested by an external reviewer or divided and sent to multiple laboratories. This solution is difficult to apply within forensic anthropology, because our testing sample almost always consists of the entirety of the recovered decomposed or skeletal remains of a decedent. Furthermore, once our testing is completed, the remains must be immediately returned to the medical examiner's office and, hopefully, to the bereaved family of the decedent. While other disciplines may withhold submitting their test reports until an independent colleague can retest the sample, time constraints most often preclude this option for forensic anthropologists. It is difficult to justify to a bereaved family that they must wait until a second examination can be conducted to confirm the identity of their family member, particularly if it requires coordinating the schedule of personnel from another laboratory. Therefore, external reviews in the field of forensic anthropology will likely be based on photographs, analytical notes, and reports—and not on actual reexamination of skeletal remains. If, on the other hand, a second series of tests on a human skeleton is required during the legal proceedings (i.e., a defense expert wants to examine the remains), it almost always requires an exhumation.

When two scientists examine the same sample, there may be a difference in interpretation and conclusions. Conflicts between an analyst and an internal peer reviewer can be resolved by referring the case to laboratory management, particularly if the management is comprised of at least one forensic anthropologist. Differences in conclusions or interpretations between an analyst and an outside reviewer have no such arbiter. This essentially limits external peer reviews to comparing the procedures, methods, and techniques used in a single case against the home laboratory's codified standard operating procedures. Again, the fact that the forensic anthropologist is examining a complete set of human remains instead of a small sample is problematic in that it limits possibilities in terms of retention and retesting.

3.5.3 Multiple tests to reach a single conclusion

Forensic anthropology practitioners perform multiple tests in sequence to arrive at a conclusion, as opposed to some forensic disciplines that conduct a single repeated test. For example, anthropologists might examine the pubic symphyseal face, the auricular surface of the ilium, the right fourth rib, and the medial clavicle when assessing age at death. If they perform their first test on the pubic symphysis, an experienced practitioner may well know the mean age and range for that phase. If the test indicates a young individual, it may bias their interpretation of each successive test.

Anthropologists also consider nonmetric morphological traits when assessing biological sex and ancestry. Practitioners perform these tests when they visually examine the skeleton and document their scores and observations of traits in their analytical notes. However, it is difficult to not casually observe morphological traits while handling the cranium prior to formal testing and therefore form an initial assessment of aspects of the biological profile. One colleague's advice was to "not look at" the skull before measuring it, but it is difficult for trained observers to filter out such easily visible and recognizable traits. Examination of the skeleton formally begins after placing the remains in anatomical position on a table prior to analysis. But it seems likely that most experienced practitioners have already conducted at least some informal nonmetric "testing" prior to picking up the calipers. Whether one measures the skull first, or performs nonmetric assessment first, each type of testing unavoidably informs subsequent tests. In other words, if metric analysis classifies the cranium as male, the analyst has that knowledge in hand prior to their nonmetric assessment, which has the potential to bias each successive observation.

The simple solution is to have one analyst conduct the first test and conceal their score and conclusions from subsequent analysts (each of whom conduct another single test, with the results of all prior tests remaining unknown to them). This solution would, of course, require a large number of in-house analysts—a rarity in the world of forensic anthropology laboratories. However, in an internal peer review, the reviewer's initial blind analysis can serve as a spot check of the primary analyst's assessment, as the reviewer's first conducted test will be the least biased and serve as an appropriate comparator.

3.6 An example of how bias affects procedures

The analysis of the biological profile will serve as an example of how aspects of the forensic anthropological practice can be subject to various types of bias and external pressure that can affect both the process of the analysis and the results. This example highlights important practical issues that forensic anthropologists must contend with, potential solutions, and challenges with implementing these solutions.

The pressure to produce a test result quickly is cited as one of the most common external influences that leads to shortcuts in analysis. An anthropologist should not yield to pressure from law enforcement, attorneys, funeral homes, or family members to rush their science. Our job is to insure that we use a careful, measured approach to our work; however, we must also acknowledge that time is of the essence to investigators. While this acknowledgment cannot be allowed to diminish the care we exercise in the normal course of an anthropology examination, it may impact the sequence of tests performed and, in some cases, alter the measures taken to reduce bias error such as sequential unmasking or peer review. Many possible questions can be raised in these types of circumstances: When radiographs of a putative decedent accompany human remains, should the antemortem–postmortem radiographic comparison wait until all skeletal analysis is finished so as not to influence our analyses? Or should analysts other than those primarily responsible for working on the case compare the radiographs to postmortem radiographs as soon as possible so that the identity of the decedent is confirmed?

It is difficult to justify waiting until the analysis is complete to inform the pathologist or investigator of a match or exclusion. Investigators need this information as soon as possible so that they can proceed with their case. The identification is central to the investigation, whereas other types of scientific tests are merely contributory. This begs the question of whether, once the identification is made, the analyst continues to assess the biological profile of the decedent. If not, then the necessity of performing one test quickly has altered the sequence of, or necessity for, subsequent testing in the forensic context.

Many, if not most, of the skeletal remains that are examined in a typical forensic anthropology laboratory are unidentified when analysis of the remains begins. The remainder have been identified by other means. In some cases, we know how the decedent was identified (e.g., via DNA or fingerprints); in others, we do not. For example, some medical examiners are willing to accept a driver's license found at the scene or the presence of a tattoo on the right arm as conclusive evidence of identity. Therefore, it seems to be a good practice to assess the biological profile in every case as a matter of policy. A forensic anthropologist's acceptance of the personal identification of a decedent based on the work of another scientist certainly introduces bias, as we are accepting *a priori* information as fact and making decisions about further testing based on this information.

Conversely, when the anthropologist establishes the identity of the decedent based on antemortem–postmortem radiographic comparison, it seems good practice to support that identification by also performing DNA testing. Genetic tests can be performed while the investigation proceeds based on the initial identification. This is important because genetic testing may take weeks, during which time the case is growing cold. Multiple forms of testing bolster the probability that we have accurately identified the decedent, particularly when scientists in other domains are using other independent methods to reach their conclusions.

If the forensic anthropologist's assessment of the biological profile and radiographic comparison significantly differ from that of the "identified" decedent, there are at least four potential reasons that the two assessments are incongruent:

- The identification was in error. The DNA sample was contaminated or a latent print examiner made a mistake that led to a wrong conclusion.
- There may have been a clerical error and the pathologist sent the laboratory the incorrect set of remains.

- The forensic anthropologist's assessment is wrong because of poor science or a faulty interpretation.
- The anthropologist applied the appropriate tests and correctly interpreted the results of the tests, but there is a research gap that needs to be addressed (e.g., the decedent was a member of a population for which we have no data).

A secondary reason to perform the biological profile, despite a previously established identification, is pedagogical. A university-based laboratory must fulfill a teaching mission in addition to research and service; graduate students require experience assessing the biological profile from skeletal remains. Provided that the initial identification is correct, the biological profile will, in most cases, match the known demographic information of the decedent. This is a clear signal to a student that they are applying the correct tests and that they are proficient in the technical skills required. When their assessment does not match the known biological profile of the decedent, students are tasked with understanding why, based on the scenarios listed earlier. Dror and colleagues (2013) are correct in their opinion that forensic analysts are not trying to provide the "right answer." We are, instead, trying to provide the best test result based on available objective evidence. When assessing the biological profile on "identified" decedents, we often find that our science produces a "wrong" answer. It is possible that we report a prediction interval of skeletal age as 35–45 years when the decedent was reported to be 28 years of age. Our primary concern should be that we practiced good science, not that the result was a "wrong" answer. We explain the disjunction to the jury by discussing the limitations of the science, human variation, and morphological outliers, hopefully with some statistics to quantify variances and error rates. In other words, does our age assessment preclude the fact that the remains are of a 28-year-old? No, and it is our job to explain this and not be pressured by investigators or prosecutors to produce the "right answer."

Of course, when our findings differ significantly from the known demographic information for the putative decedent, then we begin to question whether the initial identification is correct. Bias arises when we believe without question that all of the information provided to us is factual. Proper scientific method requires that researchers seek to test their hypotheses without a stake in the outcome. In cases for which the sex of the decedent has been determined to be male, we should ideally be testing two relatively equally likely hypotheses of a male or female biological sex. Good researchers, scientists, and investigators do not look for confirming evidence, but instead are open to all potential avenues of evidence. If we begin with the assumption that *a priori* information may be incorrect, or place no probative value on what is told to us, then we are on our way to a less biased analysis. Students can be taught that belief in any extraneous information is potentially biasing. In addition, experience will teach them that the correct approach is to assume that prior information provided may be wrong. Over their careers, they will learn that there will be many instances of incorrect information being relayed during an investigation for a variety of reasons.

A policy that requires an assessment of the biological profile in "identified" cases increases the workload and the turnaround time on casework, despite its potential utility for mitigating bias and serving as a teaching tool. It would be much more time-efficient to forgo the assessment of the biological profile and concentrate solely on trauma assessment and interpretation in these particular circumstances. Even though budgetary, time, and/or dictated policy constraints are important considerations, pure convenience should not be a primary motivating factor for laboratories' operating procedures.

3.7 Workable solutions

A primary safeguard against any type of error in a laboratory is a surety-based quality assurance program and a comprehensive laboratory manual based on a standard. If policies and procedures are written down and followed closely, it is more difficult for bias to alter testing procedures, sequence of testing, and conclusions (Haber and Haber, 2013). As mentioned earlier, if the standard operating procedure is to assess the biological profile, then no prior information should alter that policy.

Each laboratory must decide which standards to use. In the forensic sciences, some of the most commonly used standards are ISO 17025 and supplemental standards upon which accreditation is based. Additional laboratory protocols may also be written for the sole purpose of combating bias, with the knowledge that some biasing information may be useful for laboratory management, if not scientific testing. These measures will be different depending upon variations in the physical laboratory, personnel, and other resources. They should reflect what is practical and possible, not necessarily the idealized scenario.

Perhaps the best step toward combating bias is to acknowledge potentially biasing information received relative to each specific case. By recording any potentially biasing *a priori* information in your analytical notes, there is complete transparency to all interested parties, and the jury is made aware that the scientist recognizes, and tried to mitigate, bias in their work. This acknowledgment should be a formal operating procedure, preferably using a form or checklist designed for that purpose. This seems to be a relatively simple and honest response to Kassin *et al.* (2013), who stress the importance of legal experts understanding how forensic examiners reached their conclusions, based on available evidence.

3.8 Summary

Cognitive bias exists as part of the human condition. It shapes our perceptions and influences our decision making. Cognitive bias should be considered separately from instances in which a scientist forces a test result to match a target (e.g., providing a stature estimate that lies outside the 95% prediction interval in order to fit the identified individual's reported height). Those affected by prejudice and preconceived theories often do not know that their perceptions have been altered or influenced. This chapter acquaints the reader with some basic information about the various types of biases negatively affecting scientific testing and practical solutions to minimize error. Some solutions seem relatively simple to implement, while others may be quite difficult to apply in all contexts. Kassin *et al.*(2013) point out that every safeguard to reduce bias does not need to be applied in every case. Forensic labs should work wisely and apply different protocols depending on the complexity of the case. Blind analysis—the most effective policy—may not always be possible and practical, nor is it always desirable. In some cases, knowing the context of evidence increases efficiency, saves resources, and quickens the pace of an investigation. As such, forensic anthropologists must be cognizant of potential sources of bias and implement the most practical solutions for both the particular laboratory and case in question.

References

Bieber, P. (2012) Measuring the impact of cognitive bias in fire investigation. *Proceedings of the International Symposium on Fire Investigation, Science and Technology,* Adelphi, MD, October 15–17, 2012, 3–17.

Burke, A. S. (2005) Improving prosecutorial decision making: Some lessons of cognitive science. *William & Mary Law Review,* **47**, 1587–1631.

Dror, I. E. and Charlton, D. (2006) Why experts make errors. *Journal of Forensic Identification,* **56**, 600–616.

Dror, I. E. and Hampikian, G. (2011) Subjectivity and bias in forensic DNA mixture interpretation. *Science and Justice,* **51**, 204–208.

Dror, I. E., Charlton, D., and Péron, A. E. (2013) Contextual information renders experts vulnerable to making erroneous identifications. *Forensic Science International,* **156**, 74–78.

Found, B. and Ganas, F. (2013) The management of domain irrelevant context information in forensic handwriting examination casework. *Science and Justice,* **53**, 154–158.

Haber, R. N. and Haber, L. (2013) The culture of science: Bias and forensic evidence. *Journal of Applied Research in Memory and Cognition,* **2**, 65–67.

Hagan, W. E. (1894) *A Treatise on Disputed Handwriting and the Determination of Genuine from Forged Signatures.* Banks & Brothers, New York.

Kassin, S. M., Dror, I. E., and Kukucka, J. (2013) The forensic confirmation bias: Problems, perspectives, and proposed solutions. *Journal of Applied Research in Memory and Cognition,* **2**, 42–52.

Kerstholt, J., Eikelboom, A., Dijkman, T., *et al.* (2012) Does suggestive information cause a confirmation bias in bullet comparisons? *Forensic Science International,* **198**, 138–142.

Koppl, R. G., Kursbn, R., and Kobilinsky, L. (2008) Epistemics for forensics. *Episteme,* **5**, 141–159.

Nakhaeizadeh, S., Dror, I. E., and Morgan, R. M. (2014) Cognitive bias in forensic anthropology: Visual assessment of skeletal remains is susceptible to confirmation bias. *Science and Justice,* **54**, 208–214.

National Research Council (2009) *Strengthening Forensic Science in the United States: A Path Forward.* National Academies Press, Washington, DC. http://www.nap.edu/catalog/12589.html (accessed August 3, 2017).

Page, M., Taylor, J., and Blenkin, M. (2002) Context effects and observer bias—implications for forensic odontology. *Journal of Forensic Sciences*, **57**, 108–112.
Risinger, D. M., Saks, M. J., Thompson, W. C., and Rosenthal, R. (2002) The Daubert/Kumho implications of observer effects in forensic science: Hidden problems of expectation and suggestion. *California Law Review*, **90**, 1–56.
Simon, P. (1970). The Boxer. In *Bridge Over Troubled Water*. Columbia Records.
Thompson, W. C., Ford, S., Gilder, J. R., *et al.* (2011) Commentary on: Thornton J.I. Letter to the Editor—a rejection of "working blind" as a cure for contextual bias. *Journal of Forensic Sciences*, **56**, 562–563.
Thornton, J. I. (2010) Letter to the Editor—a rejection of "working blind" as a cure for contextual bias. *Journal of Forensic Sciences*, **55**, 1663.

CHAPTER 4

Theoretically interesting: Different perspectives of the application of theory to forensic anthropology practice and research

Soren Blau

Victorian Institute of Forensic Medicine/Department of Forensic Medicine, Monash University, Monash, Victoria, Australia

4.1 Introduction

The word 'theory' is derived from a technical term used in ancient Greek philosophy – *theōriā*, meaning 'a looking at', 'viewing' or 'beholding' – and referred to contemplation or speculation rather than action (*Chambers English Dictionary*, 1990). The development of a theory, which is a broad explanation of a phenomenon (or phenomena) that is testable and falsifiable and has multiple lines of evidence, together with a hypothesis, forms an integral part of the practice of both natural ('hard') and social science (Heger, 2012; DiGangi and Moore, 2013). Anthropology is the study of humans and is an umbrella term that includes social (cultural) anthropology, archaeology, linguistics and biological (physical) anthropology. Anthropology has never been defined as a hard science (Grivas and Komar, 2008; Adovasio, 2012). The discipline of anthropology has its origins in the humanities and social sciences. It is not surprising, therefore, that the development of forensic anthropology as a subdiscipline of physical anthropology and archaeology has involved incorporation of an array of scientific techniques into aspects of practice but does so within a broad social framework. The aim of this chapter is to examine the details of forensic anthropology education, practice and research as a means of better understanding current forensic anthropological theory and where the development of theories are needed and how they should be developed.

Over the past 30 years, anthropology (including archaeology) has become established as an effective forensic science tool (Blau and Ubelaker, 2016). Forensic anthropologists may be employed by an institute or facility that provides forensic

---

Forensic Anthropology: Theoretical Framework and Scientific Basis, First Edition.
Edited by C. Clifford Boyd Jr and Donna C. Boyd.

medical services. In domestic contexts, forensic anthropologists typically undertake the analysis of complete or partial remains of a single individual (e.g. Steadman, 2016) or multiple individuals in the case of mass disasters resulting from natural and human-induced incidents (e.g. Mundorff *et al.*, 2015). Some governments and non-government organisations employ the services of a forensic anthropologist to locate and identify the remains of servicemen and women missing in action (e.g. Holland *et al.*, 2008). International government and non-government organisations also employ forensic anthropologists in investigations involving cases of enforced disappearances and/or the concealment of large numbers of bodies following periods of political, ethnic and/or religious violence (e.g. Fondebrider, 2012). The extent to which a forensic anthropologist becomes involved in a case will alter depending on the nature of the case and the specific questions that require answering. The information provided by the forensic anthropologist may:

- Be pivotal: The skeletal and/or dental fragments are all that survive and there is no other information about the individual(s).
- Be supportive: The physical evidence, regardless of preservation, supports information provided in, for example, a witness statement or confession.
- Exclude a hypothesis, for example, in the investigation of unidentified human skeletal remains where the biological profile developed by the forensic anthropologist indicates the individual was an elderly Asian male but the missing person is a young Caucasian female.

Anthropologists and archaeologists choosing to engage in the 'forensic' field have found themselves interacting with law enforcement personnel, medical practitioners, forensic scientists and people from the legal community (including prosecutors, defence lawyers and judges), all of whom are concerned in one way or another with the nature and provision of expert evidence. As a result of this interaction, the discipline of forensic anthropology has had to confront the confusion often associated with the terms 'forensic' and 'science' in terms of redefining itself (Hunter and Cox, 2005). Forensic anthropology has attempted a shift to become a 'scientific study' by addressing a range of issues, most notably its perceived lack of theoretical foundations (Boyd and Boyd, 2011) and more particularly the validity and reliability of its interpretations.

The most significant reflection made by forensic anthropology practitioners in some contexts has been the examination of the theories that underpin the formation of conclusions. This has occurred in light of the fact that some of the techniques used by practitioners are quantitative and empirically testable, while others are qualitative, relying on observation and the experience of the practitioners (Grivas and Komar, 2008). These considerations have included discussions about how forensic anthropology should be taught and what qualifications and experience are required to practise as a forensic anthropologist. While initial postgraduate degrees in forensic anthropology have typically been Master of Science (rather than Arts) degrees, there have been increasing moves in some countries to include undergraduate forensic anthropology programmes within medical schools (anatomy departments) rather than from within Arts faculties (archaeology departments). There has also been an increasing need to recognise that as part of education in forensic anthropology, students need to be fully informed about the medico-legal and judicial systems in which they may practise (Komar and Buikstra, 2008; Steadman, 2013:144). Appreciating the need for a theoretical framework and having the skills to develop suitable theories are influenced by the type of training received.

Forensic anthropology has carefully monitored the ways in which forensic science interacts with the law. Although not identified overtly as a reflection of interpretive theory (i.e. how the static record is interpreted as dynamic actions – Boyd and Boyd, Chapter 1, this volume), the implementation of major changes in the US Supreme Court concerning the admittance of expert testimony following the *Daubert v Merrell Dow Pharmaceuticals, Inc.* (1993) and *Kumho Tire Company, Ltd. v Carmichael* (1999) cases was exactly that – a questioning of how experts examined, for example, a static body and reached specific opinions about areas such as cause of death, degree of force, time since death and so on. This questioning filtered through to all of the forensic sciences (Baran, 2012; Edmund, 2015). There have been disproportionate high numbers of false convictions based on serological analysis and hair, bite mark, shoe print, soil, fibre and fingerprint comparisons, as well as DNA testing as documented in the United States, Canada, the United Kingdom and Australia (Saks and Koehler, 2005; Garrett and Neufeld, 2009; Etter, 2013; Murray, 2015). These false convictions have resulted in an ongoing widespread shake-up of forensic science in general and the need for stringent criteria regarding the detail of the science (including the formation of theories) and the admissibility of scientific evidence in courts. In 2009, the US National Academy of Sciences (NAS) released a report that scrutinised the forensic science community. The report confirmed that, with the exception of DNA evidence, much of what is presented as forensic science is not really science at all (National Academy of Sciences (NAS), 2009; Gabel, 2010).

While there have been no reported false convictions based entirely on forensic anthropology evidence and forensic anthropology was not specifically mentioned in the NAS report, forensic anthropology practitioners recognised the importance of attending to the issues raised in the report. Problems identified in forensic science testimony included the misuse of empirical population data and conclusions regarding the probative value of evidence that were unsupported by empirical data (Garrett and Neufeld, 2009:9). The misuse of empirical population data includes the interpretation of non-probative evidence as inculpatory evidence, discounting of exculpatory evidence (an example in forensic anthropology is the degree to which emphasis in an investigation is placed on using attributes such as age and sex, which are estimates and therefore of investigative and not probative value), inaccurate frequency or statistics presented (statistics provided without empirical support, non-numerical statements provided without empirical support), and the lack of definition of terms such as 'could have', 'is consistent', 'is not consistent', 'more likely than not' and 'quite large probability', which without empirical evidence cannot be used (Garrett and Neufeld, 2009; see also McQuiston-Surett and Saks, 2007–2008).

While some early studies examined the method and theory associated with the process of identification in forensic anthropological practice (e.g. Skinner, 1988), it was not until the recognition of problems associated with expert testimony (see previous text) that there was a widespread discussion about how forensic anthropology should be taught and practised (Grivas and Komar, 2008). As a result, more recent publications have focused on the need for statistics, for example, in identification (Steadman *et al.*, 2006) and evidentiary standards (Christensen and Crowder, 2009). While disciplines such as forensic odontology have started to examine what practitioners mean by terminology such as 'consistent', 'likely', etc. (see preceding text) (e.g. Higgens and James, 2006), forensic anthropology is yet to address these questions.

Forensic anthropology practitioners in different countries have sought to develop professional standards through the creation of scientific working groups (SWG) (e.g. in the United States – Christensen and Crowder, 2009; Australia – Donlon, 2016), and establish accreditation systems to provide rigor to what it means to be able to call oneself a 'forensic anthropologist' (Blau, 2016). There are of course large differences between the teaching and practice of the discipline across the globe (Blau and Ubelaker, 2016), and consequently, the application of theory to forensic anthropology practice and research has to be observed in specific geographical contexts.

4.2 Practising in context

The extent to which the theoretical premise of forensic anthropology is considered is influenced by the context in which the discipline is practised. Forensic anthropology practitioners are typically employed by forensic medical institutes or universities rather than based in forensic science or police laboratories. While independence from forensic science/police laboratories is positive in terms of the examination of evidence being structurally independent of police and therefore of the police investigation, the place of employment influences how the discipline is practised.

In some contexts, there is no dedicated forensic anthropologist employed by a forensic medical service provider. There may be a piecemeal integration of a university-based forensic anthropologist (or archaeologist) with the police and/or coroner/medical examiner's office (e.g. Skinner *et al.*, 2010; see also Groen *et al.*, 2015; Blau and Ubelaker, 2016). While such arrangements are usually functional, their *ad hoc* nature often results in non-standardised practice between practitioners.

It has been argued that university-based practitioners should have more time and resources to address specific hypotheses and undertake research that informs practice (Skinner *et al.*, 2010). Some may argue that there should be no limits to research as it is not possible to understand the significance of something until a theory is presented and tested. In reality, however, there is often a disjuncture between academics and service providers. There are many examples where research and development of theoretical frameworks are undertaken for academic purposes only (e.g. to increase publication output) rather than being informed by problems observed by practitioners. This is compounded by the fact that many real-life problems are prosaic and their solution is often not provided by a new technology or novel technique that will appear attractive to granting agencies.

The choice of a suitable theory should begin with identifying the problem. It can be argued that, academically, the development of a theory, for example, that metatarsals are sexually dimorphic, is a worthwhile research endeavour because there may be cases where sexually dimorphic bones (the pelvis and skull) may be poorly preserved or absent (e.g. Robling and Ubelaker, 1997). Some may argue that there should be no limits to research on such questions, as it is not possible to understand the significance of something until such a theory is presented and tested. However, in practice, the legitimacy of the problem/question in terms of its application in the real world (i.e. in court) is questionable. It is then up to the practitioner to decide whether the results have a strong theoretical premise and demonstrate statistical rigor and, even if they do, whether it is actually appropriate (from a biological perspective) to draw conclusions from the data. Are such theories even practically relevant in light of the development of DNA evidence? In reality, if all that remained of an individual was, for example, a metatarsal, then identification would ultimately be concluded based on DNA evidence (assuming the appropriate family members could be located and the capacity to undertake DNA analysis was available, which is certainly not the case in many cities throughout the world).

In contrast to some university-based forensic anthropologists, practitioners based in forensic medical institutes are exposed to a wide range of cases involving both soft and hard tissue in different states of preservation and therefore have access to a vast pool of data for potential research. Unfortunately, the reality is that practitioners in these situations generally have a high caseload and either do not have time or do not have the interest or academic skills required to undertake research using the data to test and confirm or deny current hypotheses. Understanding and developing the nexus between service providers and academics is crucial to augmenting critical thinking and the development of theory in forensic anthropology. It would be useful, for example, if issues identified by practitioners as problematic and that are raised in OSAC meetings (typically held as a means of developing a discipline to improve service provision to stake holders) were developed into a series of research questions. It is no longer useful to state, for example, that 'age estimation' is an issue. Practitioners need to develop questions about what specifically in age estimation needs to be addressed. Such questions could then be shared with academics who could undertake targeted research, feeding results back to the practitioners and building applicable theory through this research.

4.3 Ethical considerations for the development of theory

Increasingly, the courts are arguing for forensic science (including forensic anthropology) to develop an evidence-based approach to underpin the theoretical basis of techniques that are employed. While undertaking experiments that are repeatable so other scientists can verify or nullify the results is the basis of robust science, it must be remembered that forensic anthropology involves the analysis of the actual physical remains (as opposed to other disciplines that analyse remnants of humans such as hair or fingerprints). From this arises an ethical issue: who is undertaking the research and what resources (human or non-human) are being used?

A range of theories have been explored using animal models (e.g. decomposition studies – see Stokes *et al.*, 2013 for a review; and mechanisms of trauma – Wheatley, 2008; Baumer *et al.*, 2010; Prat *et al.*, 2012), not only because of the ethical issues associated with using human samples but also because until recently (e.g. with the development of taphonomic research facilities in the United States (Steadman, 2013; Christensen *et al.*, 2014), Australia (Brennan, 2014) and Italy (Cattaneo *et al.*, 2016)), body donation programmes were restricted to use in medical schools. While it has been demonstrated that there are some similarities between the decomposition of human and non-human (porcine, bovine and ovine) skeletal muscle tissue, the extent to which the animal models represent the human process, and therefore the conclusions drawn from such research, is still in question (Stokes *et al.*, 2013; Dautartas *et al.*, 2016). Practitioners may increasingly need theories to be tested solely on research that uses human remains (hence the move towards undertaking decomposition research at so-called body farms – e.g. Power, 2016) and as such may look to other technologies such as computed tomography (CT) when investigating areas such as age estimation (e.g. Boyd *et al.*, 2015) and the analysis of skeletal trauma (e.g. Polacco *et al.*, 2013). While still requiring research ethics applications, the increasing use of CT data (acquired as part of the routine forensic medicine autopsy – e.g. Brough *et al.*, 2012) may lead to a revolution in the development of robust theory for forensic anthropology.

The importance of working with population-specific reference collections (Ubelaker, 2014) to develop standards for biological profiles is now well recognised (DiGangi and Moore, 2013). Undertaking work on human remains recovered from mass graves in post-conflict areas (where typically little relevant reference material is available) therefore draws into question the appropriateness of undertaking research on remains from these contexts in order to test theories forming the basis for biological profiles (e.g. Durić *et al.*, 2005). Is such practice ethical, and have families of the victims been consulted and provided informed consent (Hunter and Cox, 2005:215)? Is it different if local rather than international practitioners undertake the research?

4.4 Can theories be applied universally?

Along with the forensic sciences, forensic anthropology continues to reflect on its role in the Western legal system. Increasingly, however, there is a role for forensic anthropology in contexts where the rule of law and the state are still in construction and religion/traditional beliefs continue to permeate all aspects of people's lives (e.g. the investigation of large-scale killings resulting from periods of political, ethnic and/or religious violence – Ferllini, 2007; Fondebrider, 2012; Kimmerle, 2014). In such contexts, the challenges to the findings of forensic anthropologists may be made by reference to attacking the theoretical premises of the discipline (Blau *et al.*, 2011): answers to 'why' (e.g. the body is not located in the area the family thought it would be, or the missing person is not your relative) as developed by Western scientific logical theory may not be universally satisfactory. The use of science, often perceived as being rigorous, independent and objective, is seen as an important part of 'being modern'. However, in contexts where traditional faiths remain prominent, the concept of scientific knowledge and proof may collide with traditional spiritual beliefs (*cf.* Fuller, 2007). While many would argue against the notion that there can be no objective truth (as purported by the fifth-century BCE Greek group of teachers known as the Sophists, which formed the foundation of Western philosophy – Downs, 2012:8), contesting the identification of a family's loved one following a death in extremely traumatic circumstances requires forensic anthropology practitioners to reflect on the application of Western theory in science. Just as Western medicine was seen to have a role in the pursuit of colonialism providing 'credibility' to Europe's claim to moral superiority and to the perceived legitimacy of colonial rule in the name of the civilising mission (Ernst, 2004), it is vital that forensic anthropology does not perpetuate and/or reinforce a colonial legacy in the name of justice and democracy. In practical terms, this means an open dialogue between forensic anthropologists and families of the victims is essential so that both parties may understand the goals and perspectives of the other (Blau, 2015). In many contexts it is also important for forensic anthropologists to be aware of how the cultural and religious beliefs of people in the area they are working may impact, for example, the identification process. Forensic anthropologists may work with robust theories of identification, but if families indicate, for example, that they want the bodies left where they were found because they 'know' their relatives are dead and therefore do not need this to be confirmed, then the theoretical premise of identification becomes irrelevant to the victim's families, even though the loss of this detailed information may allow the perpetrators of the crime to go free.

4.5 Conclusion

While a 'sound theoretical foundation lies at the heart of all scientifically credible disciplines' (Boyd and Boyd, 2011:1407), it is important that theories and associated experiments are not developed purely for the sake of creating data to be seen as scientific and therefore somehow more robust and reliable. As Adovasio (2012:685) states, '[f]or a given field of inquiry to use science...does not necessarily mean that the field is a science'.

Forensic anthropologists (like other forensic experts) must continue to scrutinise their practice. The development of theory in forensic anthropology must be driven by purposeful questions, that is, questions that are relevant to the issues confronting the justice system. While empirically based hypothesis testing is vital to ensure a sound theory of practice, underpinning the formation of a sound theory is the ethical approach to practice. Like all forensic medicine and science experts, forensic anthropologists have an obligation to adhere to a professional code of ethics, the cornerstone of which is private morality (Schroeder quoted in Lucas, 1989:727; see also Jones, 2000:29 for a discussion of professional vs. personal ethics). There has been significant discussion in the academic literature and exposure in the media to expert scientific and technical testimony and claims in textbooks that 'experiential testimony is being replaced by standardized methods and realistic error rates that scientifically justify the opinion' (Steadman, 2013:138). Nonetheless, there continue to be examples of cases where highly qualified and experienced forensic anthropologists (or anatomists) provide so-called 'expert' evidence. Todd's (2011) critique of anthropological (anatomical) expert evidence provided in a case of a robbery (*Honeysett v the Queen* – see also Edmond and San Roque, 2014) highlights the fact that regardless of the set of basic premises of good forensic anthropology practice, there are still individuals who continue to disregard guidelines arising from the Daubert and Kumho decisions, many of which provide principles that have come to underpin the formation of theory. Other examples include the *Crown v Kimberly Mary Hainey* (Anon, 2013a, b) and *R v Hien Puoc Tang* (2006) (Fowle, 2010). Such examples highlight the continuing need for all forensic anthropology practitioners to understand the theoretical premises that underpin the discipline because of the serious implications of our conclusions.

A miscarriage of justice is most appalling because the legal system itself has created victims: the numerous wrongly convicted people and, in addition, actual perpetrators who are free to commit further crimes (Etter, 2013). Forensic medicine and scientific evidence (including forensic anthropology) can be powerful tools for good, but they can also be abused. The development of robust practice aims to reduce human error, misinterpretation and misconduct. As the twentieth-century philosopher Heidegger insisted, 'we are defined by our actions rather than intentions' (Downs, 2012:22). Consequently, while it is necessary to discuss the multiple levels of theory required to address the wider range of possible questions asked of the forensic anthropologist (Boyd and Boyd, 2011:1407), it is our actions as practitioners that will form the future of the discipline. Forensic anthropology practitioners must avoid being 'theoretically elegant but methodologically impoverished' (Adovasio, 2012:685). The future of forensic anthropology as a robust discipline and an effective forensic science tool will be based not only on the application of theory to determine a strong scientific base but also on the individual practitioner's decision making about how, when and what conclusions are formed.

Acknowledgements

I am grateful to Dr Melanie Archer, Professor Stephen Cordner and Dr Tania Delabarde for their comments on drafts of this chapter.

References

Adovasio, J. M. (2012) An 'outsider' look at forensic anthropology. In: *A Companion to Forensic Anthropology* (ed. D. C. Dirkmaat). Wiley-Blackwell, Chichester, pp. 683–689.

Anon (2013a) Judges apologise to Dundee academics over 'quack doctor' comment. *BBC News.* http://www.bbc.co.uk/news/uk-scotland-tayside-central-22281798 (accessed 8 July 2013).

Anon (2013b) Judge misdirected on undermined expert evidence: Appeal court. *The Journal of the Law Society of Scotland.* http://www.journalonline.co.uk/News/1012500.aspx (accessed 8 July 2013).

Baran, M. (2012) Lawyers get crash course to avoid wrongful convictions. *MPR News.* http://www.mprnews.org/story/2012/06/14/crime/lawyers-return-to-classroom-to-prevent-wrongful-convictions (accessed 11 January 2016).

Baumer, T. G., Passalacqua, N. V., Powell, B. J., *et al.* (2010) Age-dependent fracture characteristics of rigid and compliant surface impacts on the infant skull – a porcine model. *Journal of Forensic Sciences*, **55**(4), 993–997.

Blau, S. (2015) Working as a forensic archaeologist and/or anthropologist in post-conflict contexts: A consideration of professional responsibilities to the missing, the dead and their relatives. In: *Ethics, Archaeology and Violence* (eds. A. González-Ruibal and G. Moshenska). Springer, New York, pp. 215–228.

Blau, S. (2016) More than just bare bones: Ethical considerations for forensic anthropologists. In: *Handbook of Forensic Anthropology and Archaeology* (2nd edn.) (eds. S. Blau and D. Ubelaker). Left Coast Press, Walnut Creek, CA.

Blau, S. and Ubelaker, D. (eds.) (2016) *Handbook of Forensic Anthropology and Archaeology* (2nd edn.). Left Coast Press, Walnut Creek, CA.

Blau, S., Fondebrider, L., and Saldanha, G. (2011) Working with families of the missing: A case study from East Timor. In: *We Need the Truth: Enforced Disappearances in Asia* (eds. K. Lauritsch and F. Kernjak). ECAP, Guatemala, pp. 136–144.

Boyd, C. B. and Boyd, D. C. (2011) Theory and the scientific basis for forensic anthropology. *Journal of Forensic Sciences*, **56**(6), 1407–1415.

Boyd, K. L., Villa, C., and Lynnerup, N. (2015) The use of CT scans in estimating age at death by examining the extent of ectocranial suture closure. *Journal of Forensic Sciences*, **60**(2), 363–369.

Brennan, B. (2014) Local 'body farm' to allow Australian researchers to study decomposing human corpses. *ABC News*, 19 November. http://www.abc.net.au/news/2014-11-19/body-farm-to-study-decomposing-human-corpses-set-up-in-sydney/5904394 (accessed 11 June 2015).

Brough, A. L., Rutty, G. N., Black, S., and Morgan, B. (2012) Post-mortem computed tomography and 3D imaging: Anthropological applications for juvenile remains. *Forensic Science, Medicine and Pathology*, **8**, 270–279.

Cattaneo, C., Gibelli, D., and Salsarola, D. (2016) Forensic anthropology and archaeology: Perspectives from Italy. In: *Handbook of Forensic Archaeology and Anthropology* (eds. S. Blau and D. H. Ubelaker). Left Coast Press, Walnut Creek, CA, pp. 42–48.

Chambers English Dictionary (1990) W & R Chambers, London.

Christensen, A. M. and Crowder, C. M. (2009) Evidentiary standards for forensic anthropology. *Journal of Forensic Sciences*, **54**(6), 1211–1216.

Christensen, A., Passalacqua, N. V., and Bartelink, E. J. (2014) Forensic taphonomy. In: *Forensic Anthropology: Current Methods and Practice* (eds. A. Christensen, N. V. Passalacqua, and E. J. Bartelink). Elsevier, London, pp. 119–147.

Daubert v. Merrell Dow Pharmaceuticals, Inc. (1993) 509 U.S. 579.

Dautartas, A. M., Steadman, D. W., Mundorff, A. Z., *et al.* (2016) A comparison of seasonal decomposition patterns between human and non-human animal models. *Proceedings of the 68th American Academy of Forensic Sciences*, Las Vegas, NV, February 26, 2016, **XXII**, 180.

DiGangi, E. A. and Moore, M. K. (eds.) (2013) *Research Methods in Human Skeletal Biology*. Academic Press, New York.

Donlon, D. (2016) The development and current status of forensic anthropology: An Australian perspective. In: *Handbook of Forensic Anthropology and Archaeology* (2nd edn.) (eds. S. Blau and D. Ubelaker). Left Coast Press, Walnut Creek, CA, pp. 104–114.

Downs, J. (2012) A brief history of ethics. In: *Ethics in Forensic Science* (eds. J. C. Upshaw Downs and A. R. Swienton). Academic Press, Amsterdam, pp. 1–26.

Durić, M., Rakocević, Z., and Donić, D. (2005) The reliability of sex determination of skeletons from forensic context in the Balkans. *Forensic Science International*, **147**(2–3), 159–164.

Edmond, G. and San Roque, M. (2014) Before the High Court – Honeysett v The Queen: Forensic science, 'specialised knowledge' and the Uniform Evidence Law. *Sydney Law Review*, **36**, 323–344.

Edmund, G. (2015) What lawyers should know about the forensic 'sciences'. *Adelaide Law Review*, **36**, 33–100.

Ernst, W. (2004) Colonial psychiatry, magic and religion. The case of Mesmerism in British India. *History of Psychiatry*, **15**(1), 57–71.

Etter, B. (2013) The contribution of forensic science to miscarriage of justice cases. *Australian Journal of Forensic Sciences*, **45**(4), 368–380.

Ferllini, R. (2007) Human rights violations, past and present: Consequences and interventions. In: *Forensic Archaeology and Human Rights Violation* (ed. R. Ferllini). Charles C. Thomas, Springfield, IL, pp. 3–23.

Fondebrider, L. (2012) The application of forensic anthropology to the investigation of cases of political violence. In: *A Companion to Forensic Anthropology* (ed. D. C. Dirkmaat). Wiley-Blackwell, Chichester, pp. 639–648.

Fowle, K. (2010) The science, the technology, the law. *Australian Digital Forensics Conference*. http://ro.ecu.edu.au/cgi/viewcontent.cgi?article=1077&context=adf (accessed 1 January 2016).

Fuller, S. (2007) *Science v. Religion? Intelligent Design and the Problem of Evolution*. Polity Press, Cambridge.

Gabel, J. D. (2010) Forensiphilia: Is the public fascination with forensic science a love affair or a fatal attraction? *New England Journal on Criminal and Civil Confinement*, **36**, 233–262.

Garrett, B. L. and Neufeld, P. J. (2009) Invalid forensic science testimony and wrongful convictions. *Virginia Law Review*, **95**(1), 1–97.

Grivas, C. R. and Komar, D. A. (2008) Kumho, Daubert, and the nature of scientific inquiry: Implications for forensic anthropology. *Journal of Forensic Sciences*, **53**(4), 771–776.

Groen, M., Márquez-Grant, N., and Janaway, R. (eds.) (2015) *Forensic Archaeology: A Global Perspective*. Wiley-Blackwell, Oxford.

Heger, M. (2012) *What Is a Theory? Life's Little Mysteries*. http://www.livescience.com/32390-what-is-a-theory.html (accessed 1 October 2015).

Higgens, D. and James, H. (2006) Classification used by Australian forensic odontologists in identification reports. *The Journal of Forensic Odonto-Stomatology*, **24**(2), 32–35.

Holland, T., Byrd, J., and Sava, V. (2008) Joint POW/MIA Accounting Command's Central Identification Laboratory. In: *The Forensic Anthropology Laboratory* (eds. M. W. Warren, H. A. Walsh-Haney, and L. E. Freas). CRC Press, Boca Raton, FL, pp. 47–63.

Hunter, J. and Cox, M. (2005) Social and intellectual frameworks. In: *Forensic Archaeology: Advances in Theory and Practice* (eds. J. Hunter and M. Cox). Routledge, London, pp. 204–225.

Jones, D. G. (2000) *Speaking for the Dead: Cadavers in Biology and Medicine*. Ashgate, Dartmouth.

Kimmerle, E. H. (2014) Practicing forensic anthropology: A human rights approach to the global problem of missing and unidentified persons. *Annals of Anthropological Practice*, **38**(1), 1–6.

Komar, D. A. and Buikstra, J. E. (2008) *Forensic Anthropology. Contemporary Theory and Practice*. Oxford University Press, New York.

Kumho Tire Company, Ltd. v. Carmichael (1999) 526 U.S. 137.

Lucas, D. M. (1989) The ethical responsibilities of the forensic scientist: Exploring the limits. *Journal of Forensic Sciences*, **34**(3), 719–729.

McQuiston-Surett, D. and Saks, M. J. (2007–2008) Communicating opinion evidence in the forensic identification sciences: Accuracy and impact. *Hastings Law Journal*, **59**, 1159–1189.

Mundorff, A. Z., Black, S., Blau, S., *et al.* (2015) Disaster victim management – the role of the anthropologist. In: *Encyclopedia of Forensic and Legal Medicine* (2nd edn.) (eds. J. Payne-James and R. Byard). Elsevier, London, pp. 288–304.

Murray, E. A. (2015) *Overturning Wrongful Convictions. Science Serving Justice*. Twenty-First Century Books, Minneapolis, MN.

National Academy of Sciences (NAS) (2009) *Strengthening Forensic Science in the United States: A Path Forward*. National Academies Press, Washington, DC. http://www.nap.edu/catalog.php?record_id=12589 (accessed 4 August 2017).

Polacco, M., D'Alessio, P., Ausania, F., *et al.* (2013) Virtual autopsy in hanging. *The American Journal of Forensic Medicine and Pathology*, **34**(2), 107–109.

Power, J. (2016) Mass graves to be studied at new Sydney body farm. *Sydney Morning Herald*. http://www.smh.com.au/nsw/mass-graves-to-be-studied-at-new-sydney-body-farm-20160208-gmp3az.html (accessed 11 February 2016).

Prat, N., Rongieras, F., de Freminwille, H., *et al.* (2012) Comparison of thoracic wall behavior in large animals and human cadavers submitted to an identical ballistic blunt thoracic trauma. *Forensic Science International*, **222**, 179–185.

R v Hien Puoc Tang (2006) NSWCCA 167. http://www.austlii.edu.au/cgi-bin/viewdoc/au/cases/nsw/NSWCCA/2006/167.html (accessed 8 July 2016).

Robling, A. G. and Ubelaker, D. H. (1997) Sex estimation from the metatarsals. *Journal of Forensic Sciences*, **42**, 1062–1069.

Saks, M. J. and Koehler, J. J. (2005) The coming paradigm shift in forensic identification science. *Science*, **309**, 892–895.

Skinner, M. (1988) Methods and theory in deciding identity of skeletonised human remains. *Canadian Society of Forensic Science Journal*, **21**(3), 114–134.

Skinner, M. F., Clegg, L., Congram, D., *et al.* (2010) Taking the pulse of forensic anthropology in Canada. *Canadian Society of Forensic Science*, **43**(4), 191–203.

Steadman, D. W. (2013) The places we will go: Paths forward in forensic anthropology. In: *Forensic Science: Current Issues, Future Directions* (ed. D. H. Ubelaker). John Wiley & Sons, Ltd, Chichester, pp. 131–159.

Steadman, D. W. (2016) *Hard Evidence: Case Studies in Forensic Anthropology* (2nd edn). Routledge, London.

Steadman, D. W., Adams, B. J., and Konigsberg, L. W. (2006) Statistical basis for positive identification in forensic anthropology. *American Journal of Physical Anthropology,* **131**, 15–26.

Stokes, K. L., Forbes, S. L., and Tibbett, M. (2013) Human versus animal: Contrasting decomposition dynamics of mammalian analogues in experimental taphonomy. *Journal of Forensic Sciences,* **58**(3), 583–591.

Todd, I. (2011) Body mapping evidence. Questions of admission and reliance. http://www.elizabethstreetchambers.com.au/wp-content/uploads/2016/05/Body-Mapping-Evidence-Paper-by-Iain-Todd-2011.pdf (accessed 29 August 2017).

Ubelaker, D. H. (2014) Osteology reference collections. In: *Encyclopedia of Global Archaeology* (ed. C. Smith). Springer, New York, pp. 5632–5641.

Wheatley, B. P. (2008) Perimortem or postmortem bone fractures? An experimental study of fracture patterns in deer femora. *Journal of Forensic Sciences,* **53**(1), 69–72.

PART 2

The theory and science behind biological profile and personal identification

CHAPTER 5

From Blumenbach to Howells: The slow, painful emergence of theory through forensic race estimation

Stephen Ousley[1], Richard L. Jantz[2] and Joseph T. Hefner[3]

[1] *Department of Anthropology/Archaeology, Department of Mathematics and Information Technology, Mercyhurst University, Erie, PA, USA*

[2] *Department of Anthropology, University of Tennessee, Knoxville, TN, USA*

[3] *Department of Anthropology, Michigan State University, East Lansing, MI, USA*

5.1 Introduction

So much has been written about human races that one could argue that another book is needed to adequately address the subject. But another book would not bridge the huge gaps between drastically opposed opinions and viewpoints, especially among anthropologists, largely due to the ambiguous use of a number of terms, including foremost, "race." In this brief chapter we will concentrate on how anthropologists have approached the study of human variation. We find that anthropologists have frequently depended on nebulous or nonscientific theories and questionable methods to justify what seem to be foregone conclusions, more often reflecting the contemporary views of society or strong personal opinions, rather than using empirical data and the scientific method. As a result, earlier racist pseudoscience gave way to modern antiracist pseudoscience that has prevented further discussion. Until recently, American forensic anthropologists used race to help identify discovered skeletal remains and were simply doing their work with little thought to race theory. Few anthropologists in any discipline examined humans and human races scientifically, which should involve formulating and testing theories and hypotheses, but instead relied on confirmation bias in publications intended for like-minded audiences. More recently, however, the accumulation of a mountain of morphological and molecular evidence shows an association between traditional human races and patterns of human variation, reflecting the interplay of historical, cultural, and evolutionary factors. If more anthropologists can

Forensic Anthropology: Theoretical Framework and Scientific Basis, First Edition.
Edited by C. Clifford Boyd Jr and Donna C. Boyd.

start investigating race and other folk taxonomies as biocultural phenomena, instead of forbidding their discussion, a powerful new paradigm can emerge.

5.2 Race as a concept and theory

The number of articles and books published on race is staggering, and we cannot provide a comprehensive review of the many twists and turns in the role of race in anthropology and society in this chapter or even in one book. We can only encourage you to read as many original publications as you can. An excellent starting point is Volume 139 of the *American Journal of Physical Anthropology*, published in May of 2009 and edited by Heather Edgar and Keith Hunley. The nine articles in the special issue were the result of a remarkable symposium titled "Race Reconciled? How Biological Anthropologists View Human Variation," which brought together a wide variety of specialists in human biology, paleoanthropology, anthropological genetics, forensic anthropology, and bioarchaeology in 2007. Other especially valuable articles are Caspari (2003), Lieberman *et al.* (2003), and Pigliucci (2013). Equally important is a recent critique of the voluminous work done on human races, which concludes that far too much heat has been generated, but with little light:

> We waste our expertise endlessly attempting to adjudicate cultural mores with biological data, debating whether "race" is "real" when we know that the social reality of race, whatever race is, is mediated by the distribution of genetic variation but not determined by it (Weiss and Fullerton, 2005:169).

Instead of a comprehensive review, we will focus on the major tenets of what has become the dominant view in anthropology, repeated numerous times in the last few decades by numerous authors and in the American Anthropological Association (AAA) Statement on Race adopted in 1998, and most recently in the book *Race: Are We So Different?* (Goodman *et al.*, 2012):

1. Evolution, rather than race, explains human biological variation. Race-as-biology is based on the false idea of fixed, ideal and unchanging types.
2. Human variation is continuous. Allele frequencies, or variations in DNA, tend to vary gradually. Therefore, there is no clear place to designate where one race begins and another ends. Skin color, for example, the physical characteristic we most often use to distinguish "races," slowly changes from place to place and person to person.
3. Human biological variation involves many traits that typically vary independently. Skin color, for example, is only correlated with a few other traits such as hair and eye color, leaving unpredictable the huge number of other traits… Thus, it is a truism that "race is only skin deep."
4. Genetic variation within so-called races is much greater than the variation among them. One might assume that genetic variation among races is great; however, there is actually little genetic variation among the groups we have come to call races. For example, two individuals who might identify as "white" might well be far more genetically different from one another than from someone self-identified as "black."

5. There is no way to consistently classify human beings by race. Race groups are impossible to define in a stable and universal way, and if one cannot define groups one cannot make scientific generalizations about them. Race groups are unstable primarily because the socially determined color line changes over time and place. Someone considered "white" in Brazil can be considered "black" in the United States; someone who lives as "white" in the United States today might have been considered "Mexican" a generation earlier (shortened from Goodman et al., 2012:97–98).

In evaluating these statements and their supporting evidence, we must keep in mind that theories depend on the scientific method, which requires hypothesis testing. Scientific theories are always important even if implicit or unacknowledged. A scientific theory is an explanation or summary of a phenomenon based on a series of noncontradictory facts and non-falsified hypotheses. A hypothesis is a statement or explanation that is testable and falsifiable; in other words, it is possible to show that it is incorrect. The null hypothesis is always defined in general terms that all things are equal; for instance, there is no difference in the responses of a treatment and control group in an experiment involving drug efficacy. In the most basic comparisons in the study of human variation, the null hypothesis would be that human groups, however defined, by race, region, language, and so on, show no differences, for example, in genetic or morphological traits. In other words, human variation is insignificant, random, and unpredictable. In terms of testing for biological races in humans, the null hypothesis is that there is no patterning in human variation; humans do not cluster into more or less discrete groups. Even more specifically, one null hypothesis could be that there is no association between social races and human variation. It is also important to recognize that there are numerous alternate hypotheses that could be valid, and falsifying a null hypothesis does not prove that any particular alternate hypothesis is true. Also, we are doing inductive reasoning, meaning that samples and statistics are used, and probabilistic conclusions are the outcome, rather than arriving at some universal truth as in deductive reasoning, in which if the premises are true in a valid argument, the conclusion must be true.

Hypothesis testing involves trying to falsify the null hypothesis, and we can either reject hypotheses or fail to reject them. We cannot prove them. Hypothesis testing of this type was only recognized, accepted, and practiced after Karl Popper published books and articles in English in the 1950s and 1960s. Previously, testing a theory or hypothesis was done through verification, the attempt to assemble sufficient evidence from observational data to support the theory in order to prove it. Popper recognized that it was very often possible to assemble sufficient evidence for *any* theory or hypothesis if one looked for it. Emphasizing verification empowers confirmation bias because there is almost always some evidence for nearly any theory, especially when post hoc interpretations are allowed. Researchers could simply ignore or discount contrary evidence, thanks to greater weight of evidence that supported a theory. As Popper pointed out, the logic of verification was flawed because, while a sufficient number of observations are necessary to formulate and support a theory or hypothesis, a single observation or counterexample can disprove it (Popper, 2002). "All swans are white" was disproven when black swans were discovered in Australia. Because a hypothesis must be testable and falsifiable, it cannot be proven because one counterexample can disprove.

5.2.1 Evolution, rather than race, explains human biological variation

We agree in principle to the idea that analyzing human data at the most specific level, using relevant labels such as nationality, language, tribe, or geographic location, and time period for each group, is much more informative than pooling samples under a heading such as "race" at the start. But, right off the bat, we must recognize that much confusion has been generated due to using the word "race," which has social, biological, and anthropological meanings. Some authors either are confused or want to spread confusion: "Race is a biological category, yet it is socially constructed" (Blakey, 1999:29). In biology, "race" is a taxonomic label for a within-species variety distinctive enough, but not quite at the subspecies level, and is often used with species variants showing ecological adaptations and/or geographic limitations. However, there is no consistent standard for what qualifies as a race or even subspecies in biology. We will use the term "biological race" to represent this concept. "Race" is also used for the classification of citizens of the United States, which has legal and social consequences. The choice of using "race" for people in the United States linked classifications based on biology and society: In a young country made up of predominantly light-skinned western Europeans and dark-skinned eastern Africans, the connection between the biological and social was obvious. As Americans, we understand race, and race is a part of our individual identity, whether we like it or not. In this chapter, to avoid confusion, we will use the term "social race" when referring to the labels of the American folk taxonomy, which also encompasses "forensic race" or "bureaucratic race" in terms of the US census and government laws and regulations. Returning to our example of analyzing a number of groups, it is important to remember that analyzing them using labels based on nationality, various linguistic hierarchies, tribe, or even social race is arbitrary. In each case we can explore the relationship between group labels and biological data. Grouping by social race can be used to explore patterns of variation, as can nationality or language; all are cultural constructs. Any kind of grouping can muddle underlying biological relationships among them, but some will show more group differences than others. The only nonarbitrary labels must be based on time and/or place. Biological information can include various genetic or morphological features. Once again, we would divide the total sample into groups and look at associations with biological data. Another approach would be to conduct a cluster analysis at the front end on the biological data and then look for associations with arbitrary ways of characterizing the clusters.

In biological anthropology, "race" in humans usually refers to the idea that humanity can be divided using biological traits into a discrete number of groups, usually between three and six, which usually correspond to regions of the world. In this sense, race corresponds to the concept of biological race. However, Goodman, a one-time president of the AAA, and many other anthropologists equate biological race in humans with extreme typology, involving the "fixed, ideal, and unchanging types" that were popular before Mendelian genetics was appreciated and before numerous other scientific advancements in the first half of the twentieth century. But even staunch defenders of the existence of biological races, such as Blumenbach (the father of anthropology), Carleton Coon, and others, had acknowledged variation within them and overlap among them since the 1950s, introducing the ideas of local races and microraces (Boyd, 1950; Coon *et al.*, 1950; Garn and Coon, 1955) and later accommodating clinal variation (Coon, 1965). In using the extreme and outmoded typological definition of biological races, Goodman and others force a false dichotomy: either typology or no biological races. Goodman even seemed to dictate how assertions of human variation corresponding to races must be interpreted:

> There is no half way between seeing race as biologically valid or not. *Any reformation of race as biology will simply be interpreted as race in the older typological paradigm* (Goodman, 1998:53; emphasis added).

Characterizing biological race as extreme typology has been used repeatedly by others as well, and is easily falsifiable, forcing someone to conclude that the choice is either typological races or no biological races, a Straw Man argument. As has been pointed out by a bioethicist, this dichotomy not only forces the reader to one conclusion, forgetting that there are other alternate hypotheses, but also obfuscates the issues and hinders discussion:

> To be effective, challenges raised against research that treats race as biological or genetic need to stop relying on rhetorical or formulaic arguments and instead examine such research empirically (Sankar, 2008:280).

Empirical data should be the basis for establishing scientific theories; theories cannot rely exclusively on thought experiments. Typology was based on cherry-picked data and anecdotal observations, reflecting verification and confirmation bias, but more recent work by most anthropologists has not risen above subjective biases. For instance, Brown and Armelagos (2001) acknowledged that defining biological races should be based on multiple traits to be more objective, but for them that was impossible:

> Add another trait and classification becomes a more difficult task, and there usually are groups that cannot be classified. As you increase the number of traits, the problems in racial classification become insurmountable (Brown and Armelagos, 2001:34).

We know this is true logically, but only when we use an outmoded idea of what a trait is. Brown and Armelagos (2001) are refuting typological essentialism, the idea that all members of a race are required to have a specific complement of trait states. It was actually a forensic anthropologist, Joseph Hefner, in his sample of over 300 crania, who found that five "typical" nonmetric traits diagnostic for race defined by Rhine (1990) were found in only 51% of the "Mongoloids," 17% of the "Negroids," and 33% of the "Caucasoids" (Hefner, 2003). It is important to recognize that a forensic anthropologist performed this test using the latest methods of forensic anthropology, and his test easily falsified the theory of extreme typology. Importantly, however, Hefner (2009) and Hefner and Ousley (2014) emphasized that multiple nonmetric traits are much more informative in a statistical framework and can classify groups accurately.

In a rare empirical test for human biological races, testing the false dichotomy and defective data did not stop the following authors from reaching grandiose and incorrect conclusions. Williams *et al.* (2005) used 10 measurements and discriminant function analyses to classify a sample of 42 Nubians into 27 groups from around the world in the Howells craniometric database and concluded, "The possibility that skeletal material could be sorted by geographic origin, at any other level than geographic extremes, is quite small" (Williams *et al.*, 2005:345). Their null hypothesis was that 100% of their Nubians would be classified into the closest geographical group, Howells' Egyptians. Because 100% did not classify into Howells' Egyptians, they concluded that regional variation in humans is minimal or nonexistent. Their conclusion comes from the false dichotomy. But as we know, the null hypothesis should be that groups show no differences or no geographic patterning—both of which can be clearly falsified: Classification into groups and regions increases in accuracy with more measurements, and, in using 24 measurements, 68% of individuals from the 27 groups were classified into their own group and 95% of individuals were classified into a group from the same region as the group they came from (Ousley *et al.*, 2009). Naturally, all data used in an analysis must be accurate. If the Williams *et al.* (2005) study proved anything, it is that one should study measurement definitions before collecting and analyzing metric data. An independent classification using measurements from other Nubians showed regional affinities, and an examination of the data that Williams *et al.* (2005) used in their analysis, which they refused to share, revealed serious measurement errors. Even with considerable measurement errors, the authors did not acknowledge or recognize that their Nubians actually classified into the Howells Egyptian group more than into any other group.

With this important background information on hypothesis testing, we can evaluate the claims of Goodman *et al.* (2012).

5.2.2 Human variation is continuous

We agree that much of human variation in DNA and morphology is roughly continuous, reflecting patterns of gene flow and selection gradients that can be seen in clinal distributions of traits. Trait clines were a nonracial alternative for explaining variation and were explained by gene flow. Livingstone's (1962:279) quote "There are no races, there are only clines" is often used. Humans, though, are not continuously distributed but are usually concentrated in settlements of various distances from other settlements, and the distance between settlements has dictated the opportunity for mating. For instance, data from one nineteenth-century Massachusetts town showed that the majority of marriages were to people who lived within 10 miles (Swedlund, 1972). Differing migration patterns and local populations allow genetic drift to become a factor and make certain settlements relatively distinct. Settlements further afield from regional centers experience less gene flow from their regional neighbors and are more likely to encounter peoples from different regions. Also, in terms of human phylogenies, it is a mistake to compare an analysis of alleles that are relatively neutral to alleles under clear selection, such as those for skin color, which clearly reflect exposure to ultraviolet light, which is also clinal (Brace, 1995; Jablonski and Chaplin, 2000). Variation due to selection will not often reflect variation due to population histories. Also, different neutral traits can show different clines, meaning that multiple traits should be examined. Most importantly, we know that genes covary (see the following text), meaning that combinations of neutral alleles will provide more information and structure to variation that appears strictly clinal when only one trait is analyzed. As Lieberman (1997:4–5) noted, "New data indicate that traits are distributed in geographic gradations and each gradation for a particular trait varies in different geographic patterns consistently; if they do not covary, then the boundary lines for races cannot be identified."

5.2.3 Human biological variation involves many traits that typically vary independently

While it is debatable what "many" and "typically" mean, we disagree in theory and in fact with the implication that traits vary independently, especially among groups. This claim from Goodman effectively nullifies comparisons among groups using multiple loci or traits, instead limiting comparisons to one trait at a time: If all traits are inherited independently, no trait can give more information than any other trait, and multiple single-trait comparisons using frequencies will likely produce different results when comparing groups. But many genes show linkage disequilibrium, and many combinations of specific genes need to work together for the survival of the organism. In more or less neutral traits, combinations of traits show strong geographic patterning that reflects population genetics and population histories. For example, Novembre *et al.* (2008) examined over 500 000 SNPs from 3000 Europeans and found that the variation in the SNPs corresponded very well with geography and in fact in many cases could estimate where someone was born to within a few hundred kilometers. Most European borders were relatively restricted until recently and reflect language differences as well as nationality. Studies using a single locus at a time, like Lewontin's (1972; see below), are not as meaningful as those using more loci because more loci better reflect more of the total genetic makeup. There is a parallel in using one versus multiple morphological traits or measurements, revealing the importance of covariation in studies of human variation (Ousley *et al.*, 2009). All traits obviously under selection, like skin color, will reflect the combination of appropriate environmental conditions, so comparisons with neutral systems, which reflect gene flow and drift, can vary a great deal. It is a mistake to expect neutral alleles to be highly correlated with alleles clearly under selection.

5.2.4 Genetic variation within so-called races is much greater than the variation among them

We agree with this statement, as is, but with a few further implications. This has been the mantra ever since another rare study involving empirical data—Lewontin's (1972) publication examining genetic variation in 17 polymorphic loci. Lewontin divided his worldwide data into seven regions corresponding more or less with traditional human biological races. He found that in terms of average variation across these genetic systems, 85% was present within individuals no matter where they came from, 8% was present within each region, which left only 6% present among regions, representing differences among approximate biological races. Based on these results, Lewontin (1972) concluded that the actual differences among humans based on genetics are far smaller than their perceived differences. Thus, we are all much more similar than we think, and 6% leaves little to distinguish humans from different regions. Lewontin's results and conclusions have been repeatedly relied upon by Goodman, Armelagos, and the AAA in stressing the non-reality of traditional races: How could 6% possibly be significant?

The main problem with Lewontin's analysis is that he analyzed the genetic markers one at a time and ignored linkage disequilibrium and covariance, which reflects the combination of markers unevenly distributed among regional groups. Edwards (2003) reexamined Lewontin's methods and showed that analyzing one locus at a time can show great overlap among groups, but analyzing multiple loci simultaneously, that is, appreciating covariation, produces a more realistic picture of among-group variation and produces less overlap among groups. Ousley *et al.* (2009; figure 1) illustrated that when using multiple traits, groups can have a great amount of within-group variation yet show large differences among them. The AAA *Statement on Race* also relies on Lewontin's results and states on several web pages (e.g., Public Broadcasting System, 2003; American Anthropological Association, 2016) that race has no genetic basis, based on the fact that there is not **one** trait that defines a race perfectly—as they demonstrate through blood types and fingerprint types. More recently, there was an ad campaign using a poster with the slogan "There is no gene for race" using morphed images of human faces (Wallace, 2012; Tumbler, 2013). To our knowledge, no one, not even among the typologists, insisted that there was one trait that characterized an entire race. The importance of covariation is easily seen in Novembre *et al.*'s (2008) analysis of Europeans and in more recent molecular analyses of worldwide human data, which always use multiple traits. Since Lewontin's study, genetic analyses have become much more sophisticated and precise. Molecular analyses utilizing SNPs, STRPs, VNTRs, Alu inserts, and other neutral DNA features indicate strong geographic patterning and accurate classifications by region (Pritchard *et al.*, 2000; Rosenberg *et al.*, 2002; Bamshad *et al.*, 2003; Allocco *et al.*,

2007; Algee-Hewitt *et al.*, 2016) despite large amounts of within-region variation (Jorde and Wooding, 2004; Hunley *et al.*, 2016).

To be sure, humans are far more similar than they are different, and most variation in humans is among individuals, each of whom is genetically unique, but there is plenty of regionally-specific variation that distinguishes most humans. These three facts may seem counterintuitive at first, but all three are true. A parallel finding is seen in men and women, who share nearly all genetic material, yet have enough genetic differences to distinguish each sex. If we ignore the 23rd pair of chromosomes, the sexes are virtually identical, though each individual is unique. Once again, this finding is not typological; it is statistical and probabilistic, which is necessary when dealing with intraspecific variation. While "two individuals who might identify as 'white' *might* well be far more genetically different from one another than from someone self-identified as 'black'" (Goodman *et al.*, 2012:98, emphasis added), two random people from the same region are much more likely to share more loci than two random people from different regions, *contra* Goodman and the AAA (Bamshad *et al.*, 2003; Bamshad and Guthery, 2007; Novembre *et al.*, 2008; O'Rourke, 2010).

5.2.5 There is no way to consistently classify human beings by race

We agree, more or less, with the statement but without further implications or assumptions. In *any* collection of organisms, if one analyzes different genetic systems, it is true that different results can be produced, especially if heavily selected traits and neutral traits are combined in various ways. In animals, we know this is true in among- and within-species studies, even with neutral traits. So inconsistency in classification cannot be used to argue against the existence of biological races. If biological races and subspecies can exist in nonhuman animals, they can exist in humans as well. Within-species variation is a biological reality, but Goodman *et al.* (2012) once again obfuscate understanding through the ambiguous use of "race." Their argument, amazingly, is based on the fact that the same person can be assigned into a different social race depending on where he or she is: "Someone considered 'white' in Brazil can be considered 'black' in the United States" (Goodman *et al.*, 2012:97). Goodman is merely stating that folk taxonomies differ, which we know, and illustrates an irrelevant and merely rhetorical argument (Sankar, 2008). Munich, Germany, is the same city as München, Deutschland. Inconsistent folk taxonomies cannot be used to disprove the existence of biological races, which are defined using biological criteria. Further, if we concentrate on social race, there can be disagreements as to how someone is classified within a society. Social races can be ambiguous, depending on the person's phenotype and local folk taxonomies, yet social races are real and have clear consequences. People can self-identify in various ways, but there are limits to how someone self-identifies in regard to their legally recognized race, and the legal definitions of race are poorly defined. When applied to individuals, legal race is most often based on community perception; in other words, it depends on the perceptions and opinions of others (Wright, 1995). Inconsistencies in opinions on biological race, social race, and legal or bureaucratic race are the norm and do not prevent us from studying them as phenomena. Due to anthropologists largely refusing to discuss and investigate race neutrally, most research in perceived race has been conducted by psychologists and sociologists, and the results are far-reaching and somewhat disturbing. The sense of self—"us" and "them"—is present even in infants, who react more positively to people who are like them, as opposed to not like them, for example, in skin color or race (Kelly *et al.*, 2005; Banaji and Greenwald, 2013). Some aspects of races and racism are likely, therefore, due to predispositions for social group preferences, which are reinforced through interpreting later personal experiences with confirmation bias.

We should also recognize that within-species variation has always been challenging to evaluate objectively, even in nonhumans, because of the absence of reproductive isolation with speciation: with sufficient movements or migration, animals can interbreed with others of the same species who may be different. Comparing different species is much easier—in most cases. The genus *Papio* has a taxonomic identity crisis, interpreted by various researchers as having one species with several subspecies or semispecies, as representing up to five species, or as being a superspecies that can mate with *Theropithecus,* as seen in multiple hybrid zones and intergenic hybrids (Jolly *et al.*, 1997; Jolly, 2003). Within-species variation in humans is especially difficult because of their small- and large-scale movements, widespread geographic distribution, differentiation due to gene drift and natural selection in different areas, and, until recently, gene flow among groups that was limited much more by geographic distance.

In examining the assertions of Goodman and the AAA, we have found that their conclusions are unjustified based on their arguments. They begin either with untrue or misleading statements of "fact," or begin with accepted facts, then draw unjustified conclusions or write true but misleading conclusions seemingly written with the help of a lawyer using words such as "can," "may," "might," "many," or "could." Notably, the nineteenth century typology forms their null hypothesis. A lack of empirical data pervades most arguments, and when data are used they are cherry-picked, reflecting confirmation bias. Finally, they test their hypotheses using verification. They seem stuck in the nineteenth century. How have their arguments been so vacuous yet come to dominate anthropology? We agree with what many anthropologists maintain: that scientific views are influenced by contemporary societal and political views and personal opinions. We assert that many recent anthropologists and the AAA have been trying to make up for anthropology's racist past through a moral commitment to combating racism. Instead of scientifically investigating biological race, social race, and racism as biopsychosociocultural phenomena, anthropologists have become propagandists, using pseudoscience and repeating dogmatic statements to try to change public opinion in racist America. While the goal is admirable, the approach is indefensible, has not been successful, and has hindered progress in understanding the phenomenon of race.

There is no doubt that racism is bad, and recent events and the Black Lives Matter movement provide ample evidence that Americans still live in a racist country. Unfortunately, some instruments of institutional racism are alive and well. However, racists are morally as well as scientifically deficient, and it is doubtful that racists read anthropology journals. Goodman, other anthropologists, and the AAA apparently believe that racists do but also that racists can be enlightened by reading a publication with moral overtones. Also, Goodman and others emphasize that it is the moral obligation of *every* anthropologist to combat racism. For instance, Goodman (1998:52) wrote, "...educating that biological differences between groups are not deep, hereditary and fixed eliminates a major weapon in the racist's arsenal. It exposes racism as the human social evil that it is." It was already clear that racism is evil because it is a moral failure, even if there are deep differences among groups. With a more specific target, Turner *et al.* (2006:207) wrote that:

> Forensic anthropologists have a moral and professional responsibility as scientists, civil servants, and teachers to use theoretical models that reflect the limited utility of assigning individuals to races based on type specimens and typical features (Armelagos and Goodman, 1998; Goodman, 1997).

and

> Armelagos and Goodman (1998) have argued that nothing is to be gained by using a model that is known to be unsupported by data and socially divisive. The choice to identify or not to identify races is therefore not only a matter of good science, but also a matter of ethics and politics,

illustrating the tendency in many authors of self-referencing or restating the same dogma from the same papers over and over to make them "true."

Above all, Armelagos and Goodman (1998:364) believe that the use of biological race in science is a precursor to racism and cite other opinions in support:

> As Crick (1996) has said, if race is not a sufficient cause of racism, it is a necessary cause. In addition to scientific critique of the idea of race, particularly the notion of fixed and hierarchically arranged types, Boas (1911, 1940) suggested that the idea of race contributed to racism.

Evidently, even a suggestion is enough if it came from Boas. Armelagos and Goodman (1998) echoed a sentiment expressed by Lewontin, whose conclusions on human variation were clearly influenced by his views of science and society:

> Human racial classification is of no social value and is positively destructive of social and human relations. Since such racial classification is now seen to be of virtually no genetic or taxonomic significance either, no justification can be offered for its continuance (Lewontin, 1972:397).

Once again, ideas of "us" versus "them" are already present in infants (Banaji and Greenwald, 2013), and racists do not need scientific justification to hate, as if science would justify any such opinion. As evolutionary biologist Pigliucci (2014) has noted, researching human races scientifically has nothing to do with ethics or morality, because scientific results do not dictate action: we all believe that mentally disabled and handicapped persons deserve rights as human beings despite being clearly inferior in some capacities. In a similar vein, supporting equal rights for men and women does not depend on ignoring any biological difference between them.

Further, Goodman *et al.* (2012:95) assert melodramatically:

> Race is like a gun. One could say it is not the gun that maims and kills, but the gun is a powerful ideological tool; it is a threat of violence and control. Like a gun in the hands of an angry man, race in the hands of a racist does harm.

What audience is that intended for? One audience must be anthropologists, who need to be reminded that they are fighting the good fight. Could another audience be the rational and intellectual racists who read such books? Maybe there are a handful in the world.

Another audience could be medical practitioners and genetic epidemiologists who use social race in some professional capacity. The use of social race in medicine is still a hotly debated topic and will continue to be until personalized medicine is realized (Gravlee, 2009). Some doctors use social race as a proxy for expected genetic features and vigorously defend the use of race in interpreting illnesses and prescribing treatments, while others point out the uncertain link between social race and genetic variation. Of course, social race, which is discrete and subjective, is only a proxy for human variation, which is continuous and overlapping. Assessing an individual for medical purposes can be objective only if the DNA sequence of the individual is known as well as the many factors that affect gene expression. Social race also has consequences for the individual, and the lived experiences can influence the presence of certain diseases and illnesses (Gravlee, 2009). The real question is how well the proxy of social race actually "works." Harm can be done by assuming certain genetic variants as well as by completely ignoring them. Individualized medicine is still decades away, and social race classification in medicine can have great consequences.

Another target audience for the antiracist anthropologists is apparently students, whose opinions are to be molded to prevent racism in the future. But the arguments that race does not exist falls flat for many students, and for laymen, because they see differences in humans easily, while overlooking the similarities. As Obach (1999:252) idealistically wrote,

> ...students often resist the idea that 'white' or 'black' or the other racial classifications, as they are commonly conceived, are not objective, scientific, biological categories, but rather, that they represent notions that developed historically and that have no biological significance beyond the meaning attributed to them by the members of society.

Unfortunately, the meaning attributed to social race by the members of society has tremendous consequences, and social race is based to a large degree on biology, especially skin color, which is determined by relatively few genes. Thinking that "race is only skin deep" does not help much; race is still just as real outside of the classroom. As Edgar and Hunley (2009:3) admit,

> Although we have now been teaching for generations that races do not exist, these naïve [more or less typological race] notions persist and they continue to have social and scientific consequences. This may be because we have failed to offer a clear and satisfactory explanation that meshes with students' lived experience.

It would seem that merely refuting typology with pseudoscience and propaganda, as Goodman and others have done, without acknowledging human differences and their consequences, does not enlighten anyone or improve the situation.

Unfortunately, the overarching emphasis on antiracism in anthropology has swamped the need for a more objective approach to race. Many anthropologists have become propagandists rather than scientists, telling students, other academics, and the public how and what to think instead of better assessing and recording how and what people are thinking, much less why they think that way. Anthropologists have abandoned the scientific method in favor of the rote method. As a result, sociologists and psychologists, not anthropologists, have done far more research into the effects of racial identity and stereotyping, most notably demonstrating that racial stereotypes about IQ and other test performance can greatly affect individual test performance. For instance, African Americans score lower on tests, even on tests unconnected to ability, after being reminded of negative test performance stereotypes (Steele and Aronson, 1995). Instead of studying folk taxonomies as a part of culture, how they function, and what their consequences are, many anthropologists simply dismiss them as unjustified and refuse to discuss them. How did we get here?

5.3 Anthropology and race

Anthropology has often reflected contemporary societal opinions on race. In the nineteenth century, anthropologists, the public, and the country's leaders were not shy about voicing racist opinions. President Andrew Johnson, who took over after Lincoln was assassinated, was clearly a racist, vetoing civil rights acts and blocking the 14th amendment extending rights to former slaves. In 1867, he vetoed a reconstruction bill and was quoted as saying, "It is vain to deny that [American blacks] are an inferior race—very far inferior to the European variety. They have learned in slavery all that they know in civilization" (Feagin, 2001:84). Similar opinions of white racial superiority were even expressed by Abraham Lincoln, opinions that would be considered racist today. In anthropology, typology was the norm, with races based on morphology, and interpreted as discrete and unchanging. The United States was an ideal location to appreciate human variation because of concentrations of American Indians, Europeans, and Africans in various parts of the country. American physical anthropologists Giddon and Morton, on examining morphological differences between black and white Americans, linked them to levels of intelligence and racial superiority, reflecting contemporary American society's views justifying slavery and genocide in the United States. But physical anthropologists were not alone in these views: Daniel Garrison Brinton, the leading linguist of his day, wrote that in comparing primitive and advanced peoples, the linguistic, anatomical, and mental characteristics in "primitive" peoples reflected their lower evolutionary development, where they would remain (Brinton, 1895; Bunzl, 1996). Many other contemporary linguists agreed, as did most anthropologists—all aspects of humans aligned with Morgan's deterministic and evolutionary view of human societies (Stocking, 1982). Boas was out of step with contemporary social scientists and one of the first to argue against tying "primitive" language to "primitive" societal development, presaging his later dictum that biology, language, and culture are independent phenomena. Most quotes related to this theme come from Boas's 1896 "The Aims of Anthropology," in response to Brinton (1895) and his 1911 introduction to Volume 1 of the *Handbook of American Indian Languages.*

Most importantly, Boas (1911) reviewed how race (biology), language (linguistic classifications), and culture show an inconsistent relationship with each other in mankind, in contrast to Brinton and most contemporary writers. Similar cultural phenomena could arise from different historical developments. Importantly, Boas was pointing out that a general law could not be applied to biological, linguistic, and cultural development and differentiation because they have developed independently and in different ways around the world. Boas (1911:14) concluded,

> If we...eliminate the hypothetical assumption of correlation between primitive type, primitive language, and primitive culture, we recognize that any attempt at classification which includes more than one of these traits cannot be consistent.

In other words, Boas tested and rejected determinism and stressed that the study of mankind should *not* be focused on finding human similarities and universality but on studying all aspects of human variability and how they came about (Bunzl, 1996). Boas did not mean that all three could not affect each other, that they must be studied separately, or that some aspects should not be studied. Boas further emphasized that all anthropological classifications are "artificial," but "the essential object in comparing different types of man must be the reconstruction of the history of the development of their types, their languages, and their cultures" (Boas, 1911:14). Boas used "types" and "races" throughout his career not as typologists did, but rather as minor variants and major subdivisions of humans, respectively. In modern terms, Boas was advocating a holistic approach for studying mankind and did not exclude the study of how cultural, linguistic, and biological factors have influenced each other.

In the first half of the twentieth century, anthropologists accepted the existence of discrete races largely on faith, though some clearly wanted to prove their existence, as exemplified by Earnest Hooton in his *Indians of Pecos Pueblo* (1930).

Hooton divided individuals into racial groups by eyeballing cranial morphology and then validated their existence by finding statistically significant differences in their measurements. His theory of race was the lens through which his interpretations came about, as theories are for all of us. As a result, he named some of the groups "pseudo-Negroid," "pseudo-Alpine," "pseudo-Australoid," and "long-faced European," because he was describing their morphology in racial terms (Hooton, 1930). Here was a clear example of forcing humans into a limited number of predefined boxes rather than hypothesis testing. But in a review published in *American Anthropologist,* Woodbury (1932:143) praised it: "The Indians of Pecos, both in its material and its treatment, represents one of the great publications on the physical anthropology of the American aborigines." Hooton's view of human variation was typological and thoroughly influential (Howells, 1992).

Race, especially in physical anthropology, became a less popular research topic after World War II, when the Nazis put pseudoscientific racism and eugenics into practice through genocide. The study of race in many of the sciences was likewise affected. As Provine (1973) has pointed out, many geneticists who believed that race crossing was detrimental before the war believed that there was no evidence for detrimental effects after the war, without any significant intervening studies. The change in scientific opinions and the resulting UNESCO statement on race in 1951 clearly reflected the world's reaction to genocide.

America's opinions on race were changing during the civil rights movement in the 1960s under President Lyndon Johnson, whose policies were diametrically opposed to those of President Andrew Johnson some 100 years earlier. Ashley Montagu had been writing about the fallacy of biological race in books, concentrating on disproving aspects of the typological race concept (Montagu, 1942, 1964). Washburn (1951) proclaimed a "new physical anthropology" centered on treating human groups as populations subject to evolutionary forces rather than categorizing them *a priori* into races; a view echoed in many other publications in physical anthropology (Birdsell, 1951, 1952; Stewart, 1951; Long, 1966). One physical anthropologist who was out of step with the times was Carleton Coon, who published *The Origin of Races* in 1962. The problem with Coon's work was not so much that it was neo-typological, incorporating findings from genetics, but that it had a heavy deterministic component from the nineteenth century as well. Biological determinism in humans, which is essentialist and reductionist, explains observed cultural and intellectual achievements as due to genetics or biological race; superiority of certain peoples is inherent. Biological determinism was a feature of classical typology and nineteenth century anthropology and asserted the congruence of variation in humanity in language, culture, and biology. Coon's atavistic conclusions that some races (Europeans) were more evolved and more intelligent than others (Africans) sounded like Brinton's. As a book for a general audience, it was read by many Americans at a time of social upheaval, with racial desegregation being an especially divisive undertaking (Jackson, 2001; Marks, 2010).

Coon's emphasis on biological determinism inspired a number of critical discussions and publications from many anthropologists, including those from the AAPA, but especially from the AAA (Caspari, 2003; Patterson, 2001). Washburn, president of the AAA in 1963, published an article based on his presidential address during the previous year's AAA meeting covering "the modern concept of race, the interpretation of racial differences, and the social significances of race" (Washburn, 1963:521). He stressed that science offers no justification for racism and that racism is based on misunderstanding human culture and biology. While acknowledging that human variation was no longer typological, Washburn mentioned "races" of humans repeatedly (e.g., "Mongoloid" features), and stressed that patterns of human variation, even in those terms, was worth studying, especially in relation to human culture and with the new tools of genetics. Washburn's (1963) main target was biological determinism, expressed in racial superiority and racial discrimination. Caspari (2010) also equates biological race with determinism and essentialism, and there have been a few recent examples cloaked within the veil of science: *The Bell Curve* (Herrnstein and Murray, 1994) and *Race, Evolution, and Behavior* (Rushton, 1995). Both books asserted links between social/biological race and violence and intelligence (IQ) and provided suggestions for changes to federal social policy and curtailing programs such as affirmative action. In the determinist view, improving the environment will not improve intelligence or performance in humans; the genes dictate everything.

Combating this biological determinism is clearly a motivator for Goodman. In 1995, Goodman suspected an uptick in the use of race among biological anthropologists, interpreting it as evidence that "the revolution is incomplete" and:

> ...there is no scientific reason to continue using the concept of race in biological anthropology. It should be eradicated from our scientific vocabularies. Thus, the re-emergence of race in biological anthropology must be tied to extra-scientific issues (Goodman, 1995:223).

Yet Goodman claimed to want to open a dialog with biological anthropologists, while stressing "...all of us need to consider how, by keeping alive the myth of race, we might maintain and support subtle forms of racism" (237) and "A great deal of uneasiness and testiness is evident when one tries to discuss the validity of the concept with a group of biological anthropologists" (236), no doubt due in part to the lurking threat of being called a racist. Goodman expresses a zero-tolerance policy on biological race because of a perceived slippery slope:

> It is an easy step from the misuse of race in studies of skull shape or hemoglobin levels to its misuse in studies of intelligence (Goodman, 1998:52).

As if equating human variation with biological determinism were not enough, Goodman (1995; Goodman and Armelagos, 1996) equated studying human variation with being a racist:

> Muir (1993) has recently made the distinction between 'mean racists' and 'kind racists.' Mean racists aim to hurt whereas kind racists do not. However, kind racist, or racialists, continue to define humanity in racial terms. By doing so, kind racists leave the door open for mean racists (Goodman and Armelagos, 1996:184).

No scientist wants to be accused of being a racist (let alone a "mean" one), so the effect of such a quote can be intimidating. However, the acceptance of such an argument, which in this case refers to social or biological race, means *every one* of us may be a "kind racist," because racists could misuse virtually *anything* we write. For instance, racists could cite the widespread use of the phrase "races don't exist" to argue against affirmative action, preference for minority groups underrepresented in universities, or Head Start programs aimed at correcting social inequalities. If we all followed Goodman's recommendations, there would be no room for dialog or discussion about *any* aspects of race.

As a result of changes in society and within the discipline and as a reaction against Coon's book, biological race was thrown out and the mantras of "race doesn't exist" and "race is just a social construct" became more widespread (Lieberman and Kirk, 2004). Human variation was downplayed, with a token few sentences in publications, such as, "The denial of race is not a denial of human diversity" and "A goal of physical anthropology should be explaining biocultural complexity" (of which human variation and social races are part) (Goodman and Armelagos, 1996:183), outweighed by the volume of antiracist messages. Following the tradition of Montagu, many published extensively on the misuse of biological race (because it does not exist) in all branches of anthropology and continued to criticize forensic anthropologists specifically for doing something that should be theoretically impossible. For instance, Turner *et al.* (2006:207) wrote,

> Indeed, forensic anthropologists are rare among anthropologists in that they continue to recognize identifiable racial traits in skeletal remains (Gill, 1998; Sauer, 1992), despite clear evidence that race is not a biological category (Brown and Armelagos, 2001; Lewontin, 1972).

They called into question the scientific integrity and honesty of forensic anthropologists who did use race.

Of course, Turner *et al.* (2006) cited arguments against biological race that we know are deficient, assuming that they did not know they were, and that they were being honest. Other criticisms (e.g., Armelagos and Van Gerven, 2003) concentrated on the debunked typological concept of race, a false dilemma, and did not address the question of whether or not humans show patterned variation or acknowledge recent advances in assessing human variation (Stojanowski and Buikstra, 2004). Forensic anthropology was an especially easy target because many forensic anthropologists were "determining" race in skeletal remains using the same typological labels that had been used since the 1900s. In fact, Armelagos and Goodman (1998:370) claimed that "...we have shown that misidentifications are likely to be highly common, much more common than proposed (Goodman, 1997). The use of race in forensic research has probably led to countless misidentifications." While not countless, Goodman (1997) did provide four cases in which forensic anthropologists had incorrectly estimated race. He concluded, "At best, in other words, racial identifications are depressingly inaccurate. At worst, they are completely haphazard" (Goodman, 1997:22).

Indeed, forensic anthropology in the 1990s was stuck in the past, still using terms Hooton and other physical anthropologists had adopted after the racial classifications of Linnaeus, Blumenbach, and Hooton ("Caucasian," "Mongoloid," and "Negroid") or the equivalent translations in America's folk taxonomy, social race ("White," "Black," "Asian;" Sauer, 1993; Hefner *et al.*, 2012). The 1992 catalog of France Casting, which provided casts of skulls to anthropologists, illustrated traits typical of "Caucasoid," "Mongoloid," and "Negroid" individuals until the labels were changed to equivalent regional labels as a reaction to criticisms published by Goodman and Armelagos (1996). Nearly all practicing forensic anthropologists were part of academic departments and knew about the biological race debate. Meanwhile, studies in the *Journal of Forensic Sciences* and several books shared various techniques, or at least lists of traits, for distinguishing American blacks from American whites especially.

Forensic anthropologists could likely "confirm" biological races in forensic cases because most American forensic cases were a question of white versus black or, depending on location, non-forensic American Indian remains. Importantly, forensic anthropologists always made discrete race estimates that corresponded more or less to the traditional races and the American folk taxonomy. To forensic anthropologists, there appeared to be a clear link between the biological races inherited from physical anthropology and American social races; explicit hypothesis testing and theory building was not necessary. Alice Brues summarized the outlook of many forensic anthropologists:

> We need not emphasize any single technique because of its theoretical attractiveness: that may be done when we want to 'advance the science,' not when we merely want to know who it was that was dug up in the back forty (Brues, 1990:7).

Such an atheoretical view is not unusual in an applied science that seems to work. But there should have been greater recognition of the scientific obligation to use explicit and replicable methods, even before the *Daubert* decision. There was apparently little criticism and debate within forensic anthropology. To her credit, Brues also understood the need for theory. She wrote a prescient article on the fact that there is a lot of variation within the traditional races and that forensic anthropologists should be estimating ancestry as finer-grained population affinities more objectively using computers (Brues, 1992). Brues (1990) praised Hooton for collecting nonmetric skeletal trait data from thousands of skeletons from around the world. But no one, including Hooton or Brues, bothered to analyze the data beyond a few short descriptive publications. Finnegan and Cooprider (1978) and Finnegan and McGuire (1979) published analyses of cranial and postcranial nonmetric traits from different populations, but no one followed up on them.

5.4 Forensic anthropology and race

If biological races don't exist, and biological data were not being used, how was race, using information from the skeleton, estimated? Most contemporary forensic anthropology texts (Bass, 2005; Byers, 2002) and especially publications similar to those seen in Gill and Rhine (1990) adopted what we have called the "trait list" approach, listing nonmetric traits or skull morphologies traditionally associated with certain races, which was a corruption of Hooton's approach that involved using more data (Hefner *et al.*, 2012; Hefner and Ousley, 2014). Races were seen as intuitive or obvious units that one could recognize with enough experience. Explicit methods were rarely provided, but high accuracies were claimed, supported by anecdotal cases, revealing their subjective nature and lack of replicability (Gill *et al.*, 1988; Gill, 1998, 2009). In a highly influential book (Gill and Rhine, 1990) that went through three printings (pers. comm., Heather Edgar), Rhine (1990:18) called the estimation of race "as much art as science" in his chapter, which contains trait lists from different biological races. Especially shocking about Rhine's work is the paucity of data, though he did provide results—frequencies—based on a sample size of three "Negroids." More shocking is the recognition that there is actually no method for estimating race in his chapter. Instead, Rhine emphasized that experience was necessary to judge a skull with diverse traits, along with further musings. There were no classification statistics used and no method described to use multiple traits. As a result, there was a subtle shift in interpretation. The trait became the race, which is a gross simplification, but was probably what Rhine had been doing all along: Post-bregmatic depression means black; Carabelli's cusp means white. However, the differences between races are not based on one trait identified here and there, but rather on differences in the expression (frequency) of a suite of traits (gene expressions), assessed quantitatively and consistently. As mentioned, Hefner (2003, 2009) showed that the most commonly listed traits were not found in large group samples. Later, Hefner *et al.* (2007) demonstrated that forensic anthropologists scored nonmetric traits inconsistently, with inconsistent terms, with inconsistent interpretations, and with incorrect results largely because the traits were poorly described. There was no explicit method to use with nonmetric traits, and their utility was uncertain. But the trait list approach persists and is very appealing for teachers: If one knows the race of a skull, one can find some of the numerous traits that are supposed to be there, thanks to confirmation bias. Also, forensic anthropologists writing case reports can find those traits after an identification is made, and the race of the deceased is known. So on these levels, the traits will *seem* valid; however, the approach is insidious. The trait list approach illustrates the problem of confirmation bias: if you expect to find something, you will.

It was not until Sauer's publications (1992, 1993) that a relevant, modern, and critical theory regarding race in forensic anthropology started emerging. Sauer asserted that forensic race estimation involved an association between skeletal morphology and the individual's social race. In other words, there was a positive correlation between biological race and social race. All along, forensic anthropologists had been exploiting a high correlation between biological race labels and social race labels; any experience with remains from blacks and whites, even if they were called "Negroids" and "Caucasoids," translated to the same conclusions using social race labels. It was not, and is not the case, that "laws of inheritance and population genetics underlie studies of ancestry" (Komar and Buikstra, 2008:119), because assessing genetic ancestry has not been as important as estimating the relevant "folk taxonomy" for identification. Studies involving forensic anthropologists were using relevant social/bureaucratic labels (most often "white" or "black") to identify remains in working with law enforcement. The subtleties of human biological variation are not likely to be appreciated by law enforcement officers and legal experts, who want an unambiguous assignment of a given individual to a particular social race for the purpose of identification (Sauer, 1992; Ousley *et al.*, 2009). Likewise, many forensic anthropologists worked within the historical concept of discrete races. The forensic anthropologist contributes to identification in the medicolegal context by describing an individual's ancestry using the vocabulary of self-designated and peer-perceived designations of social race, often available in missing persons' databases, whether or not there is a clear connection to biological race.

Of course, as Sauer (1992) pointed out, if there were no differences between American blacks and whites, forensic anthropologists would not be able to identify their skeletons. In some ways, forensic anthropologists had been "affirming" biological race but, importantly, without a trace of biological determinism. No one tested Sauer's assertions directly until recently, thanks to the establishment of the forensic data bank (Jantz and Moore-Jansen, 1987; Ousley and Jantz, 1998) and the use of better statistical methods. An explicit test of Sauer's assertion confirmed the association: skeletal morphology is strongly associated with social race, at least in the United States (Ousley *et al.*, 2009). The reasons are simple: white and black Americans arrived to this continent biologically different, and institutional racism prevented large amounts of gene flow, which would have made them more similar, so they have remained different enough. Social race has structured mating in the United States; Americans are not panmictic, though the Supreme Court's 1967 ruling overturning the prohibition of interracial marriage and other social changes have changed mating behaviors (Ousley *et al.*, 2009).

Worldwide regional variation in humans is also real, as Sauer (1992, 1993) has maintained, but importantly regional variation does not prove the existence of typological races. Ousley *et al.* (2009) demonstrated the geographic patterning to human craniometric data, echoing earlier investigations by Howells (1973, 1989, 1995). Howells' publications, in fact, illustrate the evolution of physical anthropology thought from the influence of Hooton in the pre-genetic days to his pioneering work of 1973 and continued activity in the 1990s. In the 1940s, Howells thought in terms of traditional races and discussed the origin of races and collecting measurements of "natural groups of people" to describe and compare "racial types" (Howells, 1942, 1943:357). After genetics was used to study human variation and morphology was *passé*, anthropologists were still using genetic data to ascertain the antiquity of traditional races and their number (Boyd, 1950; Garn and Coon, 1955). Howells saw not only differing results from genetics but also a new way to interpret traditional races:

> This leads us back to the general question of human variability and its meaning. Perhaps it is possible to avoid opposing "genetic" concepts of race to "old-fashioned" concepts, and instead, to expand the latter *since races, after all, do exist*—by taking a more general viewpoint based upon the former. This again is not a new suggestion, but the emphasis has been modified from year to year, and that is what we may anticipate in the future. For the present, we may emphasize the universality of the human genetic heritage and explore it most usefully by using race as one way...of studying its dimensions. The change in viewpoint lies in trying to view the total range at once, in appreciation of the variation within it, rather than trying to isolate a race here or a race there, as the taxonomic equivalent of a cigar-store Indian (Howells, 1955:231, emphasis added).

Howells had shifted his belief system somewhat to recognize traditional races as simply one way to approach human variation, to be compared to genetic subdivisions because much more variation was seen in biological races, as opposed to homogeneous entities waiting to be discovered or *a priori* typological units for analysis. In 1976, Howells analyzed and reinterpreted publications from the Pacific and described migrations, acknowledging that human variation was more complex than first believed:

> This is not the same as migrations of different racial types. I once professed this latter view ('43) in a day when nothing was known about time depths and anthropologists had little comprehension of genetic variation and its distribution (Howells, 1976:642).

In this same publication, though, he did use the terms "Mongoloid" and "'typical' Mongoloids" to describe Asian groups with certain morphological affinities. In Howells' later publications (1970, 1973, 1989, 1995), he was able to explore human variation using far more data, including a worldwide database, and came to the conclusions that humans show regional variation, with overlap, and individuals can more often than not be reassigned to the groups that they came from. By the 1995 publication, Howells had come quite far, as seen in his update to Livingstone's (1962) quote: "There are no races, only populations" (Howells 1995:103). Howells recognized the population as the unit of analysis, and populations can be designated by rather arbitrary labels. Plus, we must start with population *samples*. If we were to modify Howells' statement just a bit, we would say that there are no races, only samples. Thus, there is individual variation, though individuals are similar to others in their population (to whom they are more closely related), and populations, represented by samples, are usually most similar to other population samples from the same world region due to historical patterns of gene flow. It is important to recognize that Howells came to his later conclusions by using a large database and modern, multivariate statistical methods that provide more objective, simultaneous analyses of multiple measurements.

Howells' empirical approach was the inspiration for Richard Jantz to establish the forensic data bank. Howells and Jantz have inspired many others to assemble databases from modern humans for greater understanding of human variation, for the forensic goals of personal or ethnic identification, and to examine changes over time within groups. Cranial and postcranial secular changes have been observed in Americans born between the early nineteenth century and since the mid-twentieth century (Meadows Jantz and Jantz, 1999; Wescott and Jantz, 2005) and in other groups (Weisensee and Jantz, 2011). White admixture in American blacks has been estimated as high as 23% in some regions of the United States based on genetic data (Parra *et al.*, 1998), and incorporating admixture in clustering models provides a better fit to morphological data. This indicates increasing white admixture over time, despite institutional racism (Algee-Hewitt, 2016, 2017).

Regional genetic and morphological variation in Spanish-speaking peoples of the new world, labeled as "Hispanic" by the US census, is being explored and monitored (Ross *et al.*, 2004; Spradley, 2013). Hispanics are the fastest growing ethnic group in the United States, and Hispanic immigrants show secular changes due to various reasons, although the changes are less pronounced than those observed in American whites or blacks (Spradley *et al.*, 2016). Some research is explicitly examining the relationship between self-identified individuals who use labels such as "Mexican," "Spanish," "Hispanic," "Chicano," and DNA markers and facial morphology (Lee *et al.*, 2010; Hughes *et al.*, 2013; University of New Mexico, 2016). Recognizing variation within Native American groups in comparison to East Asian groups has also been essential for repatriation obligations (Ousley and Billeck, 2001; Ousley *et al.*, 2003; Ousley *et al.*, 2005).

We now realize that ancestry estimation is the most tenuous assessment in forensic anthropology, with an indirect connection to biology, and the reasons are simple: In stature estimation, we can measure a person's stature multiple times and have an up-to-date stature to compare to stature estimates from long bones. Sex estimation using various methods is either right or wrong based on a comparison to DNA. We can estimate age at death from the skeleton, and, in many cases, we know how old someone was *in days* when he or she died. Thus, all three of these facets of the biological profile have objective measures. Ancestry estimation, however, is inherently disconnected from an independent and objective assessment of human variation. There is no way to tell whether an ancestry assessment is in the strictest sense correct, in contrast to stature, sex, and age estimation. What forensic anthropologists have been using all along were the social classifications, the folk taxonomy. As it turns out, there was a strong enough association between the biological indicators and the social labels, as Sauer (1992) suggested. Estimating ancestry in forensic anthropology is similar to estimating forensic stature, the kind of stature that is self-reported and most often recorded on a driver's license. Forensic statures can be imprecise and rather inaccurate, but almost never change, are recorded somewhere, and are highly correlated with long bone lengths and living stature, which varies throughout the day and over time in adults (Ousley, 1995).

There is still considerable disagreement about whether or not patterns of biological variation seen in humans qualify as biological racial variation. Some believe they do; others believe they do not. Some believe that regional variation in humans reflects ecological factors and thus human ecotypes, which are nonexclusive and can be based on any number of adaptive features (Pigliucci and Kaplan, 2003). While many have found geographically-clustered variation, there is plenty of diversity among groups within regions, so arriving at an exact number of races, or variants, is impossible (Ousley *et al.*, 2009). What is most important for learning more about human variation, despite differences of opinion, is that the patterns of human variation are discussed at all levels and by specialists from many areas, including anthropologists, as opposed to the moratorium that Goodman and others have imposed in the name of antiracism.

Investigating human variation and testing hypotheses about human biological races are not moral decisions: nothing related to action follows from the results, as Pigliucci (2014) noted. Determinists and essentialists like Rushton cherry-pick many kinds of data from races and see races and behavior as highly correlated, ignoring important research from nonanthropologists showing that those connections are virtually meaningless. Further, it is only the determinists who, in light of racial differences, demand that social action is needed, act accordingly, and qualify as racists. Of course, there are plenty of racists who could not care less about science. Thus, there is a broad spectrum of beliefs about human variation and race and what, if anything, we should do based on those beliefs. Figure 5.1 shows our assessment of some of the anthropologists and other scientists we have mentioned, as well as others, contrasting the different beliefs in biological race and whether the authors used scientific methods (gathered empirical data to test hypotheses), as opposed to pseudoscientific methods (cherry-pick data to verify hypotheses). Both axes are continuous, and some individual positions were adjusted for sake of clarity. A principal coordinate analysis based on qualitative and quantitative measures from publications will produce a more objective plot, but we believe the figure more or less accurately represents the practices and views of those authors.

Those on the right side are the biological determinists, with some believing that social action is needed in light of the inherent inferiority of some races; at the extreme right are eugenicists. The right side includes nineteenth-century extremes in pseudoscience, with Brinton and Morton in contrast to Galton; twentieth-century determinists also show a divergence between Rushton and Shockley. Most anthropologists are nearer the middle as far as the biological race (*x*-) axis is concerned, but in the middle are extremes on the scientific (*y*-) axis, ranging from the very empirical Boas, Jantz, and late Howells, to the pseudoscience of Gill and Rhine. Hooton was a professor and mentor to many of the anthropologists shown, but his

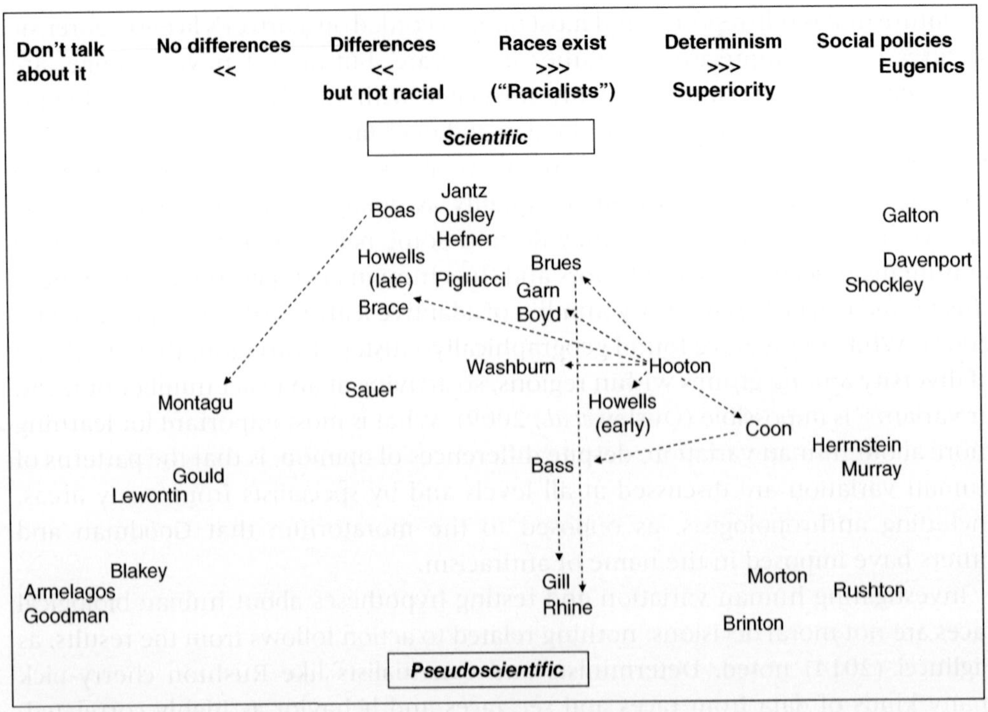

Figure 5.1 Biological race beliefs of some American anthropologists and scientists. The *x*-axis is a continuum from not discussing biological race on the far left, believing in human differences in the middle, to eugenics on the far right. The *y*-axis represents a scale from scientific at the top to pseudoscientific at the bottom–arrows show the connections between professor and student.

views differed a good deal from theirs. The left side shows a concentration of authors who use pseudoscientific methods; the extreme views of race on the left are associated with the greatest use of pseudoscience and other nonscientific arguments.

In general, it is important to note that views on human biological races are largely independent of whether or not someone uses scientific methods. Many authors believe that there is some evidence for human variation in human biological races, as in animals. Most are not determinists and do not associate human biological variation with differences in intelligence or human potential. Most of them believe that human biological variation should be investigated and that investigations so far show meaningful patterns. Most current researchers recognize an association between biological and social race.

5.5 Race and the future

We can now see that it is forensic anthropologists, many of whom analyzed forensic cases in a field that was not theoretically self-aware, that are now at the forefront of gathering and analyzing data for understanding social races and biological variation, especially in relation to phenotypic variation. As far as social race and molecular variation, many geneticists and genetic epidemiologists are conducting research into the connections between social race, environments, economic disparities, and molecular variation (Sankar, 2008). As Gravlee (2009:51) remarked,

> Epidemiologic evidence shows that, in a very certain sense, race is biology. There are, in fact, well-defined differences between racially defined groups for a range of biological outcomes—cardiovascular disease, diabetes, renal failure, cancer, stroke, and birth outcomes, to name a few. In the face of this evidence, the refrain that [social] race is not biology is impotent at best, counterproductive at worst. The challenge is to move beyond the pat assertion that [social] race is not biology to explain how [social] race becomes biology.

In this new light, social race is another classification or explanatory variable to be investigated, rather than something to be avoided. "Race is just a social construct" should be amended with the important rejoinder "with biological and social consequences." "There is no gene for race" should be amended with "but there is human variation and it is not random." As Marks (2010:203) noted, "Biological anthropology's major contribution to the study of race…[is] mediating the cultural and natural realms," and there is greater value in recognizing "that race is itself the result of a constant negotiation between objective patterns of difference (i.e., biology) and subjective perceptions of otherness (i.e., culture)." Social race is associated with genetic variation, but more importantly, with social and economic stresses, including racism, which depends on an individual's perceived social race. There is ample room to expand interdisciplinary studies of ethnogenesis and identity, the basis for various folk taxonomies around the world, their functions in societies, and their consequences (Sankar, 2008). Such studies have great potential to explore the connections between social and biological races as biocultural phenomena and the far-reaching influences they have on humans.

There are recent signs of change in the AAA attitude toward race as well, hopefully signaling a more introspective, investigative, and collaborative role for biocultural researchers. Jason Antrosio, coeditor of *Open Anthropology*, a publication of the AAA, recently wrote,

> Anthropologists have used a critique of racialized biological determinism—by either emphasizing cultural explanations or attempting to deconstruct the very notion of a biological basis for racial classifications—as a means to confront the structured racism of American society… While anthropology has therefore often been used to protest structured racism, its institutional position as an anti-race science has often also insulated it from a necessary self-critique of the discipline's own silences, exclusions, and practices around race (Antrosio, 2015).

We sincerely hope that a new era of collaborative, critical, and insightful study of human variation and social races can begin.

Acknowledgments

The authors thank Cliff and Donna Boyd for their invitation to participate in the symposium, their encouragement to write the chapter, and their patience in waiting for the final product. This publication was improved through discussions with Dr. Pamela Sankar, Department of Medical Ethics at the University of Pennsylvania. Special thanks also go to Bridget Algee-Hewitt, Department of Biology, Stanford University, and the staff of the Hammermill Library, Mercyhurst University.

References

Algee-Hewitt, B. F. B. (2016) Population inference from contemporary American craniometrics. *American Journal of Physical Anthropology*, **160**, 604–624.

Algee-Hewitt, B. F. D. (2017) Temporal trends in craniometric estimates of admixture for a modern American sample. *American Journal of Physical Anthropology*, **163**, 729–740.

Algee-Hewitt, B. F. B., Edge, M. D., Kim, J., *et al.* (2016) Individual identifiability predicts population identifiability in forensic microsatellite markers. *Current Biology*, **26**, 935–942.

Allocco, D. J., Song, Q., Gibbons, G. H., *et al.* (2007) Geography and genography: Prediction of continental origin using randomly selected single nucleotide polymorphisms. *BMC Genomics*, **8**, 68.

American Anthropological Association. (1998) *Statement on Race*. http://www.americananthro.org/ConnectWithAAA/Content.aspx?ItemNumber=2583, accessed September 21, 2016.

American Anthropological Association. (2016) *Race—Are We So Different?* http://www.understandingrace.org/home.html, accessed September 21, 2016.

Antrosio, J. (2015) The editors' note: Race, racism, and protesting anthropology. *Open Anthropology* 3, http://www.americananthro.org/StayInformed/OAArticleDetail.aspx?ItemNumber=13103, accessed September 10, 2016.

Armelagos, G. J., Goodman, A. H. (1998) Race, racism and anthropology. In *Building a New Biocultural Synthesis: Political-Economic Perspectives on Human Biology* (eds. A. H. Goodman and T. L. Leatherman). University of Michigan Press, Ann Arbor, MI, pp. 359–377.

Armelagos, G. J., Van Gerven, D. P. (2003) A century of skeletal biology and paleopathology: Contrasts, contradictions, and conflicts. *American Anthropologist*, **105**, 53–64.

Bamshad, M., Guthery, S. L. (2007) Race, genetics and medicine: Does the color of a leopard's spots matter? *Current Opinion in Pediatrics*, **19**, 613–618.

Bamshad, M. J., Wooding S., Watkins, W. S., *et al.* (2003) Human population genetic structure and inference of group membership. *American Journal of Human Genetics*, **72**, 578–589.

Banaji, M. R., Greenwald, A. G. (2013) *Blind Spot: Hidden Biases of Good People*. Delacorte, New York.

Bass, W. M. (2005) *Human Osteology*, 5th edition. Missouri Archaeological Society, Columbia, MO.

Birdsell, J. B. (1951) The problem of the early peopling of the Americas as viewed from Asia. In: *Papers on the Physical Anthropology of the American Indian* (ed. W. S. Laughlin). The Viking Fund, Inc., New York, pp. 1–68.

Birdsell, J. B. (1952) On various levels of objectivity in genetical anthropology. *American Journal of Physical Anthropology*, **10**, 355–362.

Blakey, M. L. (1999) Scientific racism and the biological concept of race. *Literature and Psychology*, **45**, 29–43.

Boas, F. (1896) The limitations of the comparative method of anthropology. *Science*, **4**, 901–908.

Boas, F. (1911) Introduction. In: *Handbook of American Indian Languages*, Vol. **1** (ed. F. Boas). Bulletin of American Ethnology, Washington, DC.

Boas, F. (1940) *Race, Language and Culture*. Free Press, New York.

Boyd, W. C. (1950) *Genetics and the Races of Man*. Little, Brown and Co., Boston, MA.

Brace, C. L. (1995) Region does not mean "race"—reality versus convention in forensic anthropology. *Journal of Forensic Sciences*, **40**, 171–175.

Brinton, D. G. (1895) The aims of anthropology. *Science*, **2**, 241–252.

Brown, R. A., Armelagos, G. J. (2001) Apportionment of racial diversity: A review. *Evolutionary Anthropology*, **10**, 34–40.

Brues, A. M. (1990) The once and future diagnosis of race. In: *Skeletal Attribution of Race: Methods for Forensic Anthropology* (eds. G. W. Gill and S. Rhine). Maxwell Museum of Anthropology, Albuquerque, NM, pp. 1–7.

Brues, A. M. (1992) Forensic diagnosis of race—general race vs. specific populations. *Social Science and Medicine*, **34**, 125–128.

Bunzl, M. (1996) Franz Boas and the Humboldtian tradition: From *Volksgeist* and *Nationalcharakter* to an anthropological concept of culture. In: *Volksgeist as Method and Ethic* (ed. G. W. Stocking). University of Wisconsin Press, Madison, WI, pp. 17–78.

Byers, S. N. (2002) *Introduction to Forensic Anthropology*, 2nd edition. Allyn and Bacon, New York.

Caspari, R. (2003) From types to populations: A century of race, physical anthropology and the American Anthropological Association. *American Anthropologist*, **105**, 65–76.

Caspari, R. (2010) Deconstructing race: Racial thinking, geographic variation, and implications for biological anthropology. In: *A Companion to Biological Anthropology* (ed. C. S. Larsen). Wiley-Blackwell, Chichester, UK, pp. 104–123.

Coon, C. S. (1962) *The Origin of Races*. Knopf, New York.

Coon, C. S. (1965) *The Living Races of Man*. Knopf, New York.

Coon, C. S., Garn, S. M., Birdsell, J. B. (1950) *Races*. Charles C. Thomas, Springfield, IL.

Crick, B. (1996) Foreword. In: *Race: The History of an Idea in the West* (I. Hannaford). Woodrow Wilson Center Press, Washington, DC, pp. xi–xvi.

Edgar, H. J. H., Hunley, K. L. (2009) Race reconciled?: How biological anthropologists view human variation. *American Journal of Physical Anthropology*, **139**, 1–4.

Edwards, A. W. F. (2003) Human genetic diversity: Lewontin's fallacy. *Bioassays*, **25**, 798–801.

Feagin, J. R. (2001) *Racist America*. Taylor & Francis, New York.

Finnegan, M., Cooprider, K. (1978) Empirical comparison of distance equations using discrete traits. *American Journal of Physical Anthropology*, **49**, 39–46.

Finnegan, M., McGuire, S. A. (1979) Classification systems for discrete variables used in forensic anthropology. *American Journal of Physical Anthropology*, **51**, 547–553.

Garn, S. M., Coon, C. S. (1955) On the number of races of mankind. *American Anthropologist*, **57**, 996–1001.

Gill, G. W. (1998) Craniofacial criteria in the skeletal attribution of race. In: *Forensic Osteology: Advances in the Identification of Human Remains*, 2nd edition (ed. K. J. Reichs). Charles C. Thomas, Springfield, IL, pp. 293–317.

Gill, G. W. (2009) Assessing ancestry (race) from the skeleton. In: *The Use of Forensic Anthropology*, 2nd edition (eds. R. B. Pickering and D. Bachman). CRC Press, Boca Raton, FL, pp. 103–111.

Gill, G. W., Rhine, S. (1990) *Skeletal Attribution of Race: Methods for Forensic Anthropology*. Maxwell Museum of Anthropology, Albuquerque, NM.
Gill, G. W., Hughes, S. S., Bennett, S. M., *et al.* (1988) Racial identification from the midfacial skeleton with special reference to American Indians and whites. *Journal of Forensic Sciences*, **33**, 92–99.
Goodman, A. H. (1995) The problematics of "race" in contemporary biological anthropology. In: *Biological Anthropology: The State of the Science* (eds. N. Boaz and L. D. Wolfe). Oregon State University Press, Bend, OR, pp. 221–243.
Goodman, A. H. (1997) Bred in the bone? *Sciences*, **37**, 20–25.
Goodman, A. H. (1998) The race pit. *Anthropology News*, **39**, 50, 52.
Goodman, A. H., Armelagos, G. J. (1996) The resurrection of race: The concept of race in physical anthropology in the 1990s. In: *Race and Other Misadventures* (eds. L. T. Reynolds and L. Lieberman). General Hall, Inc., Dix Hills, NY, pp. 174–186.
Goodman, A. H., Moses, Y. T., Jones, J. J. (2012) *Race: Are We So Different?* Wiley-Blackwell, Chichester, UK.
Gravlee, C. C. (2009) How race becomes biology: Embodiment of social inequality. *American Journal of Physical Anthropology*, **139**, 47–57.
Hefner, J. T. (2003) *Assessing Nonmetric Cranial Traits Currently Used in Forensic Determination of Ancestry*. Master's Thesis, the University of Florida, Gainesville.
Hefner, J. T. (2009) Cranial nonmetric variation and estimating ancestry. *Journal of Forensic Sciences*, **54**, 985–995.
Hefner, J. T., Ousley, S. D. (2014) Statistical classification methods for estimating ancestry using morphoscopic traits. *Journal of Forensic Sciences*, **59**, 1–8.
Hefner, J. T., Emanovsky, P. D., Byrd, J., Ousley, S. D. (2007) The value of experience, education, and methods in ancestry prediction. *Proceedings of the American Academy of Forensic Sciences*, **XIII**, 360–361.
Hefner, J. T., Ousley, S. D., Dirkmaat, D. C. (2012) Morphoscopic traits and the assessment of ancestry. In: *A Companion to Forensic Anthropology* (ed. D. C. Dirkmaat). Wiley-Blackwell, Chichester, UK, pp. 400–411.
Herrnstein, R. J., Murray, C. (1994) *The Bell Curve: Intelligence and Class Structure in American Life*. Free Press, New York.
Hooton, E. A. (1930) *The Indians of Pecos Pueblo: A Study of Their Skeletal Remains*. Yale University Press, New Haven, CT.
Howells, W. W. (1942) Fossil man and the origin of races. *American Anthropologist*, **44**, 182–193.
Howells, W. W. (1943) Physical anthropology as a technique. *American Journal of Physical Anthropology*, **1**, 355–361.
Howells, W. W. (1955) Universality and variation in human nature. In: *Yearbook of Anthropology* (ed. W. L. Thomas). Wenner-Gren Foundation for Anthropological Research, New York, pp. 227–236.
Howells, W. W. (1970) Multivariate analysis for the identification of race from crania. In: *Personal Identification in Mass Disasters* (ed. T. D. Stewart). National Museum of Natural History, Smithsonian Institution, Washington, DC, pp. 111–121.
Howells, W. W. (1973) *Cranial Variation in Man*. Papers of the Peabody Museum of Archaeology and Ethnology, Vol. **67**. Harvard University Press, Cambridge, MA.
Howells, W. W. (1976) Physical variation and history in Melanesia and Australia. *American Journal of Physical Anthropology*, **45**, 641–650.
Howells, W. W. (1989) *Skull Shapes and the Map*. Papers of the Peabody Museum of Archaeology and Ethnology, Vol. **79**. Harvard University Press, Cambridge, MA.
Howells, W. W. (1992) Yesterday, today, and tomorrow. *Annual Review of Anthropology*, **21**, 1–17.

Howells, W. W. (1995) *Who's Who in Skulls.* Papers of the Peabody Museum of Archaeology and Ethnology, Vol. 82. Harvard University Press, Cambridge, MA.

Hughes, C. E., Tise, M. L., Trammel, L. H., *et al.* (2013) Cranial morphological variation among contemporary Mexicans: Regional trends, ancestral affinities, and genetic comparisons. *American Journal of Physical Anthropology,* **151**, 506–517.

Hunley, K. L., Cabana, G. S., Long, J. C. (2016) The apportionment of human diversity revisited. *American Journal of Physical Anthropology,* **160**, 561–569.

Jablonski, N. G., Chaplin, G. (2000) The evolution of human skin coloration. *Journal of Human Evolution,* **39**, 57–106.

Jackson Jr., J. J. (2001) "In ways unacademical": The reception of Carleton S. Coon's *The Origin of Races. Journal of the History of Biology,* **34**, 247–285.

Jantz, R. L., Moore-Jansen, P. H. (1987) *A Data Base for Forensic Anthropology.* Final report to the National Institute of Justice, Grant No. 85-IJ-CX-0021. https://www.ncjrs.gov/pdffiles1/nij/111608.pdf, accessed September 2, 2016.

Jolly, C. J. (2003) Cranial anatomy and baboon diversity. *The Anatomical Record Part A: Discoveries in Molecular, Cellular, and Evolutionary Biology,* **275A**, 1043–1047.

Jolly, C. J., Woolley-Barker, T., Beyene, S., *et al.* (1997) Intergeneric hybrid baboons. *International Journal of Primatology,* **18**, 597–627.

Jorde, L. B., Wooding, S. P. (2004) Genetic variation, classification, and "race." *Nature Genetics,* Supplement **36**, S28–S33.

Kelly, D. J., Quinn, P. C., Slater, A. M., *et al.* (2005) Three-month-olds, but not newborns, prefer own-race faces. *Developmental Science,* **8**, F31–F36.

Komar, D. A., Buikstra, J. E. (2008) *Forensic Anthropology: Contemporary Theory and Practice.* Oxford University Press, New York.

Lee, Y. L., Teitelbaum, S., Wolff, M. S., *et al.* (2010) Comparing genetic ancestry and self-reported race/ethnicity in a multiethnic population in New York City. *Journal of Genetics,* **89**, 417–423.

Lewontin, R. C. (1972) The apportionment of human diversity. *Evolutionary Biology,* **6**, 381–398.

Lieberman, L. (1997) *"Race" 1997 and 2001: A Race Odyssey.* American Anthropological Association, Arlington, VA.

Lieberman, L., Kirk, R. C. (2004) What should we teach about the concept of race? *Anthropology and Education Quarterly,* **35**, 137–145.

Lieberman, L., Kirk, R. C., Corcoran, M. (2003) The decline of race in American physical anthropology. *Anthropological Review,* **66**, 3–21.

Livingstone, F. (1962) On the non-existence of human races. *Current Anthropology,* **3**, 279–281.

Long, J. K. (1966) A test of multiple-discriminant analysis as a means of determining evolutionary changes and intergroup relationships in physical anthropology. *American Anthropologist,* **68**, 444–464.

Marks, J. (2010) The two 20th-century crises of racial anthropology. In: *Histories of American Anthropology in the Twentieth Century* (eds. M. A. Little and K. A. R. Kennedy). Lexington Books, New York, pp. 187–206.

Meadows Jantz, L., Jantz, R. L. (1999) Secular change in long bone length and proportion in the United States, 1800–1970. *American Journal of Physical Anthropology,* **110**, 57–67.

Montagu, A. F. (1942) *Man's Most Dangerous Myth: The Fallacy of Race.* Harper, New York.

Montagu, A. F. (1964) *The Concept of Race.* Free Press, New York.

Muir, D. E. (1993) Race: The mythic root of racism. *Sociological Inquiry,* **63**, 339–350.

Novembre, J., Johnston T., Bryc, K., *et al.* (2008) Genes mirror geography within Europe. *Nature,* **456**, 98–101.

Obach, B. K. (1999) Demonstrating the social construction of race. *Teaching Sociology*, **27**, 252–257.
O'Rourke, D. H. (2010) Human molecular genetics: The DNA revolution and variation. In: *A Companion to Biological Anthropology* (ed. C. S. Larsen). Wiley-Blackwell, Chichester, UK, pp. 88–103.
Ousley, S. D. (1995) Should we estimate biological or forensic stature? *Journal of Forensic Sciences*, **40**, 768–773.
Ousley, S. D., Billeck, W. T. (2001) Assessing tribal identity in the plains using nontraditional craniometrics (interlandmark distances). *American Journal of Physical Anthropology*, **114**, S115–S116.
Ousley, S. D., Jantz, R. L. (1998) The forensic data bank: Documenting skeletal trends in the United States. In: *Forensic Osteology: Advances in the Identification of Human Remains*, 2nd edition (ed. K. J. Reichs). Charles C. Thomas, Springfield, IL, pp. 441–458.
Ousley, S. D., Seebauer, J. L., Jones, E. B. (2003) Forensic anthropology, repatriation, and the "Mongoloid" problem. *Proceedings of the American Academy of Forensic Sciences*, **IX**, 245–246.
Ousley, S. D., Billeck, W. T., Hollinger, R. E. (2005) Federal repatriation legislation and the role of physical anthropology in repatriation. *Yearbook of Physical Anthropology*, **48**, 2–32.
Ousley, S. D., Jantz, R. L., Freid, D. L. (2009) Understanding race and human variation: Why forensic anthropologists are good at identifying race. *American Journal of Physical Anthropology*, **139**, 68–76.
Parra, E. J., Marcini, A., Akey, J., *et al.* (1998) Estimating African American admixture proportions by use of population-specific alleles. *American Journal of Human Genetics*, **63**, 1839–1851.
Patterson, T. C. (2001) *A Social History of Anthropology in the United States*. Berg, New York.
Pigliucci, M. (2013) What are we to make of the concept of race?: Thoughts of a philosopher–scientist. *Studies in History and Philosophy of Biological and Biomedical Sciences*, **44**, 272–277.
Pigliucci, M. (2014) *On the Biology of Race*. https://scientiasalon.wordpress.com/2014/05/29/on-the-biology-of-race/#comments, accessed September 15, 2016.
Pigliucci, M., Kaplan, J. (2003) On the concept of biological race and its applicability to humans. *Philosophy of Science*, **70**, 1161–1172.
Popper, K. (2002) *The Logic of Scientific Discovery*. Routledge Classics, New York.
Pritchard, J. K., Stephens, M., Donnelly, P. (2000) Inference of population structure using multilocus genotype data. *Genetics*, **155**, 945–959.
Provine, W. B. (1973) Geneticists and the biology of race crossing. *Science*, **182**, 790–796.
Public Broadcasting System. (2003) *Race—The Power of an Illusion*. http://www.pbs.org/race/000_General/000_00-Home.htm, accessed September 21, 2016.
Rhine, S. (1990) Nonmetric skull racing. In: *Skeletal Attribution of Race: Methods for Forensic Anthropology* (eds. G. W. Gill and S. Rhine). Maxwell Museum of Anthropology, Albuquerque, NM, pp. 7–20.
Rosenberg, N. A., Pritchard, J. K., Weber, J. L., *et al.* (2002) The genetic structure of human populations. *Science*, **298**, 2381–2385.
Ross, A. H., Slice, D. E., Ubelaker, D. H., Falsetti, A. B. (2004) Population affinities of 19th century Cuban crania: Implications for identification criteria in south Florida Cuban Americans. *Journal of Forensic Sciences*, **49**, 11–16.
Rushton, J. P. (1995) *Race, Evolution, and Behavior*. Transaction, New Brunswick, NJ.
Sankar, P. (2008) Moving beyond the two race mantra. In: *Revisiting Race and Ethnicity in a Genomic Age* (eds. S. Soo-Jin Lee and B. Koenig). Rutgers University Press, New Brunswick, NJ, pp. 271–284.

Sauer, N. J. (1992) Forensic anthropology and the concept of race: If races don't exist, why are forensic anthropologists so good at identifying them? *Social Science and Medicine*, **34**, 107–111.

Sauer, N. J. (1993) Applied anthropology and the concept of race: A legacy of Linnaeus. In: *NAPA Bulletin 13. Race, Ethnicity and Applied Bioanthropology* (eds. C. C. Gordon). American Anthropological Association, Washington, DC, pp. 79–84.

Spradley, M. K. (2013) *Project IDENTIFICATION: Developing Accurate Identification Criteria for Hispanics*. National Institute of Justice, Rockville, MD. https://www.ncjrs.gov/pdffiles1/nij/grants/244194.pdf, accessed September 14, 2016.

Spradley, K., Stull, K. E., Hefner, J. T. (2016) Craniofacial secular change in recent Mexican migrants. *Human Biology*, **88**, 15–29.

Steele, C. M., Aronson, J. (1995) Stereotype threat and the intellectual test performance of African Americans. *Journal of Personality and Social Psychology*, **69**, 797–811.

Stewart, T. D. (1951) Objectivity in racial classifications. *American Journal of Physical Anthropology*, **9**, 470–472.

Stocking Jr., G. W. (1982) *Race, Culture, and Evolution*. University of Chicago Press, Chicago, IL.

Stojanowski, C. M., Buikstra, J. E. (2004) Biodistance analysis, a biocultural enterprise: A rejoinder to Armelagos and Van Gerven (2003). *American Anthropologist*, **106**, 430–432.

Swedlund, A. C. (1972) Observations on the concept of neighbourhood knowledge and the distribution of marriage distances. *Annals of Human Genetics*, **35**, 327–330.

Tumbler. (2013) *Science Sparks Art*. http://sciencesparksart.tumblr.com/post/44222512469/there-is-no-gene-for-race-artist-nancy-burson, accessed September 21, 2016.

Turner, B. L., Toebbe, D. S., Armelagos, G. J. (2006) To the science, to the living, to the dead: Ethics and bioarchaeology. In: *The Nature of Difference: Science, Society and Human Biology* (eds. G. T. H. Ellison and A. H. Goodman). Taylor & Francis, New York, pp. 203–224.

University of New Mexico. (2016) *Heritage New Mexico*. http://heritagenm.unm.edu/about, accessed September 20, 2016.

Wallace, K. (2012) *Nancy Burson: Morpher of the Face, Human and Divine*. https://karenwallacephotosocialchange.wordpress.com/2012/03/20/nancy-burson-morpher-of-the-face-human-and-divine/, accessed September 21, 2016.

Washburn, S. (1951) The new physical anthropology. *Yearbook of Physical Anthropology*, **7**, 144–152.

Washburn, S. L. (1963) The study of race. *American Anthropologist*, **65**, 521–531.

Weisensee, K. E., Jantz, R. L. (2011) Secular changes in craniofacial morphology of the Portuguese using geometric morphometrics. *American Journal of Physical Anthropology*, **145**, 548–559.

Weiss, K., Fullerton, S. M. (2005) Racing around, getting nowhere. *Evolutionary Anthropology*, **14**, 165–169.

Wescott, D. J., Jantz, R. L. (2005) Assessing craniofacial secular change in American whites and blacks using geometric morphometry. In: *Modern Morphometrics in Physical Anthropology* (ed. D. Slice). Kluwer Academic, New York, pp. 231–246.

Williams, F. L., Belcher, R. L., Armelagos, G. J. (2005) Forensic misclassification of ancient Nubian crania: Implications for assumptions about human variation. *Current Anthropology*, **46**, 340–346.

Woodbury, G. (1932) The Indians of Pecos Pueblo (Book review). *American Anthropologist*, **34**, 142–143.

Wright Jr., L. (1995) Who's black, who's white, and who cares: Reconceptualizing the United States's definition of race and racial classifications. *Vanderbilt Law Review*, **48**, 513–569.

CHAPTER 6

The application of theory in skeletal age estimation

Natalie R. Langley[1] and Beatrix Dudzik[2]

[1] *Department of Anatomy, Mayo Clinic School of Medicine, Scottsdale, AZ, USA*

[2] *Department of Anatomy, DeBusk College of Osteopathic Medicine, Lincoln Memorial University, Harrogate, TN, USA*

6.1 Introduction

Physical anthropology and archaeology form the basis of the applied discipline of forensic anthropology. The foundation of physical anthropology in the United States can be traced back to anatomy departments, where anatomists extended their interest in soft tissue variation to the skeletal framework of the human form. The conventional anatomist's talents lie largely in dissecting, identifying, and describing the range of human variation, but the anatomist as a researcher sets the foundation for questions about the evolutionary relationship between form and function. Early physical anthropologists expanded their anatomical training by studying variation in the context of evolutionary theory to formulate questions about human lifestyle and life history. The ability to interpret human skeletal biology in an evolutionary framework remains a trademark of physical anthropology today. This interpretive structure spans the time frame from the human fossil record to modern forensic casework. As an applied endeavor, however, theoretical foundations are often overlooked in forensic anthropology, and this has been difficult for the discipline to overcome.

This chapter seeks to rectify this issue by exploring the history and theoretical underpinnings of one aspect of forensic anthropology practice—skeletal age estimation. The beginnings of methodologies targeting the estimation of skeletal age stem from observation. Early anatomists involved in the dissection and processing of human cadavers began to document skeletal changes associated with development and degeneration. While skeletal maturation cannot be classified as a phenomenon, it is an observable, patterned process that has been described and interpreted in an evolutionary and theoretical context. Foundational theory

Forensic Anthropology: Theoretical Framework and Scientific Basis, First Edition.
Edited by C. Clifford Boyd Jr and Donna C. Boyd.

encompasses a broad interpretive approach to the natural biologic processes of the world (Mayr, 2001; Quammen, 2006), while interpretive theory involves the derivation of hypotheses based on a set of observations and period of experimental testing that supports or refutes the original statements of the observer. Thus, the chronicling of age-related changes exhibited in the human skeleton and the effort to estimate age based on described morphologies fall under the premise of interpretive theory. As with the broader discipline of forensic anthropology, observations lead to constructed interpretations based on context. The methodological approaches that have been produced in an effort to capture how the human skeletal form changes from birth to death encompass methodological theory in that the hypothesized method is evaluated in terms of accuracy. How well a model performs is dictated by its results. If an approach captures the true patterns or "phenomena" embodied in skeletal maturation and degeneration, then the precision and accuracy of the estimates will be reflected in efforts to validate the method on samples that were not used to develop the model.

The aim of this chapter is to provide a historical and theoretical context to the approaches practitioners use when estimating skeletal age. It is well known to any student or professional of physical anthropology that age estimation methods correlate known chronological ages of individuals in documented skeletal collections with morphological features of skeletal age indicators that include hallmarks of growth and development (i.e., epiphyseal union, tooth eruption) and degeneration (i.e., eburnation, osteophytic activity). The process of age estimation, from method development to implementation, combines inductive and deductive reasoning and much less thought is typically given to this process, unless one is involved in revising or creating a method. Researchers use inductive reasoning to develop hypotheses, conduct tests, and evaluate results to determine if predictions are supported or falsified (Boyd and Boyd, 2011). It should be recognized that well-trained and highly experienced skeletal biologists do not enter into the method development process blindly. They recognize morphological patterns and deduce how these patterns may be related to the aging process, then use these data for method development. Once satisfactory methods are developed and tested, practitioners use them to estimate skeletal age of unknown individuals.

Skeletal age estimation too often is taught and practiced in the absence of theoretical context. Emphasis tends to be placed on application and deriving age estimates for reporting purposes without encouraging burgeoning academics to think about how the methods were developed initially and, perhaps more importantly, under what biological framework they are appropriate. As data sets are updated and expanded, statistical analyses become more sophisticated and computer packages are available to practitioners on a global basis; we must be cautious not to lose sight of the role of theory in informing practice and medicolegal application.

Furthermore, the discussion of the theory involved with age estimation in this chapter is easily generalized to analyses of the human skeleton concerning all aspects of the biological profile, pathology, and trauma. Analytical procedures for a forensic anthropology case report are constantly evaluated in terms of accuracy and truth, that is, if the timing and mode of a skeletal perimortem injury can be correctly interpreted, yet the understanding of why each approach exhibits any accuracy is not often addressed in the literature. Building an accurate depiction of one's life and sometimes death from skeletal remains requires synthesizing a large amount of information and reducing it to a simple parameter using the theoretical premises of forensic anthropology (e.g., an age or stature range, sex or ancestry estimate, or an opinion about the cause or manner of death). The last few decades of analytical reflection have resulted in a shift to an emphasis on why predictive techniques work in the field of forensic anthropology and how and why analytical methods exist (Boyd and Boyd, 2011).

6.2 Skeletal age

To discuss the theoretical foundations for inferring biological age from skeletal characteristics, we must distinguish between chronological age at death and skeletal age at death. The former refers to a number calculated by subtracting the date of birth from the date of death. The latter refers to an age range that corresponds to a suite of morphological traits consistent with the majority of individuals at a given age. Therefore, chronological age at death is an integer (23, 35, 49, etc.), whereas skeletal age at death is necessarily an interval (35–45, 54–60, etc.). A number of factors affect skeletal age at death, including habitual activities, diet, congenital anomalies, injuries, pathologies, and genetic criteria such as sex and ancestry. Additionally, skeletal age is not a discrete variable, which can make accurate estimates immensely difficult. Teasing out these complicating factors from skeletal age indicators is the bread and butter of holistically trained forensic anthropologists who incorporate human skeletal biology, anatomy, culture, and life history into their analyses. Even with anthropological training, human variation dictates that exceptions exist as a response to a multitude of evolutionary processes, both at small and large temporal scales. Thus, although perceived as biological reality, the skeletal expression of traits is not always in perfect agreement with the methods developed to describe them. Well-rounded training in anatomy, life history, and statistics helps forensic anthropologists identify population substructures and explain how and why outliers exist.

6.3 Historical context

The anatomist T. Wingate Todd began large-scale skeletal age-at-death research in the late nineteenth century when he documented pubic symphyseal age changes in Western Reserve University anatomical donors used for gross anatomy dissection (Shapiro, 1939). Todd documented morphological patterns correlated with growth, development, and degeneration and established a phase-based method for age-at-death estimation of skeletal remains. An examination of Hamann-Todd collection skeletons, death records, and Dr. Todd's notes reveals that Todd recognized the distinction between chronological and skeletal age at death, as intrinsic factors such as a life of hard labor or poor health caused inconsistencies between these categories. Some of the drawers in the collection contain handwritten notes commenting that the skeleton looks older or younger than the reported or "stated" age at death. Suchey and Katz (1998) astutely note significant problems with what is colloquially referred to as the "Todd collection." Collection curators appeared to have a specific morphology in mind for each age group based on extensive observations of skeletal remains. Thus, the death record may state "23 years old," but the anatomist felt that the skeleton was more consistent with a 30- or 35-year-old, and the latter "observed age" was entered into Todd collection records (hence the 5-year interval age lumping noted in the collection demographics). A large number of unclaimed indigents from City Hospital, Lakeside Hospital, and Warrensville Hospital in Cleveland comprise the Todd collection, so an exact date of birth was often unknown. Lovejoy *et al.* (1985) note that only 3 of the over 3000 records in the Todd collection contain legal documentation of birth date. Ages listed in the files were estimated from soft tissue indicators during hospital autopsy, and Todd collection curators often noted discrepancies as great as 15–20 years between "stated age" at autopsy and "observed age," the latter referring to skeletal age at death (Lovejoy *et al.*, 1985). Nonetheless, a handful of age estimation methods used in forensic anthropology casework have been developed using individuals in this skeletal collection (Todd, 1920, 1921; Todd and Lyon, 1925; Lovejoy *et al.*, 1985; Meindl and Lovejoy, 1985; Passalacqua, 2009).

Thus, while early anthropologists used their anatomical knowledge of skeletal variation to develop age estimation methods, their samples were fraught with an uncontrollable source of error that created a circular logic between method and application: skeletal age was used to determine the age of the individuals, and then these estimated ages were used to develop age estimation methods. In addition to identifying problems with the accuracy of the data, critiques also exist regarding the data analysis in Todd's pubic symphyseal age estimation method. Namely, several valid issues have been identified that potentially impact the accuracy and theoretical validity of the method, including overly precise age ranges, lack of statistical analysis, and limited age distribution of the reference sample.

6.4 Forensic anthropology and evolutionary biology

Shortly after Todd completed his work on skeletal age estimation, evolutionary theory was redefined to include the genetic mechanisms responsible for population change. The "modern synthesis" united Darwin's idea of natural selection and Mendel's explanation of simple inheritance of traits with population genetics.

The term was coined by Huxley (1942) in his book *Evolution: The Modern Synthesis*, which linked the work of naturalists, paleontologists, and geneticists and advanced our understanding of how population genetics affects anatomical variation in extinct and extant species. Dobzhansky (1937) showed that natural populations are not uniform and harbor genetic variants, while Mayr (1942) defined species by their ability to mate and produce viable offspring as opposed to delineating these taxonomic groups solely on the basis of morphological similarities. Mayr (1942) also argued that evolutionary pressures work on the entire organism and its genome rather than isolated genes. Wright (1949) provided the mathematical foundation for modern population genetics, and Simpson (1942) explained evolutionary patterns identified in the fossil record.

The researchers of this time period provided mathematical models for quantifying the degrees of mutation, recombination, and selection that operate within species to account for evolutionary change. The modern synthesis explained that microevolutionary changes within populations were responsible for the macroevolution observed in the fossil record. Anatomical variation began to be interpreted and studied in a new light. Morphological variants were no longer the object of descriptive and typological treatises, but instead served as fodder for complex microevolutionary processes that provided evidence of evolutionary relationships as well as population and life histories. In 1951, Washburn launched the "new physical anthropology" in which he proposed incorporating the modern synthesis into the interdisciplinary four-field study of human biology and culture. He also predicted the dominant role that genes would eventually play in understanding and interpreting human evolution (Washburn, 1951). Washburn's (1951) call for a holistic, interdisciplinary interpretation of human biology and behavior has impacted forensic anthropology training and practice since the formal inception of the field in the 1970s.

The modern synthesis was followed by the discovery of the molecular double helix structure of DNA (Watson and Crick, 1953) and evolutionary biologists began to (over)emphasize the role of genes in phenotypic expression. While natural selection undoubtedly influences evolution, it does not account for all observable evolutionary change; however, neither do genes (Müller and Newman, 2003; West-Eberhard, 2003; Pigliucci, 2009). West-Eberhard (2003) argues that genes and the environment exert *equally* important influences on phenotypic variability. She suggests that epigenetic factors are essential for maintaining developmental plasticity and account for the production of alternative phenotypes from a fixed genome. Developmental plasticity shapes evolution in that most phenotypic change begins with environmentally mediated developmental change. This marks a departure from the modern synthesis interpretation of the environment's role in producing variation (e.g., that environmental factors do not guide the production of new variants, but rather genetic variation produced by mutations are either favorable or unfavorable with respect to natural selection). The environment is now viewed as "initiator of evolutionary novelties," with genes playing a secondary role in phenotypic evolution (Pigliucci, 2001; West-Eberhard, 2003).

West-Eberhard's influence on the interpretation of phenotypic plasticity resonated with skeletal biologists who have documented short-term changes in skeletal form due to environmental factors. Secular changes in long bone length and proportions (Meadows and Jantz, 1995; Jantz and Jantz, 1999), cranial vault size and shape (Jantz and Meadows Jantz, 2000; Jantz, 2001), and skeletal maturation (Crowder and Austin, 2005; Langley-Shirley and Jantz, 2010) have enticed forensic anthropology practitioners and researchers to examine the process of skeletal aging at a deeper level and to implement abductive reasoning to parse out how and why skeletal growth, development, and deterioration can differ in various environments (Langley *et al.*, 2016). For example, anthropologists have drawn on research documenting epigenetic markers that affect behavior and biology to formulate their hypotheses about secular change in human skeletal form, which has affected the size and shape of the human skeleton in a relatively minute temporal span (Low *et al.*, 2012; Guth *et al.*, 2013; Dias and Ressler, 2014; Langley *et al.*, 2016). Furthermore, rapid evolution in other organisms supports the possibility of single generation changes in phenotype in humans (Drake and Klingenberg, 2008; Herrel *et al.*, 2008; Pergams and Lawler, 2009; Milot *et al.*, 2011; Brown and Brown, 2013; Harris *et al.*, 2013). It is therefore no longer advisable or considered best practice to use methods developed on nineteenth and early twentieth-century populations to derive a biological profile for modern forensic cases.

This realization has led to a surge of research to develop population-specific standards for estimating the parameters of the biological profile and countless validation studies of these methods. Modern donor collections (e.g., Maxwell Museum Documented Skeletal Collection, William M. Bass Donated Skeletal Collection, and Texas State University Donated Skeletal Collection) were started to address the need for methods based on forensically-relevant samples instead of skeletal collections with birth years dating to roughly a century before the current population (Hamann-Todd Osteological Collection and Robert J. Terry Anatomical Collection) or, worse yet, prehistoric archaeological samples.

A legitimate concern of the latter was raised by Wood *et al.* (1992) in their discussion of the "osteological paradox." The authors explain that using the archaeological record to interpret past populations does not result in an accurate depiction of overall health or represent fertility and mortality rates as skeletal remains only represent the individuals that died. As such, the percentage of the population that survived is not accounted for and can skew conclusions about the demographic and epidemiological state of a civilization. While the paradox refers to inferences about health in prehistoric populations, the article illustrates how the age distribution and frequency of pathology in reference samples may not be representative of the target population. Statistical models are built using observations and can be used to estimate parameters of an independent set of observations. However, if the two sets of observations are different enough, the model will perform poorly. This is true when discussing reference and target populations in age estimation, as there are many evolutionary factors that can affect growth and development of an organism. For example, poor health and nutrition that are often correlated with lower socioeconomic status have been shown to retard the speed of skeletal growth and dental eruption in children, which is more tightly regulated by genes than is degeneration and senescence (Garn *et al.*, 1973).

6.5 Potential solutions to the problem of age estimation

One way that researchers have addressed the issue of skewed age distributions of modern donor populations is by partnering with medical examiner's and coroner's offices to expand modern samples (e.g., Broward County Medical Examiner's Office, Los Angeles County Medical Examiner's Office, Maricopa County Forensic Science Center, and Montana State Crime Lab) (Işcan *et al.*, 1984; Işcan *et al.*, 1985; Brooks and Suchey, 1990; Hartnett, 2010a, b; Dudzik and Langley, 2015). Research on international populations has also been undertaken to provide standards for international casework. For example, reliability of skeletal aging methods was questioned in trials prosecuted by the International Criminal Tribunal for the Former Yugoslavia (ICTY), leading to a body of work producing age, sex, and stature estimation criteria for the Balkan population (Berg, 2008; Jantz *et al.*, 2008; Prince and Konigsberg, 2008; DiGangi *et al.*, 2009).

The comprehensive theoretical framework provided by anatomy and evolutionary theory has identified a host of factors that can affect how, on average, an individual in a population matures into an adult organism and then slowly degenerates. These variables include diet, disease, biomechanical loading, and geographical location. However, many aging methods commonly employed in laboratories lack a rigorous statistical framework. In many studies, researchers seriated samples using a suite of morphological traits to constitute a phase, and then age ranges of individuals within each phase were analyzed to provide raw age ranges and/or summary statistics for each range. This is apparent in the work of Todd (1920, 1921), Lovejoy *et al.* (1985), Işcan *et al.* (1984, 1985), Katz and Suchey (1986), and Brooks and Suchey (1990) and has persisted in more recent publications as well (Osborne *et al.*, 2004; Hartnett, 2010a, b). Phase methods lump several morphological indicators of age into a single category with the assumption that each trait progresses in conjunction with the others at the same rate.

Researchers have questioned the biological reality of this assumption and proposed using simpler component scoring systems to address this issue (DiGangi *et al.*, 2009; Passalacqua and Uhl, 2009 Algee-Hewitt, 2011; Dudzik and Langley, 2015; Shirley and Ramirez Montes, 2015). Component scoring is nothing new to age estimation (McKern and Stewart, 1957; Gilbert and McKern, 1973), but the data are more difficult to analyze statistically, so researchers traditionally have favored phase-based methods. One attractive feature of component systems is that they are easy to apply and do not leave the practitioner deciding between two sometimes closely related phases. Another benefit is that they can be applied more reliably than phase methods regardless of observer experience (Shirley and Ramirez Montes, 2015). Component methods have been developed for the pubic symphysis (McKern and Stewart, 1957; Gilbert and McKern, 1973; Dudzik and Langley, 2015), auricular surface (Buckberry and Chamberlain, 2002; Igarashi *et al.*, 2005), sacral auricular surface (Passalacqua, 2009), cranial sutures (Meindl and Lovejoy, 1985), and acetabulum (Rissech *et al.*, 2006; Calce, 2012). In all of these, traits are treated as independent variables. Research has shown that component scoring with three or less states of expression for each variable results in good interobserver error agreement. Systems with a multitude of categorical tiers can result in significant levels of disagreement between observers (Shirley and Ramirez Montes, 2015). Component-based systems form the basis of the multifactorial transition analysis method and the accompanying ADBOU software (Boldsen *et al.*, 2002). Multifactorial aging methods use multiple skeletal indicators to arrive at an age range estimation. Criticisms of earlier approaches describe the use of single indicators (such as the pubic symphysis) or a combination of areas of the skeleton to deduce age in a nonsystematic way (Lovejoy *et al.*, 1985). Multifactorial methods have shown higher accuracies in some instances; however, results are variable in regard to the method used and the average target age range to be estimated (Franklin, 2010).

Simply employing a component system does not address the issues with statistical rigor in many age estimation methods. An important caveat to consider is age mimicry bias, in which estimated age will be biased toward the age-at-death distribution of the reference sample (Bocquet-Appel and Masset, 1982; Konigsberg and Frankenberg, 1992, 1994; Hoppa and Vaupel, 2002). Bayesian statistics have been suggested as a means of overcoming the limitations of reference sample age distributions and age mimicry bias. By choosing relevant samples, estimates are built using probabilities that an unknown is representative of whichever population was used to build the model. Inherently related to this approach is transition analysis, in which the age at which an individual moves across an age threshold is targeted (Boldsen *et al.*, 2002). These methods have been slow to be adopted, perhaps due to computational intensity and selection of appropriate priors. The ADBOU software package offers a solution to practitioners in that it does the computing and the user can select a forensic, archaeological, or uniform prior. The software is based on the pubic symphysis, auricular surface, and cranial sutures and can also handle missing data.

With new data, more rigorous statistical approaches and computer software programs make their way into age estimation. Some question if the practice will become too automated and removed from its theoretical roots. But the fact remains that forensic anthropologists do not work in a vacuum, blindly using scoring systems and software to obtain an age estimate and produce a biological profile. We incorporate information about lifestyle, health, and habitual activities that we derive from our observations of the entire skeleton because we are holistically trained. It would take a concerted effort to score the pubic symphysis and auricular surface and ignore lipping on the intervertebral and zygapophyseal joints as we gather data for our age estimate. And it may be a grave oversight to ignore indications that skeletal remains look older or younger than established methods reveal. Forensic anthropologists do not argue that humans are the product of biocultural evolution, but they are torn between making scientifically unsupported assessments of biological parameters and the strict demands of a medicolegal system with legal precedents governing our analyses, case notes, and reports (Heilbronner, 2011; *General Electric Co v. Joiner*, 1997; *Kumho Tire Company, Ltd. v. Carmichael*, 1999; *Melendez-Diaz v. Massachusetts*, 2009). So, how do forensic anthropologists provide age estimates that stand up to the rigors and ethical demands of the legal system yet remain sensitive to their holistic training?

The answer is not simple, but it must include quantification of the subjective traits that potentially influence our age estimates from other methods (Milner and Boldsen, 2012). If forensic anthropologists are to utilize the holistic toolkit that comes from multidisciplinary training and a biocultural interpretation of the human skeleton in the current legal environment (see National Research Council, 2009), we must provide a thorough analytical basis for our osteological conclusions. Researchers are beginning to make a headway in this direction (Milner, 2010; Milner and Boldsen, 2012; Milner *et al.*, 2016). Milner and Boldsen (2012) have shown that our experienced-based assessments are often more valuable than the standard set of anatomical structures typically used for age estimation. Clearly, there is something to be said for the role of the expert in any field (see Federal Rules of Evidence, 1975), but today's experts must learn to operate in a less forgiving legal system than the one 50 years ago.

6.6 Final comments

Montagu's (1941) publication eloquently describes the intertwined history between anatomy and anthropology and emphasizes that as researchers, we cannot be reductionists and hence cannot subsume the larger picture, in this case age distributions, into a few traits and tables of summary statistics. We bring a holistic biocultural approach to the table. This chapter advocates that practitioners, researchers, students, and educators incorporate theory and history into application. The foundations of evolutionary theory must not be omitted from the formation of forensically applicable methods or ignored in the education of students of the discipline. In addition, estimation of the biological profile requires an understanding of how skeletal and soft tissue morphologies of modern humans reflect both current and past microevolutionary processes. Understanding human evolution demands a working knowledge of the development and function of the skeleton and the related soft tissues. Thus, within the context of research, education, and forensic application, this chapter promotes the idea that formal training in anatomy, evolutionary theory, and statistics as well as a working knowledge of history and theory in forensic anthropology is imperative to move the discipline forward.

Today's solutions involve the use of more indicators that capture growth and degenerative patterns, multifactorial methods, more appropriate statistics, and software programs with easy to use interfaces to handle complicated multifactorial probability-based methods (such as ADBOU). Moreover, strict criteria now exist for method development that satisfy the scientific rigor required by the medicolegal community and, ultimately, the ethical demands of the criminal justice system.

While most programs of study require formal training in statistics and evolutionary theory, many do not *require* a full dissection course in gross anatomy. In fact, it is possible to earn a PhD in physical anthropology without so much as stepping foot into an anatomy laboratory in spite of the fact that physical anthropology is an extension of anatomy. As Montagu (1941) explains, the alphabet of physical anthropology is morphology, and students of physical anthropology must first be taught this alphabet before they can read, write, and speak the language of physical anthropology. We urge administrators and PhD advisors to mandate this essential component of physical anthropology training that was regrettably lost when physical anthropology departments made the transition from anatomy into departments of cultural anthropology and archaeology. We do not debate the benefits of this evolution of our discipline, but we lament that part of our foundation was somehow lost in the shuffle. Montagu (1941) brought this to the attention of the physical anthropology community in his *American Journal of Physical Anthropology* article "Physical Anthropology and Anatomy":

> ...the calipers are brought out to carry on from the point at which the scalpel can go no further. But that does not mean that one forgets about the scalpel as soon as one has taken up the calipers. That this has occurred in a contemporary phase of the development of physical anthropology we all of us know, and most of us, I believe, regret. There are some physical anthropologists who have never so much as touched a scalpel, but have gone right on to the calipers. Such men, however competent they may be at their work, can rarely succeed in becoming anything more than good technicians. At best they can accurately record end-effects, but they can never have any real understanding of the manner in which those end effects are brought about. In all this, as far as it goes, there is no harm; the place of the technician in any science is an important one, and a large part of the work of most scientists is that of the technician. The harm arises only when such technicians take it upon themselves to pronounce judgments upon the nature of the conditions underlying morphological facts with which they have, at best, no more than a bowing acquaintance. Such ungrounded pronouncements can only serve to bring physical anthropology into disrepute among scientists, and can do no one any good (pp. 261–262).

Ultimately, we must continue to use the theoretical constructs of anatomy and evolutionary theory to inform practice and research and to train future forensic anthropologists. Formal training in anatomy, evolutionary theory, and quantitative methods, as well as a working knowledge of history and anthropological theory, will move the discipline forward and concomitantly preserve our unique heritage.

References

Algee-Hewitt, B. F. B. (2011) *If and How Many Races? The Application of Mixture Modeling to World-Wide Human Craniometric Variation*. PhD Dissertation, University of Tennessee, Knoxville.

Berg, G. E. (2008) Pubic bone age estimation in adult women. *Journal of Forensic Sciences*, **53**, 569–577.

Bocquet-Appel, J.-P. and Masset, C. (1982) Farewell to paleodemography. *Journal of Human Evolution*, **11**, 321–333.

Boldsen, J. L., Milner, G. R., Konigsberg, L. W., and Wood, J. W. (2002) Transition analysis: A new method for estimating age from skeletons. In: *Paleodemography: Age Distributions from Skeletal Samples* (eds. R. Hoppa and J. Vaupel). Cambridge Studies in Biological and Evolutionary Anthropology. Cambridge University Press, Cambridge, pp. 73–106.

Boyd, C. and Boyd, D. C. (2011) Theory and the scientific basis for forensic anthropology. *Journal of Forensic Sciences*, **56**, 1407–1415.

Brooks, S. and Suchey, J. M. (1990) Skeletal age determination based on the os pubis: A comparison of the Acsádi-Nemeskéri and Suchey-Brooks methods. *Human Evolution*, **5**, 227–238.

Brown, C. R. and Brown, M. B. (2013) Where has all the road kill gone? *Current Biology*, **23**, R233–R234.

Buckberry, J. L. and Chamberlain, A. T. (2002) Age estimation from the auricular surface of the ilium: A revised method. *American Journal of Physical Anthropology*, **119**, 231–239.

Calce, S. E. (2012) A new method to estimate adult age-at-death using the acetabulum. *American Journal of Physical Anthropology*, **148**, 11–23.

Crowder, C. and Austin, D. (2005) Age ranges of epiphyseal fusion in the distal tibia and fibula of contemporary males and females. *Journal of Forensic Sciences*, **50**, 1000–1007.

Dias, B. G. and Ressler, K. J. (2014) Parental olfactory experience influences behavior and neural structure in subsequent generations. *Nature Neuroscience*, **17**, 89–96.

Digangi, E. A., Bethard, J. D., Kimmerle, E. H., and Konigsberg, L. W. (2009) A new method for estimating age-at-death from the first rib. *American Journal of Physical Anthropology*, **138**, 164–176.

Dobzhansky, T. (1937) Genetic nature of species differences. *American Naturalist*, **71**, 404–420.

Drake, A. G. and Klingenberg, C. P. (2008) The pace of morphological change: Historical transformation of skull shape in St Bernard dogs. *Proceedings of the Royal Society of London B: Biological Sciences*, **275**, 71–76.

Dudzik, B. and Langley, N. R. (2015) Estimating age from the pubic symphysis: A new component-based system. *Forensic Science International*, **257**, 98–105.

Federal Rules of Evidence 702 (1975) Publ. L No. 93-595, §1 88 Stat. 1926. Effective January 2, 1975.

Franklin, D. (2010) Forensic age estimation in human skeletal remains: Current concepts and future directions. *Legal Medicine*, **12**(1), 1–7.

Garn, S. M., Clark, D. C., and Trowbridge, F. L. (1973) Tendency toward greater stature in American black children. *American Journal of Diseases of Children*, **126**(2), 164–166.

General Electric Co. v. Joiner (1997) US, **522**, 136.

Gilbert, B. M. and McKern, T. W. (1973) A method for aging the female os pubis. *American Journal of Physical Anthropology*, **38**, 31–38.

Guth, L. M., Ludlow, A. T., Witkowski, S., *et al.* (2013) Sex-specific effects of exercise ancestry on metabolic, morphological and gene expression phenotypes in multiple generations of mouse offspring. *Experimental Physiology*, **98**, 1469–1484.

Harris, S. E., Munshi-South, J., Obergfell, C., and O'Neill, R. (2013) Signatures of rapid evolution in urban and rural transcriptomes of white-footed mice (*Peromyscus leucopus*) in the New York metropolitan area. *PLoS One*, **8**, e74938.

Hartnett, K. M. (2010a) Analysis of age-at-death estimation using data from a new, modern autopsy sample—Part I: Pubic bone. *Journal of Forensic Sciences*, **55**, 1145–1151.

Hartnett, K. M. (2010b) Analysis of age-at-death estimation using data from a new, modern autopsy sample—Part II: Sternal end of the fourth rib. *Journal of Forensic Sciences*, **55**, 1152–1156.

Heilbronner, R. L. (2011) Daubert v. Merrell Dow Pharmaceuticals (1993). In: *Encyclopedia of Clinical Neuropsychology*, vol. **1**. (eds. J. S. Kruetzer, J. DeLuca, and S. Caplan). Springer, New York, pp. 769–770.

Herrel, A., Huyghe, K., Vanhooydonck, B., *et al.* (2008) Rapid large-scale evolutionary divergence in morphology and performance associated with exploitation of a different dietary resource. *Proceedings of the National Academy of Sciences*, **105**, 4792–4795.

Hoppa, R. D. and Vaupel, J. W. (2002) *Paleodemography: Age Distributions from Skeletal Samples*. Cambridge University Press, Cambridge.

Huxley, J. (1942) *Evolution: The Modern Synthesis*. George Allen and Unwin Ltd., London.

Igarashi, Y., Uesu, K., Wakebe, T., and Kanazawa, E. (2005) New method for estimation of adult skeletal age at death from the morphology of the auricular surface of the ilium. *American Journal of Physical Anthropology*, **128**, 324–339.

Işcan, M. Y., Wright, R. K., and Loth, S. R. (1984) Age estimation from the rib by phase analysis: White males. *Journal of Forensic Sciences*, **29**, 1094–1104.

Işcan, M. Y., Wright, R. K., and Loth, S. R. (1985) Age estimation from the rib by phase analysis: White females. *Journal of Forensic Sciences*, **30**, 853–863.

Jantz, R. L. (2001) Cranial change in Americans: 1850–1975. *Journal of Forensic Sciences*, **46**, 784–787.

Jantz, L. M. and Jantz, R. L. (1999) Secular change in long bone length and proportion in the United States, 1800–1970. *American Journal of Physical Anthropology*, **110**, 57–67.

Jantz, R. L. and Meadows Jantz, L. (2000) Secular change in craniofacial morphology. *American Journal of Human Biology*, **12**, 327–338.

Jantz, R. L., Kimmerle, E. H., and Baraybar, J. P. (2008) Sexing and stature estimation criteria for Balkan populations. *Journal of Forensic Sciences*, **53**, 601–605.

Katz, D. and Suchey, J. M. (1986) Age determination of the male *os pubis*. *American Journal of Physical Anthropology*, **69**, 427–435.

Konigsberg, L. W. and Frankenberg, S. R. (1992) Estimation of age structure in anthropological demography. *American Journal of Physical Anthropology*, **89**, 235–256.

Konigsberg, L. W. and Frankenberg, S. R. (1994) Paleodemography: "not quite dead." *Evolutionary Anthropology: Issues, News, and Reviews*, **3**, 92–105.

Kumho Tire Company, Ltd. v. Carmichael (1999) 526 US 137. United States Supreme Court.

Langley, N. R., Jantz, R., and Ousley, S. (2016) The effect of novel environments on modern American skeletons. *Human Biology Special Issue*, **88**, 5–13.

Langley-Shirley, N. and Jantz, R. L. (2010) A Bayesian approach to age estimation in modern Americans from the clavicle. *Journal of Forensic Sciences*, **55**, 571–583.

Lovejoy, C. O., Meindl, R. S., Mensforth, R. P., and Barton, T. J. (1985) Multifactorial determination of skeletal age at death: A method and blind tests of its accuracy. *American Journal of Physical Anthropology*, **68**, 1–14.

Low, F. M., Gluckman, P. D., and Hanson, M. A. (2012) Developmental plasticity, epigenetics and human health. *Evolutionary Biology*, **39**, 650–665.

Mayr, E. (1942) *Systematics and the Origin of Species, from the Viewpoint of a Zoologist*. Harvard University Press, Cambridge, MA.

Mayr, E. (2001) *What Evolution Is* (Science Masters Series). Basic Books, New York.

McKern, T. W. and Stewart, T. D. (1957) *Skeletal Age Changes in Young American Males Analysed from the Standpoint of Age Identification*. Technical Report EP-45. Quartermaster Research and Development Command, Natick, MA.

Meadows, L. and Jantz, R. L. (1995) Allometric secular change in the long bones from the 1800s to the present. *Journal of Forensic Sciences*, **40**, 762–767.

Meindl, R. S. and Lovejoy, C. O. (1985) Ectocranial suture closure: A revised method for the determination of skeletal age at death based on the lateral-anterior sutures. *American Journal of Physical Anthropology*, **68**, 57–66.

Melendez-Diaz v. Massachusetts. (2009) S. Ct. **129**, 2527.

Milner, G. R. (2010) Transition analysis and subjective estimates of age in adult skeletons. In: Boldsen, J. and Tarp, P. (Eds.), *ADBOU 1992–2009*. Syddansk University, Denmark.

Milner, G. R. and Boldsen, J. L. (2012) Transition analysis: A validation study with known-age modern American skeletons. *American Journal of Physical Anthropology*, **148**, 98–110.

Milner, G. R., Boldsen, J. L., Ousley, S. D., *et al.* (2016) Improved adult age estimation using new skeletal traits and transition analysis. *Proceedings of the 68th American Academy of Forensic Sciences*, **XXII**, 57–58.

Milot, E., Mayer, F. M., Nussey, D. H., *et al.* (2011) Evidence for evolution in response to natural selection in a contemporary human population. *Proceedings of the National Academy of Sciences*, **108**, 17040–17045.

Montagu, M. (1941) Physical anthropology and anatomy. *American Journal of Physical Anthropology*, **28**, 261–271.

Müller, G. B. and Newman, S. A. (2003) *Origination of Organismal Form: Beyond the Gene in Developmental and Evolutionary Biology*. MIT Press, Boston, MA.

National Research Council (2009) *Strengthening Forensic Science in the United States: A Path Forward*. National Academic Press, Washington, DC. http://www.nap.edu/catalog/12589.html (accessed August 3, 2017).

Osborne, D. L., Simmons, T. L., and Nawrocki, S. P. (2004) Reconsidering the auricular surface as an indicator of age at death. *Journal of Forensic Sciences*, **49**(5), 1–7.

Passalacqua, N. V. (2009) Forensic age-at-death estimation from the human sacrum. *Journal of Forensic Sciences*, **54**, 255–262.

Passalacqua, N. and Uhl, N. (2009) Phase versus component systems in age-at-death estimation I: The methodology and usage of component systems. *Proceedings of the American Association of Physical Anthropologists 78th Annual Meeting*, Chicago, IL, April 2, 2009, 209.

Pergams, O. R. and Lawler, J. J. (2009) Recent and widespread rapid morphological change in rodents. *PLoS One*, **4**, e6452.

Pigliucci, M. (2001) *Phenotypic Plasticity: Beyond Nature and Nurture*, Johns Hopkins University Press, Baltimore, MD.

Pigliucci, M. (2009) An extended synthesis for evolutionary biology. *Annals of the New York Academy of Sciences*, **1168**, 218–228.

Prince, D. A. and Konigsberg, L. W. (2008) New formulae for estimating age-at-death in the Balkans utilizing Lamendin's dental technique and Bayesian analysis. *Journal of Forensic Sciences*, **53**, 578–587.

Quammen, D. (2006) *The Reluctant Mr. Darwin*. Atlas Books/W.W. Norton, New York.

Rissech, C., Estabrook, G. F., Cunha, E., and Malgosa, A. (2006) Using the acetabulum to estimate age at death of adult males. *Journal of Forensic Sciences*, **51**, 213–229.

Shapiro, H. L. (1939) Thomas Wingate Todd. *American Anthropologist*, **41**, 458–464.

Shirley, N. R. and Ramirez Montes, P. A. (2015) Age estimation in forensic anthropology: Quantification of observer error in phase versus component-based methods. *Journal of Forensic Sciences*, **60**, 107–111.

Simpson, G. G. (1942) The beginnings of vertebrate paleontology in North America. *Proceedings of the American Philosophical Society*, **86**, 130–188.

Suchey, J. M. and Katz, D. (1998) Applications of pubic age determination in a forensic setting. In: *Forensic Osteology: Advances in the Identification of Human Remains* (2nd Ed.) (ed. K. J. Reichs). Charles C. Thomas, Springfield, Ill., pp. 204–236.

Todd, T. W. (1920) Age changes in the pubic bone. I. The male white pubis. *American Journal of Physical Anthropology*, **3**, 285–334.
Todd, T. W. (1921) Age changes in the pubic bone. *American Journal of Physical Anthropology*, **4**, 1–70.
Todd, T. W. and Lyon, D. (1925) Cranial suture closure. Its progress and age relationship. Part II—ectocranial closure in adult males of white stock. *American Journal of Physical Anthropology*, **8**, 23–45.
Washburn, S. L. (1951) Section of anthropology: The new physical anthropology. *Transactions of the New York Academy of Sciences*, **13**, 298–304.
Watson, J. D. and Crick, F. H. (1953) Molecular structure of nucleic acids. *Nature*, **171**, 737–738.
West-Eberhard, M. J. (2003) *Developmental Plasticity and Evolution*. Oxford University Press, Oxford.
Wood, J. W., Milner, G. R., Harpending, H. C., *et al.* (1992) The osteological paradox: Problems of inferring prehistoric health from skeletal samples [and comments and reply]. *Current Anthropology*, **33**, 343–370.
Wright, S. (1949) The genetical structure of populations. *Annals of Eugenics*, **15**, 323–354.

CHAPTER 7
Theory and histological methods

Christian M. Crowder[1], Deborrah C. Pinto[1], Janna M. Andronowski[2] and Victoria M. Dominguez[3]

[1] *Forensic Anthropology Division, Harris County Institute of Forensic Sciences, Houston, TX, USA*
[2] *Department of Biology, University of Akron, Akron, OH, USA*
[3] *Skeletal Biology Research Laboratory, The Ohio State University, Columbus, OH, USA*

7.1 Introduction

It is believed within the broader discipline of anthropology that forensic anthropology lacks a strong theoretical foundation, a perception fueled by the seeming lack of foundational theory development within the field. Forensic anthropology tends to operate within the interpretive and methodological realm of theories, which is likely associated with the current focus on method reliability (Boyd and Boyd, Chapter 1, this volume). Furthermore, the multidisciplinary nature of forensic science lends itself to complex theory development, making it difficult to devise a comprehensive, unified theory in forensic anthropology. Regardless, when examining a method's development, one readily uncovers the theory from which it was conceived. This certainly applies when reviewing the development of histological methods within forensic anthropology.

Histological methods follow the principles of bone physiology, which describe bone structure and morphology as being controlled by intrinsic biological factors and influenced by extrinsic environmental factors. Bone's unique properties make it an ideal tissue for histological investigations in forensic anthropology since it maintains a dynamic structure throughout an individual's life, providing a time-related record of remodeling events. This continuous response allows for the maintenance of bone's microstructural organization when exposed to various physiological, mechanical, and metabolic demands. These adaptations may be aggregate or discrete changes, and inferences are made at both the individual and population level. Thus, bone microstructure provides useful indicators for an array of anthropological analyses (i.e., species differentiation, age estimation, bone biomechanics, and skeletal health).

Forensic Anthropology: Theoretical Framework and Scientific Basis, First Edition.
Edited by C. Clifford Boyd Jr and Donna C. Boyd.

In reviewing bone histology research and the methods developed within forensic anthropology, it is apparent that bone adaptation is the governing principle for anthropological analyses. Therefore, research developing these analyses is based on theories of bone adaptation in response to external and internal stimuli. It is likely that the seemingly clandestine nature of theory within forensic anthropology, in regard to bone histology, occurs because theory development involving bone physiology is mainly performed outside of the discipline and applied by researchers within the discipline. Considering that these theories are often developed and explored by researchers in the clinical research setting, it is understandable why forensic anthropology may appear to lack a strong theoretical foundation in bone histology. However, as explained by Boyd and Boyd (2011; Chapter 1, this volume), there are multiple forms of theory and bone biology theory employed by anthropologists that can be viewed as falling within the interpretive and methodological categories. This chapter discusses the theoretical approaches employed by anthropologists that influence our methods and guide interpretations in bone biology.

7.2 Foundational theory in bone biology

Schiffer (1988) described the hierarchical nature of theories and laws, with high-level theories as broad, overarching principles governing those at lower levels. Like all biological sciences, evolutionary biology is at the core of the theoretical foundations of bone biology. The theoretical underpinnings are biological evolution following the Darwinian phyletic gradualism and punctuated equilibrium models (Boyd and Boyd, 2011).

Evolutionary theory as argued by Darwin is not a single principle, but a collection of related yet independent theories, including variational evolution, gradualism, phyletic evolution, speciation, action of selective agents, and evolution of all organisms from a common ancestor (Bock, 2010). Variational evolution refers to changes in the attributes of organisms seen in successive generations. It encompasses change in which "selective agents" are one of the causes. Phyletic evolution, or anagenesis, results in modifications to existing organisms, and not in the origination of new species (Mayr, 1959). Speciation, or cladogenesis, leads to the evolution of new species (two or more) from one common ancestor. It also requires the inclusion of phyletic evolution in one of the resulting lineages and the existence of a barrier separating members of the original ancestral species for an extended period of time (Bock, 2010). Selection arises from interactions between organisms and their external environment and operates on the phenotype. The "selective agents" act to remove unsuitable individuals from a particular environment (Bock, 2009). Overall, these evolutionary frameworks form the overarching theoretical basis of bone biology, informing biological processes such as skeletal growth and bone modeling and remodeling.

Ontogeny and phylogeny are also key components in explaining bone biology. Ontogeny refers to the developmental history of an organism. Thus, the modeling of bone during growth and ongoing remodeling over the organism's life span will produce indicators of skeletal health and provide information regarding skeletal age. Phylogeny speaks to the evolutionary history of a species and genetic relatedness to other organisms. As related to bone biology, for example, phylogenetic signals may account for variation observed in bone growth rates, indicating that a portion of these patterns may be the result of shared ancestry (Cubo *et al.*, 2008). Though most work within anthropology lies in interpretive and methodological forms of theory development, an understanding of the governing principles within foundational theory is necessary to understand the evolutionary processes that affect human variation.

7.3 Interpretive theory in bone biology

Boyd and Boyd (2011) use the example of taphonomic theory as a middle-range (interpretive) theory in forensic anthropology because it attempts to connect static observations of remains (such as erosion, weathering, color change, breakage, etc.) to the dynamic environment that the remains are exposed to and likely affected by (wind, water, scavengers, and so on). Similarly, in bone biology, static observations include the macroscopic and microscopic architecture of bone, which are affected by their dynamic environment, specifically biomechanical and physiological agents. Theories derived from these observations propose explanations for which environmental factors affect bone modeling and remodeling. For example, it is well established that bone requires a certain amount of biomechanical stress/strain in order to maintain its integrity. Any reduction in stress/strain can result in loss of bone and potentially compromised form. The earliest model for attempting to understand this interplay was proposed by Wolff in 1892 and modified over time by various researchers, eventually resulting in the heavily-cited mechanostat theory (described in Section 7.3.2) introduced by Frost in 1983. The mechanostat theory has led to more recent advances in interpretive theory in bone biology, including the role of osteoblasts and osteocytes in mechanosensation and mechanotransduction. The following provides a description of several interpretive theories within bone biology that anthropologists employ in their research.

7.3.1 Form and function

Early theory development regarding bone mechanics and adaptation dates back to the nineteenth century with two researchers: Julius Wolff and Wilhelm Roux. Wolff (1986) argued that bone strives for physiological homeostasis and that its mechanical environment determines its final mass and trabecular architecture. He proposed Wolff's law, which generally states that the form and function of bone is followed by changes in internal architecture (Frost, 1998). His theory was grounded in mathematical principles referring to the mathematical relationship between trabecular architecture and stress trajectories (Forwood and Turner, 1995). However, Wolff did not devise his proposed mathematical theory, and thus the basic tenets of Wolff's law and his misconceptions regarding skeletal biology have been met with thorough critique (Dibbets, 1992; Forwood and Turner, 1995; Pearson and Liberman, 2004; Ruff *et al.*, 2006).

In 1881, Roux delved slightly deeper and explained that a bone's functional adaptation is based on the dynamic interaction between bone cells and the mechanical environment, therefore advocating that bone structure is controlled by the apposition and resorption of bone cells. During this time period, Claude Bernard proposed the concept of homeostasis to physiology, meaning that bone contains a self-regulating mechanism (Bernard, 1865; Martin *et al.*, 2015).

Thus in the nineteenth century, three concepts of bone biology were developed that focused on explaining the adaptation of bone to mechanical loading. Two involved the idea of physiologic homeostasis and the principle of bone functional adaptation based on the dynamic interaction between bone cells and the mechanical environment, and one proposed that bone's mechanical environment determines its final mass and trabecular architecture. While these three concepts could be used to predict changes in bone architecture, they did not explain how these changes occur (Frost, 1990).

7.3.2 The mechanostat and Utah paradigm

Harold Frost (1983) proposed a theory to describe the mechanical mechanism that controls modeling, remodeling, and bone mass during growth. Frost's *mechanostat theory* is based on the immensity of strain that results from mechanical loading and is responsible for controlling bone mass, bone strength, and bone reserve (Frost, 1987a, 2004). Strain thresholds were introduced to explain the activation and inhibition of modeling and remodeling. Frost (1987a) used a house thermometer as a parallel, stating that mechanisms controlling bone mass would turn off in the absence of error and turn on in response to it. He called these strain thresholds the minimum effective strain (MES) set points and argued that they can be altered by intrinsic factors. Hormones, pathological agents, and other nonmechanical factors may disrupt the mechanical feedback system (Frost, 1983, 1987a).

Bone modeling determines bone mass, strength, and architecture. During modeling, strains above the threshold of the minimum effective strain for modeling (MESm) cause modeling to turn on, increasing the amount of bone formation and, in turn, increasing bone mass (Frost, 1997). Strains below the MESm threshold keep modeling turned off, resulting in no additional bone formation. During remodeling, strains above the threshold of the minimum effective strain for remodeling (MESr) will keep remodeling static, thus maintaining bone. As strains fall below the threshold, remodeling goes into disuse mode, resulting in the removal of bone from the endosteal surface (Frost, 1997). This removal process can result in osteopenia and, in severe cases, osteoporosis (Carlson *et al.*, 1976; Frost, 1997).

Frost (1997) also described the effects of repeated bone strain in relation to fatigue microdamage. He proposed that strains could initiate microcracks, which in turn disrupt osteocyte-canalicular networks (Frost, 2000a).

The *Utah paradigm* of skeletal physiology evolved from a series of Hard Tissue Workshops sponsored by the University of Utah (Frost, 1998). The workshops were held to encourage multidisciplinary approaches to skeletal research and attempt to bridge the subfields of skeletal biology, medicine, and surgery (Frost, 1998). This theory introduced a shift from the former paradigm of skeletal physiology, which suggested that effector cells (fibroblasts, chondroblasts, osteoblasts, osteoclasts), which determine bone health, are controlled by nonmechanical agents (Frost, 2000b; Stout and Crowder, 2012).

The Utah paradigm examines load-bearing skeletal elements at the organ, tissue, and cellular levels (Frost, 1998, 2004), with a focus on the mechanical competence of bone (Frost, 1997, 1998). Frost's mechanostat is the primary concept in the Utah paradigm, since it explains how load-bearing bones achieve mechanical competence (Frost, 1983). The Utah paradigm suggests that the impelling force of load-bearing bone structure and strength are mechanical factors and that nonmechanical biological factors (i.e., hormones, minerals, sex, and age) may hinder or assist this process (Frost, 1998, 2004; Stout and Crowder, 2012).

The Utah paradigm, however, does not fully explain the forces that control the cause-and-effect relationship of muscle force and bone strength. Frost (2004) introduced an updated version of the original mechanostat theory indicating that genetic factors must play a role in the biological determinants of bone mass. Research suggests that the role of genetic predisposition, which accounts for the association between muscle and bone mass, has not been established (Parfitt, 2004; Stout and Crowder, 2012).

7.3.3 Exploring the effectors of the mechanostat

Research in bone biology has attempted to find the specific effectors or mechanisms that cause and guide bone modeling and remodeling. Although Frost's mechanostat is still at the heart of this research, scientists are now looking for the genetic or physiologic controls that initiate response to external and internal stimuli.

Studies have shown targeted remodeling occurs at the site of microcracks, indicating a cause-and-effect relationship (Burr *et al.*, 1985; Burr and Martin, 1993; Mori and Burr, 1993; Martin, 2002). Frost (1960) proposed that microcracks disrupt canalicular connections between osteocytes, thus providing the impetus, which initiates bone remodeling. The *osteocyte inhibitor theory* provides an alternative model, whereby osteocyte-canalicular systems act to inhibit osteoclastic activity. When the osteocyte network is disrupted, the constraining mechanism is released, stimulating resorption activity. Observations of bone in disuse and overload coincide with the idea that the osteocytes inhibit rather than stimulate remodeling (Frost, 1983). Strain levels are required to nourish osteocytes through interstitial fluid flow, but a lack of nutrition will cause a disruption in the osteocyte network, thus producing a signal to shift bone into disuse mode (Martin, 2000a, b). When the osteocyte network is disrupted by osteocyte apoptosis, the constraining mechanism is again released, thus stimulating resorption activity.

Alternatively, Burr (2002) suggests that only thirty percent of microdamage is targeted by bone remodeling. The remaining seventy percent that is nontargeted, or stochastic, may be associated with metabolic factors, interstitial fluid flow, and/or regions of high strain (Burr, 2002; Martin, 2002). The relationship between targeted and stochastic bone remodeling is not fully understood. As such, this theory has little supporting evidence, unlike Frost's mechanostat, and remains controversial within the scientific community.

In 1999, Turner reported that (i) the mechanostat failed to explain why non-weight-bearing bones do not completely resorb under disuse remodeling and (ii) regulation differs among skeletal sites. He further argued that Frost's mechanostat theory placed biomechanics at the center of bone biology, without acknowledging that bone is insensitive to mechanical loading when growth and/or parathyroid hormones are absent (Turner, 2000; Crowder, 2005). In response to Frost's prevailing theory, he introduced a mathematical theory of bone biology referred to as the *principle of cellular accommodation* to address the inconsistencies observed when the mechanostat does not conform to experimental observations (Turner, 1999, 2000).

Turner's principle of cellular accommodation theory states that bone cells assimilate from their biological environments and adjust to new environments, causing set points to vary among skeletal sites depending on local strain (Stout and Crowder, 2012). The set point in weight-bearing bones will be high, while the set point in non-weight-bearing bones will be low in comparison. Turner (1999) predicted that bone mass will stabilize once cells fully accommodate to the new environment. Altered hormone levels or varying mechanical loads will cause a change in bone remodeling but that reaction will change when bone cells adapt to the new environment. Turner's approach has been seen as a step toward a unified theory of bone remodeling (Stout and Crowder, 2012).

While many studies focus on the role of the bone cells, that is, osteocytes, osteoblasts, and osteoclasts, there are others that focus on the bone basic structural units (BSUs) or osteons to explain form and function. It is apparent that bone modeling and remodeling are influenced by the loading dynamics of different skeletal elements. Mechanical loading history and the general morphology and structure of individual skeletal elements are dynamically related so that each skeletal element may respond uniquely to different mechanical, nutritional, and physiological stressors. Considering the loading environment, Skedros (2012) proposed the *shear resistance-priority hypothesis* to explain the microstructure of bone. He states that since bone is weakest primarily in shear and secondarily in tension, these regions of bone will sustain more microdamage that must be accommodated. If the damage is not accommodated, the result is bone failure. Bone modeling typically cannot accommodate the accumulated damage, requiring a repair mechanism through the remodeling process and targeted bone remodeling. Therefore, regions of high strain are observed to have a higher number of remodeling units. Skedros (2012) also suggested varying osteon morphotypes, which result from distinctive variations in collagen/lamellar organization, as a possible adaptive mechanism to this load environment (Skedros *et al.*, 2013). Habitual load histories, therefore, could be elucidated by experimental studies. Skedros' hypothesis suggests that tension and shear are important in driving the ontogenetic adaptation of bone tissue.

The wide variation in the form and loading environments of different skeletal elements suggests that the dynamic relationship between form and function also varies. In essence, there is a unique "mechanostat" for each skeletal element (Skerry, 2006). Accordingly, skeletal elements that are minimally loaded are less influenced by mechanical stress than skeletal elements that are heavily loaded (Tommerup *et al.*, 1993). In turn, skeletal elements that are minimally influenced by mechanical stress may be subject to greater influence from nonmechanical agents. This is important for anthropologists choosing bone sampling regions that best fit the goals of their research. For example, a researcher developing a model for age estimation may consider selecting less-loaded skeletal elements, such as ribs, to avoid microstructural variation caused by larger amounts of mechanical loading.

7.4 Methodological theory in bone biology

All histological analyses employed by forensic anthropologists can be viewed as contributing to methodological theory. This interpretation is in keeping with Boyd and Boyd's (Chapter 1, this volume) explanation of Schiffer's (1988) *methodological theory*, which the authors view as a significant element in all forensic anthropological studies. According to Schiffer (1988), methodological theory influences the recovery, analysis, and inference techniques employed by archaeologists. Within forensic anthropology, two main areas of research have emerged in which interpretations of bone biology through histological analysis is used: estimating age at death and differentiating human from nonhuman bone. These research avenues employ methodological theoretical models based on the hypothetico-deductive method (Komar and Buikstra, 2008). Statistical induction theory, a branch of methodological theory according to Boyd and Boyd (2011), is commonly used in methods for constructing the biological profile (age, sex, ancestry, and stature). The authors state that the main goal of this theory in forensic anthropology is to collect large amounts of data from known individuals in order to increase the accuracy and reliability of statistical methods used in standard analyses. For example, Hefner (2009) conducted a large-scale study of the morphoscopic traits from African, Asian, European, and Native American skulls archived at the National Museum of Natural History. Using these data, he provided a means of classification based on the statistical models and this classification scheme can assist practitioners in estimating ancestry of an unknown skull. Similarly, statistical induction theory can be observed in histological age estimation methods developed by Kerley (1965), Stout (1986), and others who also use algorithms developed on research samples in order to predict age of a single unknown individual.

7.4.1 Histological age estimation

Early histological studies in anthropology did not focus on biomechanical adaptation as described by Wolff and Roux, but concentrated on cell accumulation over time as a factor of chronological age. In 1911, Balthazard and Labrun used quantitative bone histology to estimate age at death in a published report. Although very little information describing the method was reported, their results suggested that there was a strong relationship between histological features and chronological age. In 1916, Foote published a volume that examined cross sections of human and nonhuman bones, providing observations regarding age-related changes in the bone and microstructural changes associated with bone growth. In 1936, Amprino and Bairati examined cross sections from human femora noting that the number of osteons was progressive over time. These early studies, which were mostly descriptive, provided the framework for methodological theory applied to histological age estimation in forensic anthropology. As discussed previously, the work of Harold Frost and the Henry Ford Hospital Research Group in the 1950s and 1960s further advanced the general understanding of bone tissue and provided the basis for modern understandings of bone tissue response to mechanical stress, including data regarding osteon accumulation over time. Research produced by this working group coupled methodological theory testing with interpretive theory development, demonstrating the integrated relationship between methodology and theory in bone biology. Frost (1987b) continued this research for decades, branching into the field of anthropology with several publications.

It is apparent that histological analysis within anthropology began with the estimation of age at death and a brief examination of two key historical studies demonstrates the origin of distinct research lines that currently guide research within forensic anthropology. One research line follows the work of Ellis Kerley (1965), who is rightfully credited with developing the first histomorphometric age estimation method, although Balthazard and Labrun (1911) published on the subject approximately 50 years earlier. The second research line follows the work of Sam Stout (1986; Stout and Crowder, 2012) who is recognized for developing the first histological age estimation method using the mid-third of the sixth rib, derived from the research of Frost. While each line of research acknowledges the accumulation of osteons over time, they were developed under slightly different theoretical models.

Kerley's early research was aligned with methodological theory considering the impetus was to achieve more accurate age estimates in forensic casework by examining the relationship of histological variables with chronological age.

Several studies derived from the original Kerley research tended to not subscribe to a specific interpretive theory or focus on explaining theoretical models of bone biology but rather improve sampling techniques and variable selection and increase the accuracy of age estimates for the individual. On the other hand, Stout's early research encompassed methodological theory with identifiable relationships to interpretive theory, particularly those developed by Frost. Research following Stout (Stout and Crowder, 2012) tends to interpret results in accordance with the mechanostat theory and bone biology, focusing less on technical changes to improve accuracy of methods and more on making population-level inferences. In a sense, these are slightly overgeneralizations and definitely opinions of the authors; however, sample and variable selection appear to coincide with the differing approaches taken by these studies. Regardless, future research in bone histology should couple methodological and interpretive theoretical models to enhance method development and improve interpretations of histological data.

7.4.2 Determining human versus nonhuman bone

The second area of research in forensic anthropology that incorporates bone histology is the differentiation of human from nonhuman bone. All histological studies within forensic anthropology developed with this analytical focus examine the differences in bone microarchitecture through the application of methodological theory. The basic premise of these studies has been to identify features that are unique enough to differentiate human from nonhuman bone, that is, they aim to provide an analytical method to address the problem. There are two main approaches to this analysis: (i) identifying bone organization by noting the presence of woven, lamellar, Haversian, and fibrolamellar bone and (ii) quantifying osteon size and shape differences.

Similar to early histological research evaluating age-related changes, early studies in anthropology examining the differences in human and nonhuman bone were descriptive, and the quantitative histomorphometric approach was investigatory (Foote, 1916; Enlow and Brown, 1958; Jowsey, 1966, 1968). This early research differed from age-related studies in that its focus was often comparative histology, which examines the histological characteristics of various taxa in relation to one another. This approach explores interpretive theory, namely, growth and development, and relates it to foundational theory regarding the evolution of species and phylogenetic relationships. Therefore, the evaluation of bone microstructure for the purpose of species differentiation is tied to a broader understanding of bone biology. The following section provides examples of this interplay with bone biology concepts.

In 1966, Jowsey published a novel study addressing the histological differences between human and nonhuman Haversian bone. In this research, she established that osteon size varied across species and that there are age-related changes in Haversian canal size. Jowsey related her findings to interpretive theory by providing explanations for her findings in terms of metabolic demands. More recently, other researchers have demonstrated the utility of quantifying osteon size and shape (circularity) for distinguishing human from nonhuman bone (Crescimanno and Stout, 2012; Dominguez and Crowder, 2012). These studies relate findings to differences that might exist across cortices due to mechanical loading, which draws upon the mechanostat and the shear resistance-priority hypotheses (see Sections 7.3.2 and 7.3.3). More biomechanically-focused research conducted by Skedros and colleagues (1997, 2004; Mason *et al.*, 1995) demonstrated that osteons in compression tend to be smaller, more circular, and more numerous than those in tension cortices. These studies, performed outside of forensic anthropology, were not concerned with being able to differentiate human from nonhuman bone and instead focused on developing and testing higher level theories.

Other studies in forensic anthropology focused on the evaluation of bone organization as a means to differentiate species. For example, Mulhern and Ubelaker (2001) identified osteon banding as one feature that can assist with recognizing nonhuman bone. Osteon banding, according to the authors, is defined as a row of five or more osteons. Multiple rows of lengthy primary or secondary osteon chains have been described as diagnostic of nonhuman bone. However, research by Andronowski *et al.* (2017) documented the presence of osteon banding in cortical bone from adult human males. Thus, osteon banding alone is not diagnostic of human bone.

The presence of certain types of fibrolamellar bone, which is bone with alternating sheets of lamellar and woven bone, has long been used in forensic anthropology as a definitive characteristic of nonhuman bone. Specifically, a variant of fibrolamellar bone known as plexiform bone, which has a brick wall patterning with vascular channels separating regions of non-lamellar bone, is the most distinctive type of nonhuman bone tissue due to its extremely limited presentation in humans (Mulhern and Ubelaker 2001; Martin *et al.*, 2015). This type of bone is commonly observed in large fast-growing animals (Martin *et al.*, 2015). Again, the relationship is evident between methodological theory defining the morphology of microanatomical features and interpretive theory offering ontological explanations. For the most part, in forensic anthropology, histological research to differentiate human from nonhuman bone is associated with methodological theory, based on method development owing to the practitioner's needs. Continuing research to identify the differences between human and nonhuman bone not only contributes to interpretive theory but also helps reshape our understanding of foundational evolutionary theory.

7.5 Conclusions

The goal of this chapter is to provide a template for understanding the use of theory in forensic anthropology for histological analyses and research. It is by no means an exhaustive list of all existing bone biology theories or histological studies developed within anthropology. By defining what qualifies as foundational, interpretive, and methodological theories, researchers are better able to structure their research program within a specific framework. For example, researchers may sample non-weight-bearing skeletal elements to observe more age-related systemic-based remodeling for age estimation. Some may consider biomechanical adaptation as a contributing factor for age-related remodeling and sample cortical regions regardless of the loads the bone experiences. Similar considerations apply when comparing histological structures across species. Researchers may propose that high mechanical stress/strain results in different osteon structure, shape, and/or density patterns, while others may subscribe to the idea that microstructural differences result from variation in bone formation rates associated with phylogeny regardless of stress/strain relationships. Regardless of the approach, the theoretical models discussed provide a framework that guides data interpretation and moves us closer to a better understanding of bone biology. Our recommendation to forensic anthropologists conducting histological research is to attempt to couple methodological theory with interpretive concepts associated with interpretive theory.

Forensic anthropologists tend to focus on the specific rather than the general and the empirical rather than the theoretical; however, the argument that forensic anthropology lacks theory is nonsensical. As evidenced, researchers subscribe to different theoretical models regarding the factors governing bone histology. Despite differing views, working in the absence of theory is an untenable approach and leads to results void of real meaning or interpretive power. Inferences from results should be applied to make population-level interpretations to bridge empirical data and theory and make the discipline more scientific.

References

Amprino, R. and Bairati, A. (1936) Process of reconstruction and resorption in the compact substance of men's bones. Research department of hundred subjects from birth until old age. *Zeitschrift fur Zellforschung und Mikroskopische Anatomie*, **24**, 439–511.

Andronowski, J.M., Pratt, I.V., and Cooper, D.M.L. (2017) Occurence of osteon banding in adult human bone. American Journal of Physical Anthropology, https://doi.org/10.1002/ajpa23297.

Balthazard, M.M. and Labrun, F. (1911) Les canaux de Havers de l'os humain aux différents ages. *Annales d'Hygiène Publique et de Médecine Légale*, **15**, 144–152.

Bernard, C. (1865) *An Introduction to the Study of Experimental Medicine*. Henry Schuman, Inc., New York (Dover edition 1957; originally published in 1865; first English translation by Henry Copley Greene, published by Macmillan & Co., Ltd., 1927).

Bock, W.J. (2009) Design—an inappropriate concept in evolutionary theory. *Journal of Zoological Systematics and Evolutionary Research*, **47**(1), 7–9.

Bock, W.J. (2010) Multiple explanations in Darwinian evolutionary theory. *Acta Biotheoretica*, **58**(1), 65–79.

Boyd, C. and Boyd, D.C. (2011) Theory and the scientific basis for forensic anthropology. *Journal of Forensic Sciences*, **56**(6), 1407–1415.

Burr, D.B. (2002) Targeted and nontargeted remodeling. *Bone*, **30**, 2–4.

Burr, D.B. and Martin, R.B. (1993) Calculating the probability that microcracks initiate resorption spaces. *Journal of Biomechanics*, **26**, 613–616.

Burr, D.B., Martin, R.B., Schaffler, M.B., *et al.* (1985) Bone remodeling in response to in vivo fatigue microdamage. *Journal of Biomechanics*, **18**, 189–200.

Carlson, D.S., Armelagos, G.J., and VanGerven, D.P. (1976) Patterns of age-related cortical bone loss (osteoporosis) within the femoral diaphysis. *Human Biology*, **48**, 295–314.

Crescimanno, A. and Stout, S.D. (2012) Differentiating fragmented human and non-human long bone using osteon circularity. *Journal of Forensic Sciences*, **57**(2), 287–294.

Crowder, C. (2005) *Evaluating the Use of Quantitative Bone Histology to Estimate Adult Age at Death*. Ph.D. dissertation, Department of Anthropology, University of Toronto, Toronto, ON, Canada.

Cubo, J., Legendre, P., de Ricqlès, A., *et al.* (2008) Phylogenetic, functional, and structural components of variation in bone growth rate of amniotes. *Evolution and Development*, **10**(2), 217–227.

Dibbets, J.M.H. (1992) One century of Wolff's law. In: *Bone Biodynamics in Orthodontic and Orthopedic Treatment* (eds. D.S. Carlson and S.A. Goldstein). Craniofacial Growth Series, **27**, University of Michigan Press, Ann Arbor 1–13.

Dominguez, V.M. and Crowder, C.M. (2012) The utility of osteon shape and circularity for differentiating human and non-human Haversian bone. *American Journal of Physical Anthropology*, **149**, 84–91.

Enlow, D.H. and Brown, S.O. (1958) A comparative histological study of fossil and recent bone tissues, part III. *Texas Journal of Science*, **10**(2), 187–230.

Foote, J.S. (1916) *A Contribution to the Comparative Histology of the Femur*. Smithsonian Contributions to Knowledge, 35(3). Smithsonian Institution, Washington, DC.

Forwood, M.R. and Turner, C.H. (1995) Skeletal adaptations to mechanical usage: Results from tibial loading studies in rats. *Bone*, **17**(4), 1975–2005.

Frost, H.M. (1960) Presence of microscopic cracks in vivo in bone. *Henry Ford Hospital Medical Bulletin*, **8**, 25–35.

Frost, H.M. (1983) The skeletal intermediary organization. *Metabolic Bone Disease and Related Research*, **4**(5), 281–290.

Frost, H.M. (1987a) Bone "mass" and the "Mechanostat": A proposal. *Anatomical Record*, **219**, 1–9.

Frost, H.M. (1987b) Secondary osteon populations: An algorithm for determining mean bone tissue age. *Yearbook of Physical Anthropology*, **30**, 221–238.

Frost, H.M. (1990) Skeletal structural adaptations to mechanical usage (SATMU): 2. Redefining Wolff's law: The remodeling problem. *Anatomical Record*, **226**(4), 414–422.

Frost, H.M. (1997) Why do marathon runners have less bone than weight lifters? A vital biomechanical view and explanation. *Bone*, **20**(3), 183–189.

Frost, H.M. (1998) Changing concepts in skeletal physiology: Wolff's Law, the Mechanostat, and the "Utah Paradigm." *American Journal of Human Biology*, **10**, 599–605.

Frost, H.M. (2000a) Does bone design intend to minimize fatigue failures? A case for the affirmative. *Journal of Bone and Mineral Metabolism*, **18**, 278–282.

Frost, H.M. (2000b) The Utah paradigm of skeletal physiology: An overview of its insights for bone, cartilage and collagenous tissue organs. *Journal of Bone and Mineral Metabolism*, **18**, 305–316.

Frost, H.M. (2004) A 2003 update for bone physiology and Wolff's Law for clinicians. *Angle Orthodontist*, **74**(1), 3–15.

Hefner, J.T. (2009) Cranial nonmetric variation and estimating ancestry. *Journal of Forensic Sciences*, **54**(5), 985–995.

Jowsey, J. (1966) Studies of Haversian systems in man and some animals. *Journal of Anatomy,* **100**(4), 857–864.

Jowsey, J. (1968) Age and species differences in bone. *Cornell Veterinarian,* **58**, 74–94.

Kerley, E.R. (1965) The microscopic determination of age in human bone. *American Journal of Physical Anthropology,* **23**, 149–164.

Komar, D.A. and Buikstra, J.E. (2008) *Forensic Anthropology: Contemporary Theory and Practice.* Oxford University Press, Oxford.

Martin, R.B. (2000a) Toward a unifying theory of bone remodeling. *Bone,* **26**, 1–6.

Martin, R.B. (2000b) Does osteocyte formation cause the nonlinear refilling of osteons? *Bone,* **26**(1), 71–78.

Martin, R.B. (2002) Is all cortical bone remodeling initiated by microdamage? *Bone,* **30**, 8–13.

Martin, R.B., Burr, D.B., Sharkey, N.A., *et al.* (2015) *Skeletal Tissue Mechanics* (2nd Ed.). Springer Press, New York.

Mason, M.W., Skedros, J.G., and Bloebaum, R.D. (1995) Evidence of strain-mode-related cortical adaptation in the diaphysis of the horse radius. *Bone,* **17**(3), 229–237.

Mayr, E. (1959) Where are we? *Cold Spring Harbor Symposia on Quantitative Biology,* **24**, 409–440.

Mori, S. and Burr, D.B. (1993) Increased intracortical remodeling following fatigue damage. *Bone,* **14**(2), 103–109.

Mulhern, D.M. and Ubelaker, D.H. (2001) Differences in osteon banding between human and nonhuman bone. *Journal of Forensic Sciences,* **46**(2), 220–222.

Parfitt, A.M. (2004) The attainment of peak bone mass: What is the relationship between muscle growth and bone growth? *Bone,* **34**, 767–770.

Pearson, O.M. and Liberman, D.E. (2004) The aging of Wolff's "law": Ontogeny and responses to mechanical loading in cortical bone. *Yearbook of Physical Anthropology,* **47**, 63–99.

Roux, W. (1881) *Der zuchtende Kampf der Teile, oder die "Teilauslese" im Organismus (Theorie der "funktionellen Anpassung").* Wilhelm Engelmann, Leipzig.

Ruff, C.B., Holt, B., and Trinkhaus, E. (2006) Who's afraid of the big bad Wolff? "Wolff's law" and bone functional adaptation. *American Journal of Physical Anthropology,* **129**, 484–498.

Schiffer, M.B. (1988) The structure of archaeological theory. *American Antiquity,* **53**(3), 461–485.

Skedros, J.G. (2012) Interpreting load history in limb-diaphyses: Important considerations and their biomechanical foundations. In: *Bone Histology: An Anthropological Perspective* (eds. S.D. Stout and C.M. Crowder). CRC Press, Boca Raton, FL, pp. 153–220.

Skedros, J.G., Su, S.C., and Bloebaum, R.D. (1997) Biomechanical implications of mineral content and microstructural variations in cortical bone of horse, elk, and sheep calcanei. *The Anatomical Record,* **249**, 297–316.

Skedros, J.G., Hunt, J.J., and Bloebaum, R.D. (2004) Relationships of loading history and structural and material characteristics of bone: Development of the mule deer calcaneus. *Journal of Morphology,* **259**(3), 281–307.

Skedros, J.G., Keenan, K.E., Williams, T.J., *et al.* (2013) Secondary osteon size and collagen/lamellar organization ("osteon morphotypes") are not coupled, but potentially adapt independently for local strain mode or magnitude. *Journal of Structural Biology,* **181**, 95–107.

Skerry, T.M. (2006) One Mechanostat too many? Modifications of the site-specific response of bone to mechanical loading by nature and nurture. *Journal of Musculoskeletal and Neuronal Interactions,* **6**(2), 122–127.

Stout, S.D. (1986) The use of bone histomorphometry in skeletal identification: The case of Francisco Pizarro. *Journal of Forensic Sciences*, **31**(1), 296–300.

Stout, S.D. and Crowder, C.M. (2012) Bone remodeling, histomorphology, and histomorphometry. In: *Bone histology: An anthropological perspective* (eds. S.D. Stout and C.M. Crowder). CRC Press, Boca Raton, FL, pp. 1–21.

Tommerup, L.J., Raab, D.M., Crenshaw, T.D., *et al.* (1993) Does weight-bearing exercise affect non-weight-bearing bone? *Journal of Bone and Mineral Research*, **8**(9), 1053–1058.

Turner, C.H. (1999) Toward a mathematical description of bone biology: The principle of cellular accommodation. *Calcified Tissue International*, **65**, 466–481.

Turner, C.H. (2000) Toward a mathematical description of bone biology: The principle of cellular accommodation. *Calcified Tissue International*, **67**, 185–187.

Wolff, J. (1986) *The Law of Bone Remodeling*. Springer, Berlin (translated from the original German publication 1892).

CHAPTER 8

Forensic applications of isotope landscapes ("isoscapes"): A tool for predicting region-of-origin in forensic anthropology cases

Lesley A. Chesson[1], Brett J. Tipple[1], James R. Ehleringer[1], Todd Park[2] and Eric J. Bartelink[3]

[1] *IsoForensics, Inc., Salt Lake City, UT, USA*
[2] *Unified Police of Greater Salt Lake, Salt Lake City, UT, USA*
[3] *Department of Anthropology, California State University, Chico, CA, USA*

8.1 Introduction

In a 2004 census of medical examiners and coroners, the Bureau of Justice Statistics tallied nearly 13 500 unknown human decedents in the United States (Hickman *et al.*, 2007). Approximately 4400 new cases were added to that total each year, of which roughly 1000 remained unidentified after 1 year. This large volume of unidentified decedent cases—in combination with the tens of thousands of individuals reported missing each year—represents an enormous burden to local, state, and federal law enforcement agencies (Ritter, 2007).

The types of evidence commonly used in forensic human identification include personal effects and distinctive features (e.g., birthmarks, surgical scars, etc.), DNA profiles, fingerprints, and medical and dental records. In addition, the use of news and social media is becoming an increasingly effective investigative tool to gather clues about an individual's identity, especially in cases where forensic sketches or facial approximations are available for circulation (see, e.g., the "Deer Island Baby Doe" case (Sanchez, 2015)). Additional discussion of methods used in forensic human identification can be found in Thompson and Black (2007) and Mallett *et al.* (2014).

Despite the plethora of human identification tools available to the forensic anthropologist, it is not possible to apply all of these techniques in every case. Some methods require intact remains, which may not always be available for

Forensic Anthropology: Theoretical Framework and Scientific Basis, First Edition.
Edited by C. Clifford Boyd Jr and Donna C. Boyd.

examination. Application of many forensic human identification methods can be hampered when a victim's body is badly decomposed, deliberately mutilated, or incomplete. In addition, dental identification methods require comparative records from missing person's cases, which are not always available, and DNA-based identification methods require familial reference sample data to be submitted to the CODIS database.

Are there additional investigative techniques the forensic anthropologist can use when traditional methods produce inconclusive results as to a person's identity? In these cases, isotope analysis may be helpful. The effectiveness of the technique in unidentified decedent cases is predicated on the ability to precisely measure differences in isotope "fingerprints" found within human remains. The intrinsic chemistry of these materials can then be used to understand their derivation and history. For the identification of an unknown decedent from remains such as hair or tooth enamel, isotope analysis can provide answers to two questions:

1. Are the remains consistent with the local region where they were found?
2. What are the possible locations from which the remains may have or may not have originated?

This chapter describes the use of isotope analysis—especially prediction models and isotope landscapes, or "isoscapes"—in forensic human identification. Application of the technique to human remains relies on both reconstruction (interpretive) and methodological theoretical foundations. As an example of interpretive theory, the following sections present current knowledge about the processes influencing the isotope record(s) of human tissues, which can be used to reconstruct aspects of an individual's life history. Isotopic data generated from precipitation patterns, tap water, geological records, and food provide the framework from which to predict residence patterns and/or region-of-origin for an unidentified decedent based on the isotopic signatures recorded into body tissues. Procedures for measuring the isotope record(s) of human tissues are also presented here (methodological theory), with recommendations for good practice. The chapter concludes with two casework examples of isotope analysis applied to unidentified human remains.

8.2 What are isotopes?

The word "isotope" is formed from the Greek words *isos*, meaning equal, and *tópos*, meaning position (Fry, 2006). All isotopes of the same element occupy the same position within the periodic table. Those positions are determined by *atomic number*, which represents the number of protons (and electrons) found in the nucleus of atoms of that element. In turn, *atomic mass* is the sum of all protons, electrons, and neutrons found in an atom. Isotopes are different forms of an element that contain the same number of protons and electrons, but different numbers of neutrons, thereby affecting the atomic mass, but not the atomic number. In forensic human identification, there are three elements and their isotopes that are of particular interest for reconstructing origin/travel movement history—hydrogen (H), oxygen (O), and strontium (Sr)—and three additional elements and isotopes that provide dietary information: carbon (C), nitrogen (N), and sulfur (S).

Isotopes can be stable, undergoing no radioactive decay, or radioactive. As an example, consider the element carbon. Most naturally occurring C atoms contain 6 protons (atomic number = 6), 6 electrons, and 6 neutrons. The sum of subatomic particles in the nucleus is 12 and the atom can be symbolized as ^{12}C. In some rare instances, a carbon atom contains an additional neutron in the nucleus. The atomic number is still 6. However, the sum of subatomic particles in the nucleus is 13 instead of 12 and can be symbolized as ^{13}C. Along with ^{12}C, ^{13}C is a stable isotope of carbon. In extremely rare cases, a carbon atom may contain 8 neutrons, for a sum of subatomic particles in the nucleus of 14. Symbolized as ^{14}C, this radioactive form of carbon, known as "radiocarbon," decays to ^{14}N with a half-life of 5730 years.

The isotope analysis community has adopted an accepted convention for reporting isotopic composition in a material: a ratio of ratios, whereby the ratio (R) of a rare to more abundant isotope in a sample is compared with that in a standard. For carbon, the calculation is based on the ratio $^{13}C/^{12}C$. Ratios are often small fractions—for example, <0.01. For ease of reporting, this ratio of ratios can be converted to delta (δ) notation and presented in parts per thousand (‰) as follows:

$$\delta^{13}C = \frac{R_{sample}}{R_{standard}} - 1 \quad (8.1)$$

For hydrogen ($^{2}H/^{1}H$), oxygen ($^{18}O/^{16}O$), nitrogen ($^{15}N/^{14}N$), and sulfur ($^{34}S/^{32}S$) isotope ratios, the notation is $\delta^{2}H$, $\delta^{18}O$, $\delta^{15}N$, and $\delta^{34}S$, respectively. In contrast, the isotopic abundances of strontium (Sr) in a material are typically expressed as the raw ratio R_{sample} with no comparison to $R_{standard}$ or conversion to δ-notation—for example, $^{87}Sr/^{86}Sr$. This is because the raw ratio R_{sample} is often close to 1—for example, 0.701.

The subtle mass differences resulting from variation in neutron numbers cause isotopes of the same element to behave differently in biological, chemical, and geological processes. As a result, isotope abundances within materials—the isotopic "fingerprints"—vary and are indicative of derivation and source.

8.3 Why do isotope compositions of human tissues differ?

As mentioned previously, there are six elements of particular interest for human identification: H, O, and Sr, plus C, N, and S. These *bioelements* are most useful for human identification because, through deductive reasoning, *you are what you eat and drink,* from an isotopic point of view. A person records information about inputs—for example, water and food—through the transfer of isotopes into various tissues (West *et al.*, 2006). The "snapshot" of time represented by different tissues can vary and provide information on the individual's past (tooth enamel, bones) and more recent present (body water, hair, nails).

8.3.1 Hydrogen and oxygen isotopes

The abundances of hydrogen and oxygen isotopes in human tissues are ultimately linked to water imbibed by an individual. The isotopic composition of water varies geographically in a predictable manner based on the behavior of "heavy" and "light" isotopes during evaporation and condensation processes in the global water cycle (Gat, 1996). The largest reservoir in the global water cycle is the ocean and the standard used for δ-notation of H and O isotopes is Standard Mean Ocean Water, with a defined δ-value of 0‰ for both H and O isotopes.

As water evaporates, "heavier" molecules—those containing ^{2}H or ^{18}O—are less likely to evaporate than those containing ^{1}H or ^{16}O. The result is water vapor that has lower (more negative) δ-values than the ocean. When the water vapor moves inland and cools, it forms a cloud and the water molecules more likely to precipitate are those containing "heavier" isotopes. The result is precipitation that has higher (more positive) δ-values than the cloud, yet lower δ-values than the ocean; the water vapor remaining in the cloud has even lower δ-values (Figure 8.1a).

Isotope fractionation in the water cycle creates a systematic, predictable pattern of water isotope ratios across land surfaces. In general, more positive δ-values (e.g., containing more ^{2}H or ^{18}O) are found in water at low elevations and closer to the ocean, while more negative δ-values (e.g., containing less ^{2}H or ^{18}O) are found in water at higher elevations and locations further inland. These patterns can be displayed in an *isotope landscape* or *isoscape* (Figure 8.1b) (Bowen and Revenaugh, 2003; Bowen *et al.*, 2007). Moving from the coastline, δ-values of water decrease. Although the δ-values are not specific to a city, they are characteristic of different geographic regions. These spatial variations in water δ-values are subsequently recorded in human tissues, such as hair (Ehleringer *et al.*, 2008), via drinking water consumed by an individual.

8.3.2 Strontium isotopes

Sr isotopes in human tissues are related to the age of local bedrock and the transfer of Sr from that bedrock into the surrounding ecosystem. Sr isotope abundances are typically measured and reported as the ratio $^{87}Sr/^{86}Sr$. The source of ^{87}Sr is the radioactive decay of ^{87}Rb, with greater periods of decay increasing the concentration of ^{87}Sr relative to ^{86}Sr. Strontium isotope ratios in bedrock thus vary in a predictable manner based on the initial concentration of ^{87}Rb, the decay constant of ^{87}Rb, and elapsed time (e.g., a rock's age).

In general, the Sr isotope ratios of older rocks are higher, or more "radiogenic," than those of younger rocks due to the constant decay of ^{87}Rb to ^{87}Sr. Geologic

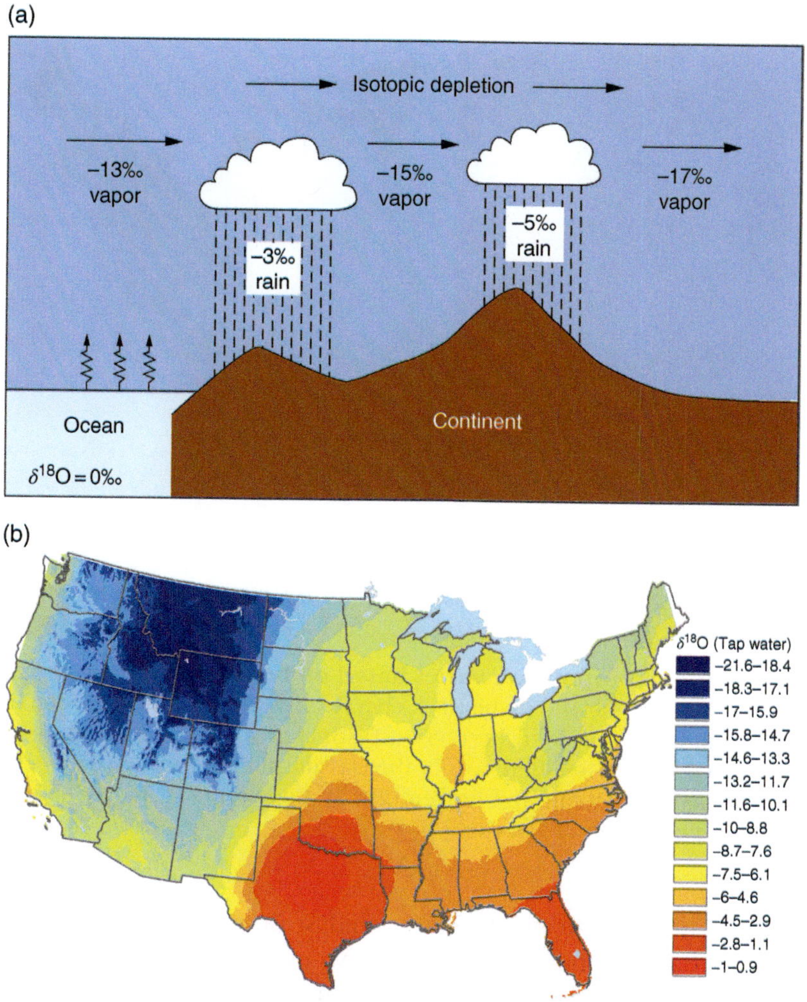

Figure 8.1 Fractionation processes affect the O (and H) isotopes of water. (a) The standard used for O isotope measurements is Standard Mean Ocean Water (SMOW), with a defined δ-value of 0‰ for O isotopes (as well as H isotopes). The ocean contains H_2O molecules comprising both "heavy" and "light" isotopes. Water molecules containing "light" isotopes (^{16}O or ^{1}H) are more likely to evaporate than those containing "heavy" isotopes, resulting in water vapor that has lower (more negative) δ-values than that of the ocean. That water vapor moves inland and cools, forming a cloud; the water molecules that precipitate from the cloud are more likely to contain "heavy" isotopes. The result is precipitation that has higher (more positive) δ-values than the cloud, but lower (more negative) δ-values that the ocean. The water vapor remaining in the cloud is characterized by even lower δ-values. (b) Fractionation processes in the water cycle create a systematic, predictable pattern of water isotope ratios across land surfaces. These patterns can be displayed in an isotope landscape or *isoscape*. As you move from the coastlines and inland or up latitudinal or elevational gradients, water isotope ratios typically decrease. Panel (b) from Bowen *et al.* (2007). Copyright © 2007 by John Wiley & Sons, Inc. Reprinted with permission of John Wiley & Sons, Inc.

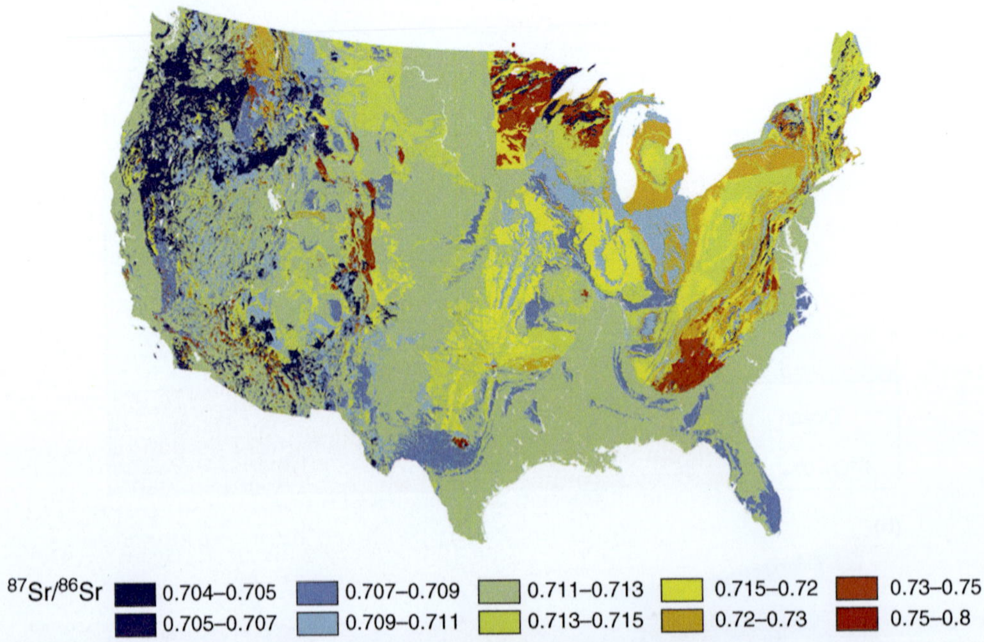

Figure 8.2 Sr isotopic composition varies based on bedrock identity. Variations in $^{87}Sr/^{86}Sr$ ratios as predicted based on bedrock characteristics (e.g., type, age, etc.) and modeled following Beard and Johnson (2000). Distinct breaks in predictions at state borders are artifacts related to differences in the classification of bedrock between state geological surveys. From Bataille and Bowen (2012). Copyright © 2012 by Elsevier. Reproduced with permission of Elsevier.

maps are useful to translate age into estimated Sr isotope abundance (Beard and Johnson, 2000; Bataille and Bowen, 2012). An example Sr isoscape is shown in Figure 8.2. The $^{87}Sr/^{86}Sr$ ratios of the underlying geology are transferred to soils and waters through chemical and physical weathering and become incorporated into biological materials, especially bone and tooth enamel where Sr can substitute for calcium (Beard and Johnson, 2000; Schwarcz *et al.*, 2010). In general, there is negligible isotopic fractionation from the strontium source into the organic tissue (Capo *et al.*, 1998).

8.3.3 Carbon, nitrogen, and sulfur isotopes

Carbon and nitrogen isotope ratio variations provide information about an individual's dietary preferences. The $\delta^{13}C$ value of a tissue is connected to photosynthesis and the discrimination of plants against atmospheric $^{13}CO_2$ during photosynthetic carbon assimilation. Discrimination against ^{13}C is larger in plants that use the C_3 photosynthetic pathway than in plants that use the C_4 pathway. Thus, C_3 plants, such as wheat, rice, and most fruits and vegetables, are characterized by $\delta^{13}C$ values ranging from −30 to −22‰. In contrast, C_4 plants, such as corn and sugar cane, are characterized by $\delta^{13}C$ values ranging from −14 to −10‰ (Tipple and Pagani, 2007).

Carbon isotope analysis of a tissue such as hair keratin or bone collagen can provide information on the types of foods consumed by an individual during life because the $\delta^{13}C$ value of a tissue reflects that of the diet. In some cases, dietary preference provides origin information as well. For example, there are differences in the carbon isotopic composition of hair from Americans and Europeans (Valenzuela *et al.*, 2012; Thompson *et al.*, 2014) due to the wide availability of C_4 plants in the American diet either eaten directly or incorporated through the consumption of animals with a particular plant diet. Carbon isotope ratio differences have also been observed in the bone apatite and collagen of individuals from the United States and countries in Southeast Asia. Recently, this difference has been used to screen remains from past wars and conflicts to aid in provenancing unidentified individuals (Holland *et al.*, 2012; Bartelink *et al.*, 2014a).

The nitrogen isotope ratios of human tissues can supply additional information about the foods consumed by an individual. There is a general increase in $\delta^{15}N$ values with trophic position due to the fractionation of ^{15}N during nitrogen assimilation and excretion (Post, 2002). As a consequence, individuals consuming large quantities of meat or seafood tend to have higher $\delta^{15}N$ values than those eating a vegetarian or vegan diet (Petzke *et al.*, 2005). This pattern has been used to estimate the diet of ancient populations, including the mummified remains of human sacrifice victims (Wilson *et al.*, 2007; Panzer *et al.*, 2014). However, nitrogen isotope abundances can also be affected by an individual's health. In cases of starvation—or even medical conditions such as anorexia (Hatch *et al.*, 2006; Mekota *et al.*, 2006)—the $\delta^{15}N$ values of an individual's tissues may increase, reflecting the recycling of protein within the body.

Sulfur isotope ratios reflect three major sources: (i) weathering of local bedrock, (ii) atmospheric deposits, and (iii) contributions of marine-derived sulfate to the landscape (the "sea-spray effect") or food web (though seafood consumption). Similar to carbon, $\delta^{34}S$ values can provide both dietary and some broad geographic origin information. For example, sulfur isotopes in human hair collected in the United States and Europe were significantly different (Valenzuela *et al.*, 2011), likely impacted by both differences in geology/geography and dietary patterns between the two regions.

8.4 How do we interpret isotope data collected for forensic human identification?

This chapter primarily focuses on relationships observed in three isotope/tissue models useful for human identification:

1. O isotopes of drinking water and hair keratin
2. O isotopes of drinking water and bone/tooth enamel bioapatite
3. Sr isotopes of the local bedrock and tooth enamel

Because O isotopes of water and Sr isotopes of bedrock vary geographically, abductive reasoning suggests that analysis of these isotopes in a tissue can be used to predict or infer potential origins for an individual. These predictions can help investigators narrow search parameters (e.g., "reduce the size of the haystack"[1]) and focus the resources being used to identify an unknown decedent.

While the models described in the following text are not the only ways to interpret isotope data in investigations of unidentified decedents, they are among the models most frequently applied because the information they provide is so valuable. These isotope/tissue models can be used to estimate an individual's origin independent of any other examination technique (e.g., DNA, dental records, etc.). In addition, they can provide information on various periods of the individual's life history—e.g., different "snapshots" of time. For example, hair records information about the weeks or months before death (Thompson *et al.*, 2014), depending on the rate of growth and length of hair strands available for isotope analysis plus the lag between a change in the isotopic composition of inputs and the incorporation of isotopes into the hair keratin. Bone remodeling at a rate of approximately 10% per year provides insight into the dietary choices and travel movements made by the individual over the last decade or so of life (Hedges *et al.*, 2007), while enamel records information about childhood through late adolescence (depending on the specific tooth[2]). Further, by using a combination of independent geospatial isotope models, multiple measurements can be combined to provide refined predictions of origin. In order to apply these prediction models to human remains, it is crucial that the isotopic composition of the tissue of interest does not change following growth and environmental exposure. The condition of the tissue to be analyzed is thus an important concern when preparing and measuring human remains for isotopic composition. Using "bad" data in a model will make it difficult (if not impossible) to produce origin predictions that are useful to an investigation. Due to space considerations, assessment of sample quality is not discussed in detail here; however, see Bartelink *et al.* (2014b) for additional information on sample screening and preparation guidelines.

8.4.1 Oxygen isotopes in drinking water and hair keratin

Hair keratin can be considered a sequential recorder of an individual's history due to the near constant rate of growth of hair (Thompson *et al.*, 2014). Analyzing short (~2.5 mm) segments of hair allows investigators to reconstruct changes in the isotopic composition of inputs to the individual at roughly weekly intervals. An example hair sequence is presented in Figure 8.3 for an unidentified female decedent discovered in Salt Lake County (Utah) in 1978. It is evident from oxygen isotope variations in the figure that Jane Doe had traveled in the 18-month period before her death. Where might those travels have taken her?

To predict drinking water $\delta^{18}O$ values—and thus potential location—from the $\delta^{18}O$ values of the decedent's hair, a model relating oxygen isotopes in drinking

[1] Public Broadcasting Service (accessed August 12, 2015)—http://www.pbs.org/wgbh/nova/tech/stable-isotopes.html.

[2] Atlas of Tooth Development and Eruption, https://atlas.dentistry.qmul.ac.uk (accessed August 8, 2017).

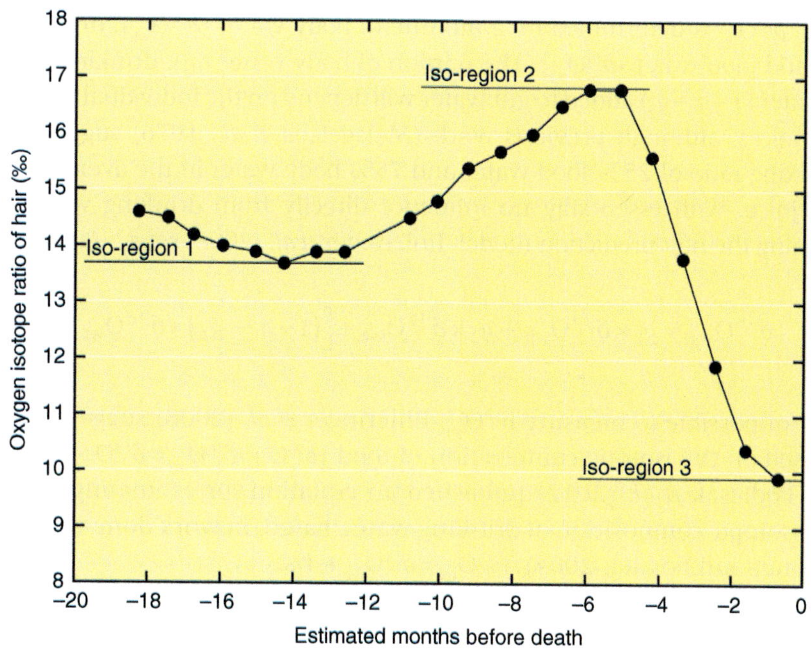

Figure 8.3 Salt Lake County Jane Doe's travel history is reconstructed using oxygen isotopes. Three distinct isotope ranges are identified in the 18-month sequence of hair strands analyzed during casework. The identified ranges suggest that the individual resided in an "iso-region" for a sufficient period of time that her hair achieved isotopic equilibrium with local drinking water.

water and hair keratin is needed. Ehleringer *et al.* published such a model in 2008, built with paired samples of hair and tap water collected from hair salons in small towns across the continental United States. The researchers observed a relationship between the oxygen isotopic composition of tap water and hair, which could be presented as a simple linear regression or as a semi-mechanistic model that considered different pools of O isotopes in the modern human.

In the semi-mechanistic model relating drinking water and hair keratin oxygen isotopes, the isotopic composition of gut water ($\delta^{18}O_{wg}$) plays a determining role in "fixing" the $\delta^{18}O$ values of amino acids used to build keratin. This is due to exchange of O atoms, which takes place when dietary proteins are cleaved at low pH in the stomach and small intestine during digestion; once absorbed across the gut wall, amino acid $\delta^{18}O$ values should not undergo further change. In the following equation, α_{ow} is the oxygen isotope fractionation associated with the carbonyl oxygen–water interaction (1.016; Kreuzer-Martin *et al.*, 2003):

$$\delta^{18}O_{hair} = \alpha_{ow} \times \left(1000 + \delta^{18}O_{wg}\right) - 1000 \quad (8.2)$$

In turn, $\delta^{18}O_{wg}$ is determined by a mixture of body water ($\delta^{18}O_{wb}$), drinking water ($\delta^{18}O_{we}$), and food water ($\delta^{18}O_{wf}$). The portion of body water (g_1), drinking water (g_2), or food water ($1-g_1-g_2$) added to gut water will depend on the individual and personal dietary choices, although previous work (Malagelada *et al.*, 1976) suggests a volumetric mixing ratio of 25% food water and 75% body water in the average human's digestive juice, with essentially no influence directly from drinking water ($g_2=0$). When tuning the hair prediction model, Ehleringer *et al.* (2008) set $g_1=0.57$ and $g_2=0$:

$$\delta^{18}O_{wg} = g_1 \times \delta^{18}O_{wb} + g_2 \times \delta^{18}O_{we} + \left[\left(1 - g_1 - g_2\right) \times \delta^{18}O_{wf}\right] \tag{8.3}$$

If it is not possible to measure $\delta^{18}O_{wf}$, Ehleringer *et al.* (2008) suggested a calculation based on the isotope composition of food ($\delta^{18}O_f$): $\delta^{18}O_{wf}=\delta^{18}O_f-27‰$. More recently, Podlesak *et al.* (2012) published an equation for estimating food water from the isotopic composition of drinking water, based on work done with German cattle (Boner and Förstel, 2004): $\delta^{18}O_{wf}=\delta^{18}O_{we}+4‰$.

Finally, body water ($\delta^{18}O_{wb}$) is influenced by a variety of factors, including the isotopic compositions of drinking water ($\delta^{18}O_{we}$), food ($\delta^{18}O_f$), and inhaled O_2 ($\delta^{18}O_{O_2}$), plus losses of oxygen through breathing/evaporation and exhaled CO_2. Following work by Gretebeck *et al.* (1997), body water oxygen isotopic composition can be described as:

$$\delta^{18}O_{wb} = \frac{a \times \delta^{18}O_{we} + b \times \delta^{18}O_f + c \times \left[\alpha_{O_2}\left(1000 + \delta^{18}O_{O_2}\right) - 1000\right] - \left[1000 \times h \times \left(\alpha_{fwlo} - 1\right) + 1000 \times j \times \left(\alpha_{CO_2} - 1\right)\right]}{h \times \alpha_{fwlo} + j \times \alpha_{CO_2} + k} \tag{8.4}$$

In Equation 8.4, *a*, *b*, and *c* represent the proportional contributions of drinking water, food, and inhaled O_2, respectively, to body water, while *h*, *j*, and *k* represent losses of body water via breathing/evaporation, CO_2, and unfractionated water excretion, respectively. The fractionations between atmospheric and absorbed O_2 (α_{O_2}), body water and CO_2 (α_{CO_2}), and water lost via breathing/evaporation (α_{fwlo}) are assigned values of 0.992, 1.038, and 0.992, respectively (see Gretebeck *et al.*, 1997; Ehleringer *et al.*, 2008; Podlesak *et al.*, 2012, for more details on the values assigned to various parameters in Eq. 8.4). The isotopic composition of O_2 is +23.5‰ (Kroopnick and Craig, 1972), while $\delta^{18}O_f$ will vary based on dietary choices and location. For simple rough-order-of-magnitude predictions, a value of +26‰ (Chesson *et al.*, 2010) can be used for $\delta^{18}O_f$.

This model—and its associated equations (Eqs. 8.2–8.4)—can be used to predict the oxygen isotopic composition of hair from drinking water, and vice versa. Water isoscapes play a key role in predictions, allowing investigators to spatially display those regions with water isotope ratios that are consistent with the isotopic composition of hair measured for an individual.

8.4.2 Oxygen isotopes in drinking water and skeletal bioapatite

Origin assignment based on oxygen isotope analyses of human bone or tooth enamel is based primarily on foundational work done in archaeological settings and pioneering research completed in the 1980s. Three of the most important publications on skeletal bioapatite $\delta^{18}O$ values from that era include Longinelli (1984), Luz *et al.* (1984), and Levinson *et al.* (1987). Generally speaking, those studies presented data from discrete populations of "modern" and "historic" samples and included both skeletal and dental remains. Additionally, measurements were made on the *phosphate* component of skeletal bioapatite.

In 2008, Daux *et al.* (2008) combined the previously published datasets of bone and tooth phosphate $\delta^{18}O$ values with analyses of teeth from modern and eighteenth century individuals to generate a "super sample set" (n=42 locations) for predicting drinking water $\delta^{18}O$ values from bioapatite phosphate using a simple linear regression model:

$$\delta^{18}O_{\text{water}} = 1.54(\pm 0.09) \times \delta^{18}O_{\text{tooth/bone}} - 33.72(\pm 1.51)‰ \tag{8.5}$$

To apply this bioapatite–water oxygen isotope prediction model (e.g., Eq. 8.5) in modern forensic cases, investigators typically first prepare ground samples of skeletal remains (Meier-Augenstein, 2010; Font *et al.*, 2015)—for example, apatite isolated from whole bone or enamel powder collected from a tooth after the organic fraction is chemically removed (using either sodium hypochlorite or hydrogen peroxide). Next, the oxygen isotope signature of *carbonate* is measured through direct reaction of powdered samples with phosphoric acid to produce CO_2 (Passey *et al.*, 2007; Kusaka and Nakano, 2014).

The analysis method used to measure oxygen isotope ratios of skeletal remains in modern forensic settings can be significantly different from the methods used in the pioneering work relating water and bioapatite $\delta^{18}O$ values. As noted previously, data used in the predictive relationship shown in Equation 8.5 came from the oxygen isotope analysis of *phosphate* in bone and teeth (Daux *et al.*, 2008). Production of silver phosphate from skeletal remains is labor intensive and involves fluorination processes that are highly dangerous. In contrast, the *carbonate* component of bone and teeth can be easily measured via acidification and collection of CO_2.[3]

Since the Daux *et al.* (2008) model used to predict drinking water was built using phosphate $\delta^{18}O$ values, forensic investigators measuring carbonate must convert $\delta^{18}O$ values to equivalent phosphate $\delta^{18}O$ values. There are multiple methods published for this conversion (Iacumin *et al.*, 1996; Chenery *et al.*, 2012;

[3]There is a fractionation between carbonate ($-CO_3$) and CO_2 that is temperature-dependent and thus temperature must be carefully controlled during sample acidification and analysis of carbonate $\delta^{18}O$ values. The $\delta^{18}O$ values measured for carbonates are typically normalized to the VPDB oxygen isotope scale. To use these data in published water prediction models, values must be converted to the VSMOW oxygen isotope scale as follows (Coplen, 1988): $\delta^{18}O_{VSMOW} = 1.03091 \times \delta^{18}O_{VPDB} + 30.91‰$.

France and Owsley, 2015), but the methods do not necessarily agree and no "super sample set" has been created that relates phosphate $\delta^{18}O$ values to carbonate $\delta^{18}O$ values. Many forensic investigators use the model of Iacumin *et al.* (1996) for carbonate–phosphate conversion (see, e.g., *Stable Isotope Forensics* (Meier-Augenstein, 2010)), which is also used in the case study examples that follow:

$$\delta^{18}O_{phosphate} = 0.98 \times \delta^{18}O_{carbonate} - 8.5‰ \tag{8.6}$$

Following the conversion of measured $\delta^{18}O$ values from carbonate to phosphate, drinking water $\delta^{18}O$ values are predicted using Daux *et al.* (2008; Eq. 8.5) or another of the models cited by those authors (e.g., Longinelli, 1984; Luz *et al.*, 1984; Levinson *et al.*, 1987). As seen for hair oxygen isotopes, water isoscapes play a key role in bioapatite origin predictions whereby regions consistent with the isotopic composition of the bone or tooth can be displayed graphically as prediction "swaths" on a map.

8.4.3 Strontium isotopes of local bedrock and skeletal remains

Measurement of $^{87}Sr/^{86}Sr$ ratios of human skeletal remains is often included in multi-isotope methods for human identification (Juarez, 2008; Kamenov *et al.*, 2014; Font *et al.*, 2015). This is because Sr isotope ratios can also provide information about an individual's local environment during the period of tissue formation. However, the information provided by Sr isotope ratios for origin attribution is independent of the information provided by oxygen isotope ratios, making the combination of oxygen and strontium isotope analyses a powerful technique for narrowing possible origins to select areas (e.g., further reducing the size of a search haystack).

Investigators typically assume a 1:1 relationship between the $^{87}Sr/^{86}Sr$ ratios measured in a bone or tooth and bioavailable $^{87}Sr/^{86}Sr$ ratios found in the individual's original location (Beard and Johnson, 2000). Based on this assumption, the strontium isotope ratios of a tissue can be directly compared with reference datasets of environmental $^{87}Sr/^{86}Sr$ ratios or to isoscape models (Beard and Johnson, 2000; Bataille and Bowen, 2012) that estimate bioavailable $^{87}Sr/^{86}Sr$ ratios (in water) by location based on bedrock type, leaching effects, and Sr transport. There are very few reference datasets or isoscapes for Sr isotope ratio variation in the environment and even fewer on Sr isotope ratio variation in skeletal remains. Most of the remains data come from archaeological settings and assemblages of unknown individuals (Hodell *et al.*, 2004; Bentley *et al.*, 2008; Chenery *et al.*, 2010; Price *et al.*, 2011).

The relationship between Sr isotope ratios in a tissue and the bioavailable $^{87}Sr/^{86}Sr$ ratios of the individual's local environment during the time of tissue formation may be complex. As a consequence, it is likely that the bedrock–skeleton strontium isotope model is not yet completely developed or understood. Not surprisingly, this is an area of active research and development (Chesson *et al.*, 2012; Tipple *et al.*, 2013; Font *et al.*, 2015; Herrmann *et al.*, 2015).

8.5 Examples of the application of isotope analysis to unidentified remains

Two case examples demonstrating the application of isotope analysis for identification of human remains from unknown decedents follow. For the first case—a Salt Lake County (Utah) Jane Doe—oxygen isotope analyses of hair keratin and tooth enamel bioapatite are used. In the second case, which focuses on a mandible found in Siskiyou County (California), oxygen isotopes of bone and tooth enamel bioapatite as well as strontium isotopes of tooth enamel are presented.

8.5.1 Jane Doe from Salt Lake County

On October 25, 1978, the body of a nude female was found wrapped in a carpet at the old Salt Lake Beach near I-80 in Salt Lake County, Utah. The date of death was estimated to be approximately one month prior to discovery. Remains included bone, teeth, and hair. No missing persons report available to police at the time fit the remains and Jane Doe remained unidentified for 30 years. In 2008, isotope analyses were conducted on the hair and three teeth to answer a series of questions that could help focus the investigation: Was Jane Doe a resident of Salt Lake City? Had she traveled to/from Utah? If yes, where had she traveled before death?

Approximately 18 months of hair growth from Jane Doe were analyzed. It was apparent based on changes in the measured δ-values of her hair that she had been moving in the year and a half before her death, potentially living in three regions of the continental US during that time period. What were those locations?

The average $\delta^{18}O$ values of analyzed hair segments ranged from 9.9 to 16.8‰ and there were clear time trends throughout the 18-month period (Figure 8.3). Previous work (Sharp *et al.*, 2003; O'Brien and Wooller, 2007) has shown that the isotopes in human hair do not achieve a steady state (i.e., equilibrium) with values expected for local conditions for a period of time of approximately 2+ months following a move. Based on these criteria, the observed sequence of hair-segment oxygen isotope data suggested that the individual may have possibly resided in three "iso-regions" during the period 18 months prior to her death. Three distinct isotope ranges in the hair-segment time sequence are indicated in Figure 8.3, where the oxygen isotopic composition of the hair segments reached relative steadiness before changing. The measured $\delta^{18}O$ values of Jane Doe's hair suggested the following:

- For the time interval of approximately 14–12 months prior to death, Jane Doe lived in a region isotopically consistent with several southeastern states, including some areas of Texas (Figure 8.4).
- For the time period of approximately 6–4 months prior to death, Jane Doe lived in a region isotopically consistent with a relatively small portion of northern Texas and southern Oklahoma.
- After the time period approximately 4 months prior to death, Jane Doe moved to a third region isotopically consistent with the Salt Lake Valley and other Intermountain West states.

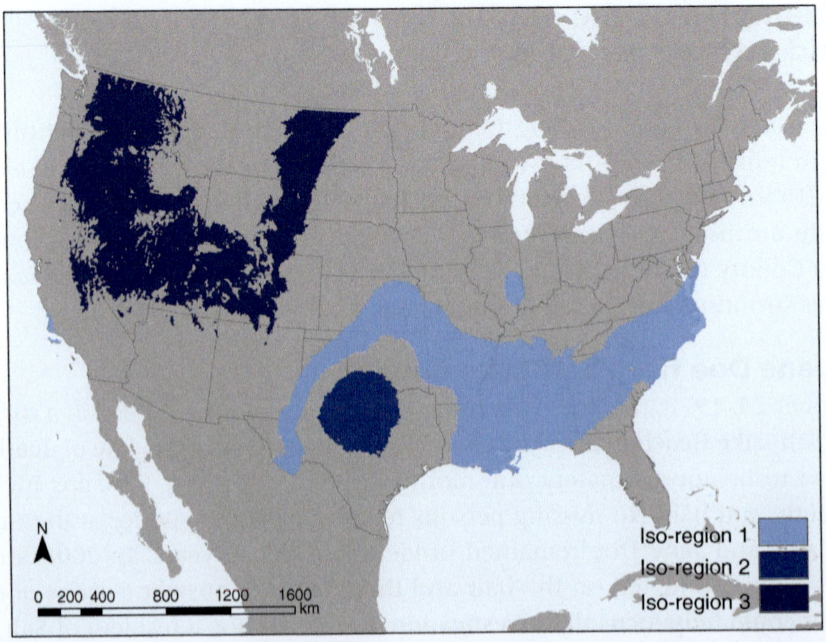

Figure 8.4 Geographic locations consistent with hair keratin $\delta^{18}O$ values measured for Salt Lake County Jane Doe. See Figure 8.3 for the identification of three "iso-regions." Geographic Information System (GIS) software was used to spatially represent drinking water predictions made from hair keratin $\delta^{18}O$ values. Data: Tap water (Bowen *et al.*, 2007).

To generate the predictions shown in Figure 8.4, Equations 8.2–8.4 were used to predict drinking water $\delta^{18}O$ values from hair $\delta^{18}O$ values in the periods of equilibrium. As a first-order approximation of uncertainty for the potential origins, an "error window" or measurement uncertainty of ±0.5‰ was applied to measured hair $\delta^{18}O$ values prior to predictions. The range in predicted water $\delta^{18}O$ values was then displayed graphically by screening a water isoscape (Bowen *et al.*, 2007) (Figure 8.1) to show just those regions consistent with the predictions. Screening was done with Geographic Information System (GIS) software.

At the time of death, the $\delta^{18}O$ values for the victim's hair were consistent with values expected for a resident of the Intermountain West region of the United States, including the Salt Lake Valley. One conclusion is that the individual may have been a current local resident at the time of her death. However, the isotope data indicated that she had likely been a resident for only a short period of time prior to death, as seen in the hair $\delta^{18}O$ values just before death (Figure 8.3).

Measurement and interpretation of the oxygen isotope ratios of tooth enamel carbonate collected from Jane Doe's teeth were consistent with the prediction that she had spent at least some years of her youth in the southeastern United States (Figure 8.5). To generate the predictions shown in Figure 8.5, Equations 8.5 and 8.6 were used to predict drinking water $\delta^{18}O$ values from tooth enamel $\delta^{18}O$ values.

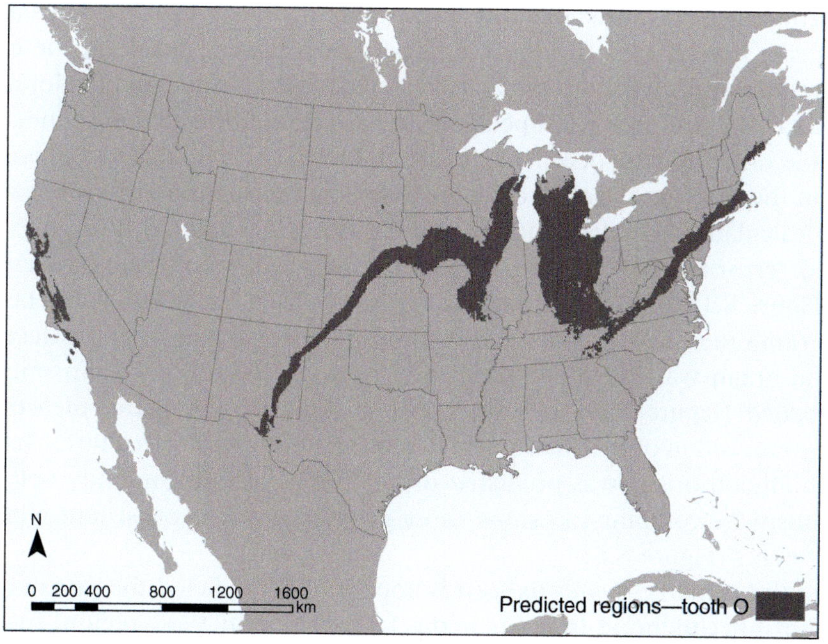

Figure 8.5 Geographic locations consistent with tooth enamel apatite $\delta^{18}O$ values measured for Salt Lake County Jane Doe. The average drinking water $\delta^{18}O$ value was calculated from the analysis of three teeth. Geographic Information System (GIS) software was used to spatially represent drinking water predictions made from enamel $\delta^{18}O$ values. Data: Tap water (Bowen *et al.*, 2007).

As for hair, an "error window" of ±0.5‰ was used, applied to predicted water. The range in predicted water $\delta^{18}O$ values was then displayed graphically by screening the water isoscape to show just those regions consistent with the predictions.

Jane Doe was identified in June 2012 when DNA testing confirmed her identity as that of Patricia Barrett. Ms. Barrett was 45 years old at the time of her disappearance and investigators believe she had been in the Salt Lake Area approximately 2 months before death. Information provided by her family, who lost contact with her in August 1978, indicated that she may have been homeless. Ms. Barrett originally hailed from Texas and still had family there. She had been wandering in the year and a half before death, potentially visiting Texas, Oklahoma, and Louisiana before traveling to Utah. The case is now an active homicide investigation.

8.5.2 Mandible from Siskiyou County

A second example of the application of isotope analysis techniques to human remains focuses on a case from Siskiyou County, California, where an isolated mandible was recovered from along a creek bank within the North Coast Range in 2012 (Bartelink *et al.*, 2016). Morphological and metric assessments suggested the decedent was an adult male, although classification of ancestry was indeterminate based on the ambiguous traits present. No other remains were recovered. The investigating agency wanted to know if the remains were possibly tied to a missing person's case from the area, a local man who never lived outside of the county. A bone sample and a left third molar were collected from the mandible for oxygen isotope analysis; strontium isotope analysis was also conducted on the molar.

Probable origin for the decedent during childhood was predicted using isotope data from the tooth analyses. Predictions were made using Equations 8.5 and 8.6 for O to calculate likely drinking water $\delta^{18}O$ values; results (with the previously described "error window") were used to screen a water isoscape (Bowen *et al.*, 2007) (Figure 8.1) to display possible origins. For Sr, a 1 : 1 relationship between $^{87}Sr/^{86}Sr$ ratios measured in the tooth enamel and bioavailable Sr of the decedent's childhood origin was assumed. Then, a Sr isoscape (Beard and Johnson, 2000) was screened (Figure 8.2) to show those regions matching the measured Sr isotopic composition of the tooth, using an estimated "error" of ±0.001. The decedent's childhood origin was predicted using O and Sr independently before the predictions were combined to show those geographic areas consistent with both measurements (Figure 8.6).

The tooth bioapatite–water oxygen isotope model predicted the decedent may have spent his childhood in or near the Intermountain West region, including

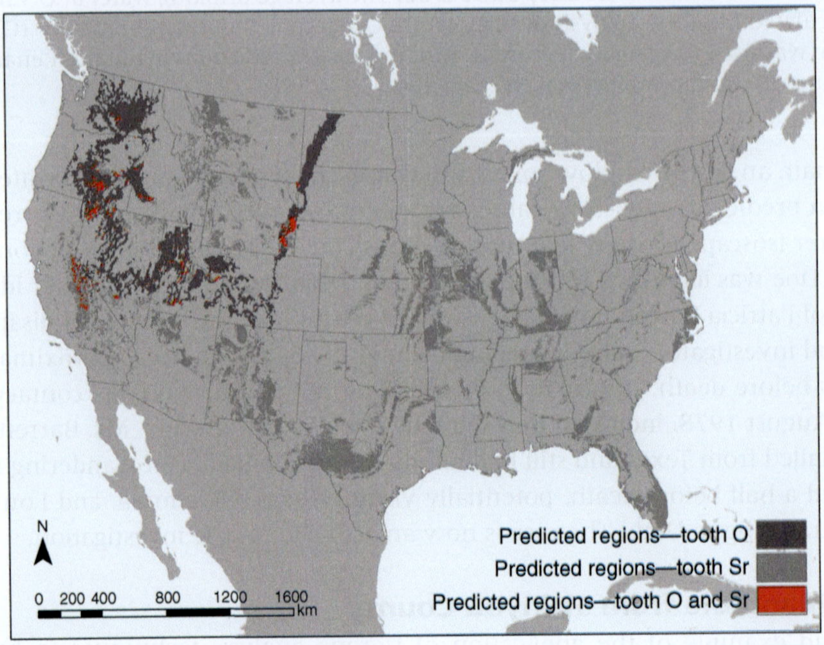

Figure 8.6 Geographic locations consistent with tooth enamel $\delta^{18}O$ values and $^{87}Sr/^{86}Sr$ ratios measured for the Siskiyou County mandible. Geographic Information System (GIS) software was used to represent geographic locations that are consistent with tooth enamel apatite $\delta^{18}O$ values (darker gray), $^{87}Sr/^{86}Sr$ ratios (lighter gray), and both isotopes (red). Data: Tap water (Bowen *et al.*, 2007). Bedrock (Bataille *et al.*, 2012).

some isolated, high elevation regions of California. As seen in Figure 8.6, the origin predictions based on tooth enamel $\delta^{18}O$ values fall within a roughly continuous "band" of potential locations, representing areas of similar climate (and thus similar water oxygen isotopic composition). In contrast, predictions based on $^{87}Sr/^{86}Sr$ ratios measured for the tooth are more discontinuous due to the discrete distributions of bedrock within the continental United States. When combined, predicted regions that fit *both* the oxygen and strontium isotope analysis results (Figure 8.6) are greatly reduced to isolated regions in South Dakota, Wyoming, Colorado, Utah, Nevada, Idaho, Washington, and Oregon, as well as northern California, where the remains were found.

Oxygen isotope analysis of bone from the mandible provided a second "snapshot" in time, representing approximately 8–10 years before the individual's death. As for the tooth, drinking water $\delta^{18}O$ values—and thus probable origin—were predicted using Equations 8.5 and 8.6, plus a water isoscape. The bone prediction was then compared with the tooth prediction to determine if the decedent spent his adulthood before death and his childhood in similar locations (Figure 8.7). Origin predictions based on bone bioapatite suggest that the decedent may have spent the years before death in or near the Intermountain West region, similar to predictions made based on tooth enamel bioapatite. Investigation into the decedent's identity is still ongoing, and DNA testing is currently underway.

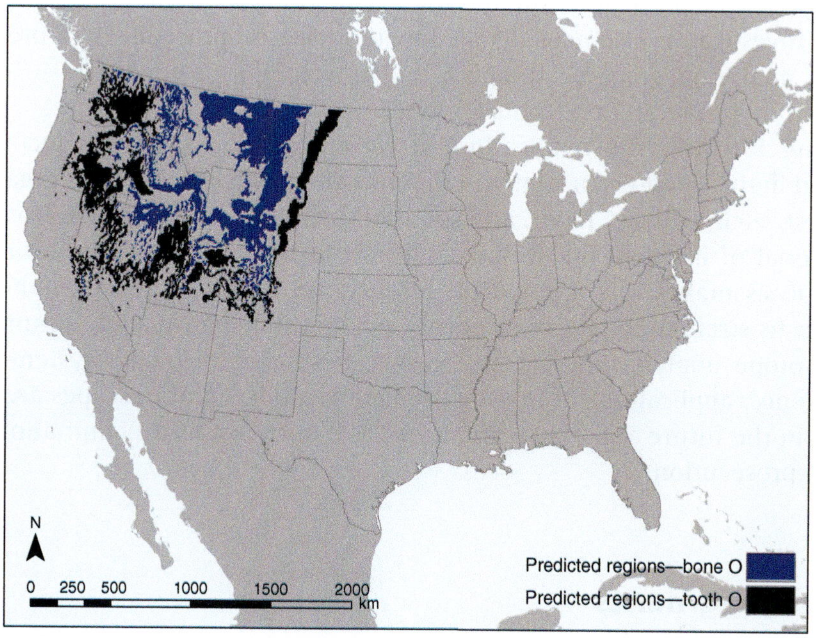

Figure 8.7 Geographic locations consistent with tooth enamel and bone apatite $\delta^{18}O$ values measured for the Siskiyou County mandible. Geographic Information System (GIS) software was used to represent geographic locations that are consistent with tooth enamel apatite $\delta^{18}O$ values (black) and bone apatite $\delta^{18}O$ values (blue). There were no regions of overlap. Data: Tap water. (Bowen *et al.*, 2007).

8.6 What are the future applications of isotope analysis?

As described in this chapter, the isotope "fingerprints" of human tissues such as hair, bone, and tooth enamel provide information on an individual's geographic life history, as well as dietary lifestyle. (Note that the dietary application was not used in the case examples). Three of the most utilized models for predicting geographic origin of unknown decedents include the relationships between the isotope signatures of tissues and the environment for the following:

1. O isotopes of drinking water and hair keratin
2. O isotopes of drinking water and tooth enamel/bone apatite
3. Sr isotopes of local bedrock and tooth enamel

In application, isotope landscapes—or isoscapes—are essential for visualizing model outputs based on naturally occurring and predictable patterns in the isotope variations of water (O isotopes) and bedrock (Sr isotopes). As demonstrated in two case study examples, prediction of potential origins using isotope models and isotope maps can help to "reduce the size of the haystack" in a forensic investigation.

The approach described here for applying O and Sr isotope analyses to human remains would work for additional elements such as lead (Pb), sulfur (S), and carbon (C). Application requires well-tested models describing the relationship between the isotopes of an input and the resultant tissue of interest (interpretive theory). Investigators also need detailed methodological procedures for preparing remains, analyzing prepared samples, and interpreting isotope data to ensure results are fit for use and not compromised.

Looking forward, the application of forensic isotope analysis techniques described in this chapter for human remains can be expanded to other materials of interest, such as drugs, foods, and spoils of the illegal wildlife trade. No matter the material of interest, the well-established theory currently supporting isotope analysis makes this a powerful forensic technique. Applied studies will continue to strengthen the theoretical and methodological underpinnings of stable isotope analysis and its application to the medicolegal system. As a consequence, applications of isotope prediction models and isoscapes are likely to grow in the future and play a greater role in both forensic examinations and criminal prosecution.

Acknowledgments

The authors would like to acknowledge Amy MacKinnon, Stefanie Kline, and Julia Prince-Buitenhuys for their assistance preparing the bone and tooth samples from the Siskiyou County Case. The authors also thank Bonnie Mortenson of Siskiyou County Sheriff's Office for permission to conduct the isotope testing.

References

Bartelink, E.J., Berg, G.E., Beasley, M.M., and Chesson, L.A. (2014a) Application of stable isotope forensics for predicting region of origin of human remains from past wars and conflicts. *Annals of Anthropological Practice*, **38**, 124–136.

Bartelink, E.J., Berry, R., and Chesson, L.A. (2014b) Stable isotopes and human provenancing. In: *Advances in Forensic Human Identification* (eds. X. Mallett, T. Blythe, and R. Berry). CRC Press, Taylor & Francis Group, Boca Raton, FL, pp. 165–192.

Bartelink, E.J., MacKinnon, A.T., Prince-Buitenhuys, J.R., *et al.* (2016) Stable isotope forensics as an investigative tool in missing persons investigations. In: *Handbook of Missing Persons* (eds. S.J. Morewitz and C. Sturdy-Colls). Springer International Publishing, Switzerland, pp. 443–462.

Bataille, C.P. and Bowen, G.J. (2012) Mapping $^{87}Sr/^{86}Sr$ variations in bedrock and water for large scale provenance studies. *Chemical Geology*, **304–305**, 39–52.

Bataille, C.P. Laffon, J., and Bowen, G.J. (2012) Mapping multiple source effects on the strontium isotopic signatures of ecosystems from the circum-Caribbean region. *Ecosphere*, **3**(12), 1–24.

Beard, B.L. and Johnson, C.M. (2000) Strontium isotope composition of skeletal material can determine the birth place and geographic mobility of humans and animals. *Journal of Forensic Sciences*, **45**, 1049–1061.

Bentley, R.A., Wahl, J., Price, T.D., and Atkinson, T.C. (2008) Isotopic signatures and hereditary traits: Snapshot of a Neolithic community in Germany. *Antiquity*, **82**, 290–304.

Boner, M. and Förstel, H. (2004) Stable isotope variation as a tool to trace the authenticity of beef. *Analytical and Bioanalytical Chemistry*, **378**, 301–310.

Bowen, G.J. and Revenaugh, J. (2003) Interpolating the isotopic composition of modern meteoric precipitation. *Water Resources Research*, **39**, 1299–1311.

Bowen, G.J., Ehleringer, J.R., Chesson, L.A., *et al.* (2007) Stable isotope ratios of tap water in the contiguous United States. *Water Resources Research*, **43**, W03419.

Capo, R.C., Stewart, B.W., and Chadwick, O.A. (1998) Strontium isotopes as tracers of ecosystem processes: Theory and methods. *Geoderma*, **82**, 197–225.

Chenery, C., Müldner, G., Evans, J., *et al.* (2010) Strontium and stable isotope evidence for diet and mobility in Roman Gloucester, UK. *Journal of Archaeological Science*, **37**, 150–163.

Chenery, C.A., Pashley, V., Lamb, A.L., *et al.* (2012) The oxygen isotope relationship between the phosphate and structural carbonate fractions of human bioapatite. *Rapid Communications in Mass Spectrometry*, **26**, 309–319.

Chesson, L.A., Podlesak, D.W., Erkkila, B.R., *et al.* (2010) Isotopic consequences of consumer food choice: Hydrogen and oxygen stable isotope ratios in foods from fast food restaurants versus supermarkets. *Food Chemistry*, **119**, 1250–1256.

Chesson, L.A., Tipple, B.J., Mackey, G.N., *et al.* (2012) Strontium isotopes in tap water from the coterminous USA. *Ecosphere*, **3**, art67.

Coplen, T.B. (1988) Normalization of oxygen and hydrogen isotope data. *Chemical Geology: Isotope Geoscience Section*, **72**, 293–297.

Daux, V., Lécuyer, C., Héran, M.-A., *et al.* (2008) Oxygen isotope fractionation between human phosphate and water revisited. *Journal of Human Evolution*, **55**, 1138–1147.

Ehleringer, J.R., Bowen, G.J., Chesson, L.A., *et al.* (2008) Hydrogen and oxygen isotope ratios in human hair are related to geography. *Proceedings of the National Academy of Sciences*, **105**, 2788–2793.

Font, L., van der Peijl, G., van Leuwen, C., *et al.* (2015) Identification of the geographical place of origin of an unidentified individual by multi-isotope analysis. *Science & Justice*, **55**, 34–42.

France, C.A.M. and Owsley, D.W. (2015) Stable carbon and oxygen isotope spacing between bone and tooth collagen and hydroxyapatite in human archaeological remains. *International Journal of Osteoarchaeology*, **25**, 299–312.

Fry, B. (2006) *Stable Isotope Ecology*. Springer, New York.

Gat, J.R. (1996) Oxygen and hydrogen isotopes in the hydrological cycle. *Annual Review of Earth and Planetary Sciences*, **24**, 225–262.

Gretebeck, R.J., Schoeller, D.A., Socki, R.A., *et al.* (1997) Adaptation of the doubly labeled water method for subjects consuming isotopically enriched water. *Journal of Applied Physiology*, **82**, 563–570.

Hatch, K.A., Crawford, M.A., Kunz, A.W., *et al.* (2006) An objective means of diagnosing anorexia nervosa and bulimia nervosa using $^{15}N/^{14}N$ and $^{13}C/^{12}C$ ratios in hair. *Rapid Communications in Mass Spectrometry*, **20**, 3367–3373.

Hedges, R.E.M., Clement, J.G., Thomas, C.D.L., and O'Connell, T.C. (2007) Collagen turnover in the adult femoral mid-shaft: Modeled from anthropogenic radiocarbon tracer measurements. *American Journal of Physical Anthropology*, **133**, 808–816.

Herrmann, N., Li, Z.-H., and Warner, M. (2015) *Isotopic and Elemental Analysis of the William Bass Donated Skeletal Collection and Other Modern Donated Collections*. NCJRS Library, Rockville, MD. Available at: https://www.ncjrs.gov/App/Publications/abstract.aspx?ID=270772 (Accessed July 14, 2016).

Hickman, M.J., Hughes, K.A., Strom, K.J., and Ropero-Miller, J.D. (2007) *Medical Examiners' and Coroners' Offices, 2004*. U.S. Department of Justice, Office of Justice Programs, Washington, DC.

Hodell, D.A., Quinn, R.L., Brenner, M., and Kamenov, G. (2004) Spatial variation of strontium isotopes ($^{87}Sr/^{86}Sr$) in the Maya region: A tool for tracking ancient human migration. *Journal of Archaeological Science*, **31**, 585–601.

Holland, T.D., Berg, G.E., and Regan, L.A. (2012) Identification of a United States airman using stable isotopes. *Proceedings of the American Academy of Forensic Sciences*, **XVIII**, 420–421.

Iacumin, P., Bocherens, H., Mariotti, A., and Longinelli, A. (1996) Oxygen isotope analyses of co-existing carbonate and phosphate in biogenic apatite: A way to monitor diagenetic alteration of bone phosphate? *Earth and Planetary Science Letters*, **142**, 1–6.

Juarez, C.A. (2008) Strontium and geolocation, the pathway to identification for deceased undocumented Mexican border-crossers: A preliminary report. *Journal of Forensic Sciences*, **53**, 46–49.

Kamenov, G.D., Kimmerle, E.H., Curtis, J.H., and Norris, D. (2014) Georeferencing a cold case victim with lead, strontium, carbon, and oxygen isotopes. *Annals of Anthropological Practice*, **38**, 137–154.

Kreuzer-Martin, H.W., Lott, M.J., Dorigan, J., and Ehleringer, J.R. (2003) Microbe forensics: Oxygen and hydrogen stable isotope ratios in *Bacillus subtilis* cells and spores. *Proceedings of the National Academy of Sciences*, **100**, 815–819.

Kroopnick, P. and Craig, H. (1972) Atmospheric oxygen: Isotopic composition and solubility fractionation. *Science*, **175**, 54–55.

Kusaka, S. and Nakano, T. (2014) Carbon and oxygen isotope ratios and their temperature dependence in carbonate and tooth enamel using a GasBench II preparation device. *Rapid Communications in Mass Spectrometry*, **28**, 563–567.

Levinson, A.A., Luz, B., and Kolodny, Y. (1987) Variations in oxygen isotopic compositions of human teeth and urinary stones. *Applied Geochemistry*, **2**, 367–371.

Longinelli, A. (1984) Oxygen isotopes in mammal bone phosphate: A new tool for paleohydrological and paleoclimatological research? *Geochimica et Cosmochimica Acta*, **48**, 385–390.

Luz, B., Kolodny, Y., and Horowitz, M. (1984) Fractionation of oxygen isotopes between mammalian bone-phosphate and environmental drinking water. *Geochimica et Cosmochimica Acta*, **48**, 1689–1693.

Malagelada, J.R., Longstreth, G.F., Summerskill, W.H., and Go, V.L. (1976) Measurement of gastric functions during digestion of ordinary solid meals in man. *Gastroenterology*, **70**, 203–210.

Mallett, X., Blythe, T., and Berry, R. (2014) *Advances in Forensic Human Identification*. CRC Press, Boca Raton, FL.

Meier-Augenstein, W. (2010) *Stable Isotope Forensics: An Introduction to the Forensic Applications of Stable Isotope Analysis*. John Wiley & Sons, Ltd: Chichester, UK.

Mekota, A., Grupe, G., Ufer, S., and Cuntz, U. (2006) Serial analysis of stable nitrogen and carbon in hair: Monitoring starvation and recovery phases of patients suffering from anorexia nervosa. *Rapid Communications in Mass Spectrometry*, **20**, 1604–1610.

O'Brien, D. and Wooller, M. (2007) Tracking human travel using stable oxygen and hydrogen isotope analyses of hair and urine. *Rapid Communications in Mass Spectrometry*, **21**, 2422–2430.

Panzer, S., Peschel, O., Haas-Gebhard, B., *et al.* (2014) Reconstructing the life of an unknown (ca. 500 years-old South American Inca) mummy—Multidisciplinary study of a Peruvian Inca mummy suggests severe Chagas disease and ritual homicide. *PLoS ONE*, **9**, e89528.

Passey, B.H., Cerling, T.E., and Levin, N.E. (2007) Temperature dependence of oxygen isotope acid fractionation for modern and fossil tooth enamels. *Rapid Communications in Mass Spectrometry*, **21**, 2853–2859.

Petzke, K.J., Boeing, H., and Metges, C.C. (2005) Choice of dietary protein of vegetarians and omnivores is reflected in their hair protein ^{13}C and ^{15}N abundance. *Rapid Communications in Mass Spectrometry*, **19**, 1392–1400.

Podlesak, D.W., Bowen, G.J., O'Grady, S., *et al.* (2012) δ^2H and $\delta^{18}O$ of human body water: A GIS model to distinguish residents from non-residents in the contiguous USA. *Isotopes in Environmental and Health Studies*, **48**, 259–279.

Post, D.M. (2002) Using stable isotopes to estimate trophic position: Models, methods and assumptions. *Ecology*, **83**, 702–718.

Price, T.D., Frei, K.M., Dobat, A.S., *et al.* (2011) Who was in Harold Bluetooth's army? Strontium isotope investigation of the cemetery at the Viking Age fortress at Trelleborg, Denmark. *Antiquity*, **85**, 476–489.

Ritter, N. (2007) Missing persons and unidentified remains: The nation's silent mass disaster. *NIJ Journal*, **256**, 2–7.

Sanchez, R. (2015) For forensic artist of "Baby Doe" image, eyes are turning point. *CNN.com* (Online). Available at: http://www.cnn.com/2015/07/09/us/massachusetts-dead-toddler-forensics/index.html (Accessed July 14, 2016).

Schwarcz, H.P., White, C.D., and Longstaffe, F.J. (2010) Stable and radiogenic isotopes in biological archaeology: Some applications. In: *Isoscapes: Understanding Movement, Pattern, and Process on Earth through Isotope Mapping* (eds. J.B. West, G.J. Bowen, T.E. Dawson, and K.P. Tu). Springer, Dordrecht, The Netherlands, pp. 335–356.

Sharp, Z.D., Atudorei, V., Panarello, H.O., *et al.* (2003) Hydrogen isotope systematics of hair: Archeological and forensics applications. *Journal of Archaeological Science*, **30**, 1709–1716.

Thompson, T. and Black, S.M. (eds.) (2007) *Forensic Human Identification*. Taylor & Francis, Boca Raton, FL.

Thompson, A.H., Wilson, A.S., and Ehleringer, J.R. (2014) Hair as a geochemical recorder. In: *Treatise on Geochemistry, 2nd ed. (Vol. 14): Archaeology and Anthropology*. Elsevier, pp. 371–393.

Tipple, B.J. and Pagani, M. (2007) The early origins of terrestrial C_4 photosynthesis. *Annual Review of Earth and Planetary Sciences*, **35**, 435–461.

Tipple, B.J., Chau, T., Chesson, L.A., *et al.* (2013) Isolation of strontium pools and isotope ratios in modern human hair. *Analytica Chimica Acta*, **798**, 64–73.

Valenzuela, L.O., Chesson, L.A., O'Grady, S.P., *et al.* (2011) Spatial distributions of carbon, nitrogen and sulfur isotope ratios in human hair across the central United States. *Rapid Communications in Mass Spectrometry*, **25**, 861–868.

Valenzuela, L.O., Chesson, L.A., Bowen, G.J., *et al.* (2012) Dietary heterogeneity among Western industrialized countries reflected in the stable isotope ratios of human hair. *PLoS ONE*, **7**, e34234.

West, J.B., Bowen, G.J., Cerling, T.E., and Ehleringer, J.R. (2006) Stable isotopes as one of nature's ecological recorders. *Trends in Ecology & Evolution*, **21**, 408–414.

Wilson, A.S., Taylor, T., Ceruti, M.C., *et al.* (2007) Stable isotope and DNA evidence for ritual sequences in Inca child sacrifice. *Proceedings of the National Academy of Sciences*, **104**, 16456–16461.

PART 3

Scientific foundation for interpretations of antemortem, perimortem, and postmortem processes

CHAPTER 9

The anatomical basis for fracture repair: Recognition of the healing continuum and its forensic applications to investigations of pediatric and elderly abuse

Donna C. Boyd
Department of Anthropological Sciences, Radford University Forensic Science Institute, Radford University, Radford, VA, USA and Department of Biomedical Science, Virginia Tech Carilion School of Medicine, Roanoke, VA, USA

9.1 Introduction: Diagnosing pediatric and elderly non-accidental injury

Evaluation and adjudication of pediatric and elderly abuse in a forensic setting can be challenging. Verification of a non-accidental origin for trauma in these types of death investigations is often complex and ambiguous because traditional forms of evidence for non-accidental trauma may not be conclusive (Abel, 2011; AMA Council on Scientific Affairs, 1987; Baker *et al.*, 2011; Brogdon and McDowell, 2003, 2011; Brogdon *et al.*, 2013; Collins, 2006; Cooper *et al.*, 2008; Cumming, 1979; Flaherty *et al.*, 2014; Griest, 2010; Jayawardena and Liao, 2006; Jenny, 1994; Lee and Lathrop, 2010; Lett, 1995; Pillemer and Finkelhor, 1988; Ragan, 2011; Reece, 1994; Ross and Abel, 2011; Salter, 1980; Wolf, 1988).

Although investigations of non-accidental injury (NAI) are typically accomplished clinically through a standard exam and radiographic and follow-up skeletal survey (Bilo *et al.*, 2010; Brogdon, 1977, 1998; Brogdon *et al.*, 2003; DiMaio and Dana, 2007; Duffy *et al.*, 2011; Gill *et al.*, 2013; Harper *et al.*, 2016; Johnson and Bache, 2008a; Kleinman, 2015; Kleinman *et al.*, 1989, 1996; Levy and Harcke, 2011; McGraw *et al.*, 2002; Merten *et al.*, 1983, 1994; Riezzo, 2010; Thali *et al.*, 2011; Thomsen *et al.*, 1997) and are mandated for suspected abuse cases involving children below the age of 2 years (American Academy of Pediatrics, 2009), many signs of non-accidental trauma may remain occult. In response to this problem,

Forensic Anthropology: Theoretical Framework and Scientific Basis, First Edition.
Edited by C. Clifford Boyd Jr and Donna C. Boyd.

Love and colleagues have recommended a pediatric skeletal examination (PSE) and accompanying methodology for evaluating all suspicious pediatric deaths (Love, 2016; Love and Sanchez, 2009; Love *et al.*, 2013, 2014; Pinto *et al.*, 2015).

A prominent method of differentiating non-accidental from accidental trauma has been the identification of unique location, type, and severity of perimortem injuries. Classic signatures of pediatric non-accidental trauma are derived from prior case studies; these "sentinel injuries" reportedly include the presence of subdural hematomas and retinal hemorrhages (Caffey, 1946; Case, 2008a, b; DiMaio and Dana, 2007; Dolinak and Matshes, 2005; Kirschner and Wilson, 1994; Lantz and Couture, 2011), first and other rib fractures, particularly at the posterior (vertebral) ends (Barsness *et al.*, 2003; Flaherty *et al.*, 2014; Gunther *et al.*, 2000; Hirsch *et al.*, 2016; Kemp *et al.*, 2008; Kleinman and Schlesinger, 1997; Kleinman *et al.*, 1992, 1995; Leventhal *et al.*, 1993; Marks *et al.*, 2006; Merten *et al.*, 1983; Ng and Hall, 1998; Offiah and Hall, 2009; Strouse and Owings, 1995; Worlock *et al.*, 1986), classic metaphyseal lesions (CMLs) or epiphyseal fractures (Kleinman, 1998a, b, c; Kleinman and Marks, 1996a, b, c, 1998; Kleinman *et al.*, 1991; Loder and Bookout, 1991; Merten *et al.*, 1981, 1983), spiral long bone fractures (particularly of the humerus) (Bilo *et al.*, 2010; Galloway, 1999; Leventhal *et al.*, 1993; Wedell and Galloway, 2014; Worlock *et al.*, 1986), or other diagnostic fractures (e.g., Kroman *et al.*, 2002; Lonergan *et al.*, 2003). In addition, many clinicians generally note a magnified Injury Severity Score (ISS) in pediatric patients with non-accidental trauma (Carter and Moulton, 2016).

Much less has been written with regard to signature non-accidental trauma in the elderly. Gironda *et al.* (2016), in a sample of aged patients admitted with fractures to Southern California hospitals over a 3-year period, identified patterned injuries highly correlated with abuse. These include fractures to the head, face, and back. Brogdon and McDowell (2003, 2011) note similarities in elderly and pediatric abuse in regard to defensive injuries and those related to "grasping, squeezing, or forcible restraint," exacerbated by the effects of senile osteoporosis (Brogdon and McDowell, 2011:288). This results in a high frequency of injuries to long bones and the maxillofacial region.

However, reliance on these sentinel fracture patterns can be problematic and ambiguous. Pathognomonic indicators of NAI are not always present—Kogutt *et al.*'s (1974) study of infant fractures in an abused population of the University of Texas Medical Center patients, for example, showed that the majority of fractures did not correspond with the classic ones previously correlated with abuse. CML fractures were not common; instead, transverse and spiral fractures predominated. And King *et al.* (1988) observed that single perimortem diaphyseal long bone fractures were more common in a sample of abused children seen at Los Angeles Children's Hospital than CMLs. For the elderly, Brogdon and McDowell (2011) advise care in interpretation of signature non-accidental fractures due to the influence of age-related deteriorative conditions of osteoporosis, chronic disease, malnutrition, and atrophy, which make their bones vulnerable to fracture in a non-abusive context. Thus, much caution is advised in the use of sentinel fracture patterns as evidence for abuse, because it is likely that no injury patterns exist that are exclusively pathognomonic for NAI (Love and Martinez, Chapter 10, this volume; Cunha and Pinheiro, 2009).

Identification and interpretation of *antemortem* fractures may be more informative in resolving suspected abuse cases through validation of patterning consistent with manner of death. Pediatric and elderly decedents with NAI typically manifest the cumulative effects of a long-term, repetitive pattern of injury. Evidence for antemortem fractures in various phases of healing document the presence of a recurring pattern of prior abuse and place an accidental etiology for the perimortem death event into question (Hilton, 1994; Klepinger, 2006; Thorpe *et al.*, 2014). Thus, our ability to recognize, interpret, and date antemortem fractures is the key to accurate resolution of many pediatric and elderly death investigations.

Yet our current understanding and interpretation of fracture healing and the ability to date it are inadequate. Estimation of time since injury (TSI) has been described as an "inexact science" (Prosser *et al.*, 2005), fraught with a "significant subjective element" (Offiah and Hall, 2009:12) because it is based on inadequate samples derived from poorly documented or non-forensic sources with little understanding of the anatomical basis for and variables affecting bone healing. This perception of our inability to accurately interpret timing of injury has oftentimes led to TSI estimation being viewed as "nonscientific" and excluded in court through *Daubert* challenges (see Chapter 16, this volume).

This chapter reviews the theoretical basis for fracture healing in those populations at most risk for abuse—children and the elderly—and its timing from a forensic anatomy perspective. It includes a review of bone growth and healing processes (which are often a recapitulation of growth) and attempts by previous researchers to place these phenomena into antemortem healing phases or stages. A new forensically-based healing model that acknowledges the healing continuum is presented. It is developed with the aid of digital light microscopy, which allows more accurate observation of the healing process, particularly when it is informed by the anatomical and theoretical basis for that process. These anatomically-informed, microscopically-based standards for assessing bone healing are presented with an eye toward developing models to evaluate TSI in pediatric and elderly non-accidental death investigations.

9.2 Theoretical basis for fracture healing and TSI estimation

TSI estimation for antemortem fractures has undergone extensive criticism because of the "unknowable" nature of the timing of the event. In examining fracture healing, we are looking at injury events that occurred before death and that progressed through at least the initial stages of healing. Thus, as with all aspects of forensic science, we are investigating and interpreting past and, in many cases, unique events. Our inductive observations of facts relating to healing of bone allow us to make inferences and develop hypotheses about the reparative process and its progress over time, even though we cannot see or replicate the initial injury or active healing. Our inferences are made more exact by knowledge of the context—temporal, locational, and environmental—of the injury. We can then test these hypotheses with new cases (or facts). Using cases with known contextual frames, we can then proceed to detail the process of healing and its physical manifestations. Since healing is a continuous process, we recognize that any defined stages or phases of healing will represent heuristic models that, if clearly delineated, can facilitate our depiction of the progression of bone repair for future cases. Ultimately, we can develop a base from which we can model the healing process from its beginning to the point at which we observe it osteologically.

This type of logic builds on inductive case studies, leading to abductive inferences to the best explanation of the healing process and its timing. With more cases of known contextual frames, our inferences will become more refined and produce empirically stronger sequences.

As in all historical sciences, we are always faced with uncertainty in the inability to "prove" our inferences but, by analyzing contextually-specific cases, such as those discussed here, we can begin to formulate the theoretical foundation for timing of the healing process and test and strengthen our explanatory inferences regarding it. The research presented here is, therefore, a starting point in that process.

9.3 Anatomical basis for fracture healing

Landmark studies by Caffey (1946), Kempe *et al.* (1962), and Silverman (1953) laid the initial groundwork for use of fracture repair observations in child abuse cases by identifying and describing the healing process associated with pediatric fractures and the "battered child syndrome." Galloway (1999), Kerley (1976), Maples (1986), Sauer (1998), and Walker *et al.* (1997) were among the first researchers to bring attention of the topic of TSI to forensic anthropology. More recently, Love and colleagues (Love, 2016; Love and Sanchez, 2009; Love *et al.*, 2011, 2013, 2014; Pinto *et al.*, 2015) have set the standards for pediatric non-accidental trauma research and clinical evaluation, while Marks and colleagues (Marks and Haden, 2002; Marks and Mileusnic-Polchan, 2007; Marks *et al.*, 2006, 2009) have pioneered histological methods for pediatric fracture analysis, and Crowder and Stout (2012) have increased our understanding of histological bone biology.

Most forensic anthropologists are familiar with the basic healing process for injured bone, involving inflammation, soft and hard callus development, and remodeling. But this process is more complex than typically represented in much of the forensic anthropology literature and is often not anatomically-informed (at least not accurately). The details of the biological process of bone healing have important implications for what can be seen and interpreted macroscopically and microscopically from traumatized bone in a clinical (forensic) context.

Many aspects of bone healing, particularly in children, mimic and mirror the normal bone growth process (Ortner, 2003). As Frick (2015:3) and Heppenstall (1980) note, the cells and mechanisms that govern bone growth and bone repair are, in large part, the same. Thus, an understanding of the normal process of bone growth is requisite to a consideration of the anatomical basis for bone healing.

9.3.1 Bone growth and development

Most bones, particularly long bones, grow through a process of both endochondral and membranous ossification. While membranous ossification occurs through the production of flat membranes, endochondral ossification depends upon the development of cartilage models (anlage). Both of these dynamic primary ossification processes are important in early (embryonic and postembryonic) bone formation. They differ, however, in both their procedural mechanisms and their end effect upon the growth of a bone (Scheuer and Black, 2004).

9.3.1.1 Membranous (intramembranous) and endochondral ossification

The first type of ossification to occur embryologically (seen in the clavicle in the 6th week *in utero*), membranous ossification is typically associated with the development of flat bones or bone segments like those in the skull, os coxa, scapula, and acromial end of the clavicle. However, this type of ossification, as an important part of bone remodeling, occurs throughout life and affects every bone in the body (Scheuer and Black, 2000). It is also the primary mechanism during development through which growth in long bone *diameter* occurs (Lindaman, 2001; Marks, 1998). It arises through direct condensation of the mesenchymal cells into flat membranous sheets (Humphries, 2011; Marks, 1998; Rosenberg, 2015). This process involves the differentiation and transformation of mesenchymal cells into osteoblasts, which, through their proliferation and enlargement, lead to deposition of an osteoid matrix that eventually becomes mineralized. In cortical bone, the early osteon system is developed from the centrifugal radiation of primary trabeculae from the center of ossification. Entrapped osteoblasts within each successively deposited bone layer become osteocytes within the lacunae in the interstitial spaces of this osteon system (Rosenberg, 2015), which, when condensed and vascularized, comprises the haversian system characteristic of cortical bone. In contrast, in cancellous (spongy) bone, the evolving bone tissue is surrounded by vascularized connective tissue (Resnick *et al.*, 2002). Regardless of osseous tissue location (i.e., cortical or cancellous), primitive bone evolves through continued transformation of mesenchymal cells into osteoblasts, leading to an expansion of the osteoid matrix and matrix entrapment of osteoblasts and conversion of them into osteocytes (Resnick *et al.*, 2002). It is this intramembranous ossification process, involving successive deposition of bone on the exterior surface of a long bone combined with resorption endosteally, that results in appositional growth in the diameter of a long bone (Marks, 1998). Bone remodeling and repair (e.g., through fracture) also is dependent upon this membranous process of subperiosteal appositional deposition and resorption (Scheuer and Black, 2000).

Endochondral ossification is typically associated with skeletal regions manifesting significant amounts of cancellous bone (Scheuer and Black, 2000). It involves the initial formation of a cartilaginous long bone model and its subsequent growth in diaphyseal *length*. Embryologically, undifferentiated mesenchymal (stem) cells organize and condense into a cartilaginous matrix that eventually becomes a model for a future long bone. Successions of chondrocytes live, die, and calcify at the center of this cartilaginous matrix, resulting in the formation of a primary ossification region in the center of a long bone shaft (Frick, 2015; Marks, 1998; Resnick *et al.*, 2002; Rosenberg, 2015). With vascularization, new mesenchymal cell transformations into osteoblasts, chondroclasts, and osteoclasts result in the deposition of bone on the cartilage anlage (Frick, 2015), producing primary cancellous bone.

This cycle of chondrocyte life, death, and calcification is progressively replayed at the ends of the primary centers, forming an "ossification front" as well as a developing physis (Dwek, 2010). Osteoblasts eventually transform the cartilage matrix through their deposition of osseous tissue. As in intramembranous ossification, trapped osteoblasts become osteocytes (Resnick *et al.*, 2002).

Progressive proliferation and calcification of this cartilaginous cellular matrix continues at the terminal ends of the long bone, resulting in growth in its proximal and distal lengths. Thinning of the cartilage postnatally between the epiphysis and diaphysis eventually results in the epiphyseal plate (Frick, 2015).

Differentiation of osteoblasts along the periphery of the developing cartilage matrix forms a perichondrium, which, upon vascularization, differentiates into a fibrovascular periosteum (Scheuer and Black, 2000). Deeper (subperichondral) cells are transformed into osteoblasts and produce, through intramembranous ossification, a subperiosteal collar around the cartilaginous primary center of ossification (Humphries, 2011; Marks, 1998), referred to as a periosteal or subperiosteal bone collar or "bone bark" (Dwek, 2010). This encloses the cartilaginous model in a shell and promotes the process of appositional (membranous) growth.

The periosteum eventually covers most all long bone portions except for the interarticular regions and the patella. In infants, it is only loosely attached to the diaphysis of a long bone (and is thus vulnerable to stripping (Rosenberg, 2015)) and is comprised of two membranous layers—an outer fibrous (collagen-based) one and an inner cambium one. While the fibrous one provides for structural integrity, it is the inner cambium layer of the periosteum that contains the osteogenic potential that is critical to bone growth, development, and repair, for this is where the osteogenic progenitors, osteoblasts, and fibroblasts reside, in conjunction with a rich vascular and neural network (Dwek, 2010). It is this cambium layer that provides for growth in diameter of long bones. In adults, the periosteum is primarily a fibrous layer comprised of fibroblasts and collagen and is contiguous with tendinous and muscular tissue (Rosenberg, 2015).

Membranous new bone formation occurring beneath the periosteum (subperiosteal new bone formation (SPNBF)) is often associated with normal bone growth in young infants (Kleinman, 1998c; Kwon *et al.*, 2002; Offiah and Hall, 2009; Shopfner, 1966; Volberg *et al.*, 1977). This occurs due to the production of excess woven bone that outpaces its rate of remodeling into more mature lamellar bone (Scheuer and Black, 2000). Kwon *et al.* (2002) note that a thin (<2 mm) layer of SPNBF is normally observed (radiographically) in infants 1–4 months, possibly as late as 6 months old. This is referred to as "physiologic SPNBF" to distinguish it from trauma-associated SPNBF. It is usually symmetrical, never extends to the metaphysis, and is generally not greater than 2 mm thick in diameter (Kleinman, 1998c; Offiah and Hall, 2009). Pergolizzi and Oestreich (1995) note that physiologic SPNBF is often observed parallel to long bone (particularly femoral and tibial) shafts, in contrast to fracture-related SPNBF that is due to separation (stripping) of the periosteum from bone and begins calcifying farthest away from the fracture site. SPNBF can also be associated with infectious, metabolic, and neoplastic disease (Offiah and Hall, 2009).

Subsequent to the postnatal appearance of secondary ossification centers (epiphyses) at the long bone ends, eventual thinning of the cartilaginous matrix between the epiphyses and diaphysis results in the development of the epiphyseal plate and additional long bone expansion in the length dimension. A periosteal collar becomes firmly attached at the physis at the zone of Ranvier and the ring of LaCroix.

These processes of bone growth (and repair) are regulated through complex mechanisms under genetic, hormonal, and mechanical control. For example, it has been estimated that there are potentially thousands of genes that influence the ossification process—more than 5000 were identified as responsive to fracture repair in a study of overgrowth of the rat femoral physis (Ashraf *et al.*, 2007; Frick, 2015). Growth-regulating hormones (e.g., estrogen, testosterone), bone morphogenetic proteins (BMPs), peptide-signaling proteins (e.g., transforming growth factor, TGF-β), and immunoregulatory cytokines have been identified as important contributors to and influencers of bone growth and development (Resnick *et al.*, 2002). Mechanical factors relating to oxygen tension at a growth site and within the periosteum also play a role in ossification.

9.3.2 Fracture healing

Although endochondral ossification and the periosteum (and its periosteal cells) are identified as the greatest contributors to bone healing, as with bone growth, membranous ossification also plays an important role. In fact, Ferguson *et al.* (1999) and Gerstenfeld *et al.* (2003) envision fracture healing as a specialized postembryonic process that "recapitulates aspects of embryological skeletal development." This process differs between diaphyseal and physeal and postcranial and cranial locations.

9.3.2.1 Diaphyseal healing

Most clinicians (e.g., Frick, 2015; Lindaman, 2001; Schiller and Teitelbaum, 1999; Sheikh, 2000a; Wilkins, 2005) divide the fracture healing process into inflammatory, reparative, and remodeling phases (although Frost (1989a) describes healing phases as "Fracture, Granulation, and Modeling/Remodeling"). Healing of the diaphysis is highlighted by the following events and processes.

Inflammation of the injured region begins immediately after trauma induction and injury to tissue. Rodriguez-Martin (2006) divides the inflammatory phase of healing into two subphases—the hematoma phase and the cellular phase. The hematoma phase is heralded by vasodilatation and bleeding from soft tissue, the periosteum, and the region around the fracture site. Fibrin-containing hematomas, both inside and outside of the bone, develop. Hematoma development acts as a "signaling agent" (Frick, 2015:4; Wilkins, 2005), stimulating the cellular phase focused on organization of the hematoma and cellular repair.

This cellular response to bone fracture occurs in the subperiosteal region of the bone within 24 hours of fracture. Because of its loose adherence to the diaphysis, stripping of the periosteum, with concomitant bleeding, is more likely to occur in injury of pediatric bone (Frick, 2015; Ortner, 2003; Rodriguez-Merchan, 2005)—thus, injury to the periosteum (e.g., disruption or elevation) can occur through the initial trauma or subsequent development of the hematoma. Osteoprogenitor cells beneath the periosteum stimulate the osteoblastic production of new periosteal bone—SBNBF—early in the inflammatory phase (Frick, 2015). Reconstitution of the fibrous layer of the periosteum also occurs early in the inflammatory response and helps to stabilize the fracture site. Thus, it is clear that the periosteum plays a significant role in very early fracture healing (Dwek, 2010; Rodriguez-Merchan, 2005).

Cellular repair is additionally promoted through the release of leukocyte and macrophage inflammatory cells. These cells, in turn, initialize the release of growth factors, immunological cytokines, and peptide-signaling proteins that lead to proliferation and differentiation of osteoblasts and chondrocytes, stimulating the process of endochondral ossification (Frost, 1989a).

Disruption of the vascular network at and near the fracture site may lead to necrotic bone in this region. The process of removal (absorption) of this necrotic bone by osteoclasts may be manifest by a widening and rounding of the fracture margin during the first week or two post-injury (Maples, 1986). Rodriguez-Martin (2006:207) describes this early bony evidence of fracture repair as "fracture margins that show some osteogenic reaction with some spiculae and small pieces of bone attached to the fracture's margins." This may also result in an appearance of sclerosis (thickening) and greater visibility of the fracture and its margins on radiographs 2–3 weeks post-injury as new bone is deposited on necrotic bone (Frick, 2015).

Reparation of the fracture site involves initial repair and bridging of the fractured region through replacement of the hematoma with a soft callus that begins as "granulation tissue"—a vascularized aggregate of fibroblasts, which eventually becomes a collagen-based scaffolding of fibrovascular tissue (Wilkins, 2005). This scaffold eventually mineralizes to become the collagen of woven bone that forms around the fracture through the previously described processes of both endochondral and membranous ossification. As Kleinman and Walters (2015) note, this process begins near fracture margins and extends away from the fracture site, with cartilage formation primarily occurring (through endochondral ossification) at the callus periphery. Formation of new blood vessels and subsequent vascular ingrowth is a very important component of this process (Frick, 2015), promoting bone formation through mineralization.

Callus formation occurs both above and below the periosteum, producing both an endosteal and periosteal (external) callus (Frick, 2015; Nightengale, 2005). Proliferation, differentiation, and eventual ossification of cartilaginous cells derived from the inner cambium layer of the periosteum occur at the center of the fracture site, mimicking the endochondral ossification process, while membranous ossification processes occur at the periphery of the fracture site, where the cambium layer of the periosteum lays down a collar of periosteal bone (Johnson and Bache, 2008b). As the periosteum produces bone beneath it, the periosteum is pushed away from the bone and forms a periosteal collar of the bone around the fracture site, comprised initially of fiber and cartilage (and thus potentially occult in radiographs). Thus, the *periosteal* callus is the (externally) most visible to forensic anthropologists (and, later, radiologists) and is formed by osteoblasts originating from the inner osteogenic cambium layer of the periosteum. This is seen at the fracture site and along the undersurface of the periosteum a distance away from the fracture site. The *endosteal* callus derives from endochondral bone formation within the medullary cavity. It is the combination of endosteal and periosteal callus formation that serves to bridge the fracture site. The bony callus surrounding the fracture fragment joins the callus coming from the other side, leading to clinical union of the bone. Endosteal callus formation (through endochondral ossification) is also important when periosteal callus formation is inhibited (Malinin and Temple, 2016).

Physiological union, however, does not occur until *remodeling*, characterized by replacement of woven by more mature lamellar bone (Campbell and Schrader, 2006; Carter and Beaupre, 2001; Lindaman, 2001; Martin *et al.*, 1998; Ogden, 1990; Shapiro, 2008; Ubelaker and Montaperto, 2011) and eventual contouring—larger-scale absorption and formation of bone around larger regions of the fracture according to biomechanical principles and influences. This process typically involves bone proliferation on the compression side of the fracture and bone resorption on the tensile side (Johnson and Bache, 2008b).

9.3.2.2 Physeal and metaphyseal healing

CMLs represent high specificity for child abuse and are the direct result of torsional or shearing forces (Brogdon *et al.*, 2013; Kleinman *et al.*, 1986, 1991; Kleinman and Marks, 1996a, b, c, 1998; Offiah and Hall, 2009). Although sometimes classified as "corner" and "bucket handle" fractures, these actually represent similar if not the same type of fracture, just visualized radiologically in different imaging projections (Offiah and Hall, 2009). For young infants, the metaphysis or primary spongiosa represents the weakest and most vulnerable part of a bone (Kleinman, 1998c) due to the absence of significant mineralization of cartilage in this region. Metaphyseal bone has no periosteal cambium layer (Sheikh, 2000a), resulting in reduced callus formation in this region (and less visualization of fractures radiographically). However, it represents an active area for remodeling due to increased vascularity and osteogenic potential (Wilkins, 2005).

Kleinman *et al.* (1986) and Kleinman and Marks (1996a, b, c, 1998) have contradicted previous interpretations of CMLs as avulsion injuries to the metaphysis. They have shown through histology that these injuries typically consist of a series of planar microfractures through the primary spongiosa of the metaphysis. The result is a fracture line extending in a plane to the periphery of the bone, away from the physis. Disruption of the subperiosteal bone collar leads to undercutting of a peripheral bony segment (Offiah and Hall, 2009).

For older juveniles, fracture vulnerability shifts to the physeal cartilage that may become separated from the metaphysis through shear and/or compressive forces (Arkader and Skaggs, 2015). Since the physis contains cartilage, it does not strictly follow the traditional endochondral healing process when fractured. Cartilage does not "heal" in the same way as bone; for example, it does not remodel (Frick, 2015). Kleinman and Walters (2015) describe the process of endochondral ossification operative in physeal injuries. Visible within the growing physis are progressively organized layers of cartilaginous cells known as chondrocytes. Histologically, there is a progression of developmental zones proceeding from this cartilaginous physis to the metaphysis. This involves resting zones of chondrocytes near the epiphysis, which are awaiting activation, as well as proliferating and hypertrophic zones of chondrocytes in the intermediate layers undergoing organization into columns. Fractures typically occur through the zones of resting or proliferative cartilage, producing little evidence of hematoma, but instead granulation tissue. Closer to the metaphysis is a calcifying zone where calcified osteoid is deposited around the cartilage matrix, while at the metaphysis, there is ossification, resorption, and remodeling of the cartilaginous matrix columns (Brogdon *et al.*, 2013; Nightengale, 2005). Proliferation of uninjured cartilage cells results in physis widening and eventual conversion of cartilage to bone. Normal endochondral ossification resumes when revascularization occurs (Frick, 2015).

The periosteum is tightly attached in this region and may not be disrupted; thus, SPNBF may not form and the periosteal reaction, if present, may be subtle (Cramer, 1996; Frick, 2015; Shilt and McPherson, 2015). Shilt and McPherson (2015) maintain that only with periosteal shearing or metaphyseal displacement will a significant periosteal reaction develop at the physis. In contrast, Kleinman and Walters (2015) note that the periosteum is easily torn on one side of the physeal region, in association with its stripping on the contralateral side of the metaphysis and diaphysis. This may result in significant SPNBF production at the metaphysis.

In general, injuries to the growth plate heal more rapidly than those in the diaphysis. Sheikh (2000a) and Frick (2015) note healing of physeal injuries in young juveniles within 3 weeks, regardless of specific location. However, fractures involving the proliferative cartilage zone are more likely to interfere with (and retard) normal growth processes, particularly in the lower limbs (Nightengale, 2005).

9.3.2.3 Cranial healing

The overwhelming majority (at least 80%) of pediatric deaths from non-accidental trauma involve cranial (subdural, subarachnoid, retinal) hemorrhaging and traumatic brain injury (TBI) (Case, 2008a, b). Cranial fractures are often (but not always) associated with TBI, primarily affecting the parietals, occipital, frontal, and temporals (Wiersema *et al.*, 2014). Since the structure and growth of the human cranium are quite different compared with that of a postcranial bone, it stands to reason that fracture healing would differ as well. Rather than a periosteum and endosteum, the mature cranium consists of a diploë surrounded by an inner and outer table. Thus, the development of a soft and hard callus and dependence on an osteogenic periosteal layer are clearly not an integral part of cranial fracture healing. Instead of an active periosteum, it is an active dura mater associated with growth and other factors that likely influence cranial healing in subadults (Greenwald *et al.*, 2000a, b; Love *et al.*, 2011).

Much of our understanding of cranial healing is derived from clinical case studies of adult cranial trauma samples. Sevitt (1981) has described the healing process of adult crania as involving the deposition of small pockets of immature bone at fracture margins. Osteoclastic activity becomes an important aspect of cortical bone healing due to the lack of space for new bone formation. Increased osteoclastic activity creates "cutting cones"—regional areas of osteoclastic bone resorption—which help make room for osteoblastic activity (also see Shipman *et al.*, 1985; Steyn *et al.*, 2014). Hassler and Zentner (1990) describe these pockets of new bone deposition as "islands" of bone developing at the fracture margins that expand to bridge these margins. Woven bone, deposited to bridge fracture gaps, will not exceed the diameter of the native *in situ* bone; therefore, healing cranial fractures are not typically associated with classic calluses. Instead, a thin layer of SPNBF oftentimes covers the outer table (Love *et al.*, 2011), or it may not form at all (Offiah and Hall, 2009).

In a study of the Civil War collection from the National Museum of Health and Medicine, Barbian and Sledzik (2008) observed (macroscopically and with the aid of a 5× magnifying lens) healing responses in the form of osteoblastic, osteoclastic, and sequestration activities in 127 adult male crania exhibiting antemortem trauma. Osteoclastic resorption was the first observation possible, as early as 6 days post-injury. A period of "latency" of a week was noted between the initial osteoclastic observation and the prevalence of osteoblastic and additional osteoclastic responses commonly seen by the 2nd and 3rd weeks. Remnants of the healing process could still be observed as long as 225 days post-injury (also see Sauer and Dunlap, 1985).

It is not known if this cranial healing process occurs similarly in juvenile bone. Infant crania do not have a well-developed diploë in the middle of an outer and inner table. It is not known exactly when this mature cranial architecture develops, although it is appears to be within the first year of life (Love *et al.*, 2013). Clearly, this is an important determinant in pediatric fracture patterning and healing which requires additional research.

In terms of timing, healing of pediatric cranial defects occurs at an accelerated rate compared with adults (Hassler and Zentner, 1990; Love *et al.*, 2011; Paige *et al.*, 2006), although this rate has yet to be quantified. Bilo *et al.* (2010) confine their observations of juvenile cranial fracture healing to the "fading" (rounding) of fracture margins, which they (also see Cameron, 1978; Kleinman and Barnes, 1998) note can be observed radiographically 4–6 weeks post-fracture. Uncomplicated linear fractures sustained through birth trauma may not be clearly defined or visible on radiographs after 2–6 months. But it may take up to a year for these fractures to become occult in older children. Ortner (2003) believes the pediatric cranial healing rate is slower than that seen with pediatric postcranial fractures. In spite of all of these observations, Bilo *et al.* (2010:192) state, pessimistically, that "it is impossible to date skull fractures."

9.4 Factors affecting the rate of bone healing

A wide range of variables has been recognized as influencing the rate of bone healing. These can be organized into intrinsic, extrinsic, and biomechanical factors and include age, fracture type, location, severity, treatment, as well as other factors.

9.4.1 The biological profile (age, sex, ancestry)

Age of the individual is recognized as one of the most important variables affecting healing rates (Frick and Jones, 2009; Heppenstall, 1980; Skak and Jensen, 1988). Time needed for fracture healing varies inversely with an individual's age, with the youngest individuals (e.g., below the age of 1 year) exhibiting the quickest healing times (Kwon *et al.*, 2002; Love *et al.*, 2011; Marks *et al.*, 2009). This is primarily because of the significantly thickened periosteum and increased vascularity (and subsequent porosity) of pediatric bone (Rang, 1983). This results in a greater ability to generate an inflammatory response to an injury and bridge the fracture with a periosteal callus well before endochondral ossification of the cartilage model underlying the hematoma begins. Osseous repair is initiated within a few hours after injury in pediatric bone and healing is estimated to proceed at a tempo at least twice the adult rate (Marks *et al.*, 2009; Ortner, 2003). This may be visible macroscopically as early as 4 days and histologically as early as 2 days in young infants (Love *et al.*, 2011; Marks *et al.*, 2009). Dwek (2010) notes that the periosteal cambium layer is thickest during the fetal period, becoming progressively thinner and losing its osteoblastic potential throughout childhood and adulthood. At an older age, periosteal thinning combined with decreased vessel density and number of fibroblasts often makes the cambium layer of the periosteum a very thin tissue indistinguishable from the overlying fibrous layer. Macroscopic evidence of healing may not be visible until 7–14 days post-injury (Mann and Hunt, 2005; Sauer, 1998). Burke (2012) notes that remodeling in pediatric fractures may remove radiographic and CT evidence of them, but this is rarely the case for adult, particularly elderly, fractures.

In the elderly, the effects of age-related osteoporosis have been well documented in the clinical literature. A meta-analysis by Chen *et al.* (2016) of 16 biomechanical studies of ovariectomized rats (those with ovaries removed, leading to reduced estrogen) examines the relationship between fracture healing and osteoporosis development. These researchers document significantly delayed fracture healing in osteoporotic rats compared with controls. Oliver *et al.* (2013) also note a delayed histological healing pattern of cellular differentiation and bone resorption in ovariectomized rats, while Namkung-Matthai *et al.* (2001) note a delay in mature bone production. However, Giannoudis *et al.* (2007) point out that the biological explanation for delayed healing of osteoporotic fractures has yet to be clarified.

Regarding other aspects of the biological profile, Hufnagl (2005) found no correlation between radiographic timing of healing and sex or ancestry. Yeo and Reed (1994) found no correlation between juvenile healing times and sex.

9.4.2 Type, location, cause, severity, and number of injuries

The amount of soft tissue injury serves as an important variable in healing outcome—if this is great, then the blood supply to the fracture site is compromised and the fracture healing schedule may be delayed or even disrupted. In greenstick fractures or other fractures manifesting minimal displacement, no or minimal hematoma develops (see Section 9.4.3). This restricts the signaling of agents that initiate and propel fracture healing on a cellular level. Damage to surrounding muscle is also an important variable in healing outcome—disruption of the muscle–periosteum interface has been shown to inhibit callus development (Malinin and Temple, 2016).

In terms of fracture location, the osteogenic potential of long bones (e.g., the tibia) has been shown to be greater than that in the cranium (Bilkay *et al.*, 2008). But even within long bones, there is variability observed. Rodriguez-Merchan (2005) notes that physeal injuries in pediatric patients heal in less than 3 weeks, regardless of location. Wilkins (2005) notes that the greater vascularity and thus osteogenic potential of the metaphysis compared with the diaphysis results in quicker healing times at the metaphysis. He describes the diaphysis as primarily an area of "dormant osteogenesis." Thus, diaphyseal fractures will likely exhibit longer healing times compared with metaphyseal fractures. Rib fractures, because they exist within a thorax focused on the dynamic movements of respiration, may exhibit delayed healing compared with long bone fractures (Bilo *et al.*, 2010).

Repetitive injury (fractures occurring serially at the same location) also significantly affects bone repair rates. Reinjury of the same fracture site may damage the newly-created vasculature, leading to the development of additional active fibrous and granulation tissue and an "exuberant callus" (O'Connor and Cohen, 1998; Wiersema and Love, 2015). This may significantly delay the healing response (Bilo *et al.*, 2010; Love *et al.*, 2011). Given that the majority of non-accidental pediatric fractures are medically untreated, O'Connor and Cohen (1998:171) note: "every [non-immobilized] fracture is subjected to repetitions of trauma." This may help explain why several researchers (Islam *et al.*, 2000; Marks *et al.*, 2009; Prosser *et al.*, 2005) have postulated healing differences in accidental versus non-accidental skeletal injury—abusive injury typically repetitively targets specific body locations (e.g., thorax and joints). Repeated, untreated trauma in these regions may result in a different healing progression compared with that observed in accidental injury. Sanchez *et al.* (2013:470) suggest that superimposition of fractures through repetitive injury may make fracture dating "impossible."

The effect of cranial injury on postcranial healing has been noted by many clinicians, most notably Perkins and Skirving (1987), Smith (1987), and Spencer (1987). Volume of callus development was significantly greater in Perkins and Skirving's sample of 22 patients with both cranial trauma and femoral fractures compared with the control group of femoral fracture patients with no cranial trauma. Healing time was quicker in those patients with head trauma (mean of 12.4 weeks compared with 15.7 weeks). However, the age of these patients is not presented; also, the mechanism for this correlation is not explained, other than the notation that there must be some kind of "centralized" control of fracture healing within the body. A similar observation in Spencer's (1987) sample of 53 patients (ranging in age from 4 to 67 years) with cranial trauma and limb fractures also supports a correlation between these variables. A rapid and mature layer of new bone is observed peripheral to the fracture site. Spencer describes this abundant healing response as "atypical" and recommends against terming it a "callus." Again, however, no specific explanatory mechanism is promulgated.

9.4.3 Injury treatment and local biomechanical factors

Biomechanical studies of bone have identified a host of intrinsic and extrinsic factors that affect its propensity to fracture and subsequent ability to heal, including type, magnitude, and rate of load, as well as material and structural properties of bone (Agnew and Bolte, 2012; Gonza, 1982; Hipp *et al.*, 1992; Ubelaker and Montaperto, 2011). Perhaps most important for fracture healing and TSI is the concept of fracture mobility and treatment.

Motion at the fracture site significantly affects the healing process in terms of both healing mechanism and timing. Fractures allowing movement after injury are described in the medical literature as "open." These allow a *secondary* healing process involving a periosteal response, abundant callus development, and *endochondral* ossification of this callus. Mobility leads to lesser oxygen tension and greater cartilage and callus formation (Frick, 2015). Sheikh (2000a:2) notes that "the greater the motion at the fracture site, the greater will be the quantity of callus." Many non-accidental fractures seen in forensic autopsy settings, by their occult nature and absence of medical intervention, fall into this category. They may also be seen in a clinical setting when treatment of displaced fractures involves the placement of casts, external fixation, or nonrigid implants such as intramedullary nails which allow some movement (Green and Swiontkowski, 2009; Johnson and Bache, 2008b; Sheikh, 2000a).

Closed fractures (incomplete fractures or those immobilized through rigid compression fixation or other processes) are most typically seen in a clinical context and result in *primary* bone healing (Johnson and Bache, 2008b; Sheikh, 2000a). Fractured ends are in direct contact with one another (or are surgically placed in contact with one another through rigid fixation) and there is limited movement potential. Immobilization of the fracture site leads to a direct attempt by the cortex to bridge the fracture gap through haversian remodeling via *intramembranous* ossification. Because the fracture margins are in contact, osteoclast cutting cones create new enlarged haversian canals through the fracture surface that cross these ends (Heppenstall, 1980; Johnson and Bache, 2008b). New osteons are then directly formed by osteoblasts. Thus, repair of fractured ends occurs through deposition of already aligned mature lamellar bone derived from haversian systems in the bony cortex. If these ends are not in contact, lamellar bone may be deposited at right angles and then remodeled afterward (Dwek, 2010). This type of fracture does *not* elicit the typical periosteal healing reaction described earlier with open fractures and secondary healing (Johnson and Bache, 2008b; Sheikh, 2000b), so significant cartilaginous, fibrous, or external callus may not be present or visible. These modifications to the bone healing process illustrate the potential of bone to heal itself in the absence of the traditional periosteal model derived from endochondral and membranous ossification (Malinin and Temple, 2016). Although this type of healing is most typically seen clinically, it may also be observed for incomplete fractures in a forensic setting. The end result is a *slower* primary cortical bone healing process (Sheikh, 2000a).

Thus, the degree of displacement and subsequent motion potential at the fracture site has direct influence on both its mechanism and rate of repair (Ubelaker and Montaperto, 2011). Recognition of these quite different healing mechanisms (primary vs. secondary) has consequences for TSI estimation. Applying TSI estimates based on medically-treated closed fractures to untreated forensic open ones is problematic and may introduce much error.

9.4.4 Systemic and other factors

Hormones play an important role in bone metabolism and affect bone healing rates. These include parathyroid hormone (important for calcium metabolism and osteoclast stimulation), calcitonin (decreases resorption potential of osteoclasts and osteocytes), and growth hormone and insulin (increase collagen synthesis in bone) (Frost, 1989b; Heppenstall, 1980; Nightengale, 2005). Cortical steroids have been shown to inhibit or retard fracture healing, while vitamin A, C, and D deficiencies have negative consequences for cartilage and collagen production and mineralization (Heppenstall, 1980; Humphries, 2011; Nightengale, 2005). A variety of metabolic diseases have been shown to either reduce or accelerate bone turnover (Resnick *et al.*, 2002); diseases such as diabetes (Kalaitzoglou *et al.*, 2016) and cancer, for example, have been shown to reduce healing potential. Other factors affecting healing rates include exercise, nutrition, irradiation, high doses of hyperbaric oxygen, electric currents, and magnetic fields (Bilo *et al.*, 2010; Brighton, 1980; Ogden, 2000). Health (e.g., bone strength and density) and nutritional status of the individual significantly influence the body's ability to heal (Galloway, 1999; Ortner, 2003; Soto Martinez and Love, 2016; Ubelaker and Montaperto, 2011), although an advanced rate of fracture healing in juveniles compared with adults has been recorded even in malnourished children (Love *et al.*, 2011). Kovaks (2005) notes slower recovery (healing) times with elderly fractures, in part due to increased levels of pro-inflammatory cytokines resulting in immunosuppression, while Meyer *et al.* (2001) attribute slower elderly fracture healing to decreased gene expression.

It is clear from this discussion that there are a multitude of factors that influence bone healing, leading to inhibited or accelerated rates of healing. Any estimation of TSI will need to acknowledge as many of these variables as possible.

9.5 Fracture healing stages and dating systems

Fracture healing stage systems that are available in the medical and forensic literature derive primarily from the clinical setting, relying heavily on radiography. While healing phase and timetable systems for adults are fairly plentiful (e.g., Bilo *et al.*, 2010; Cruess, 1984; Cruess and Dumont, 1975; Cunha and Pinheiro, 2009; Heppenstall, 1980; Maat, 2008; Maat and Huls, 2010) (see a prominent example in Table 9.A.1), given the significant effect of age on healing time, their application to juvenile and elderly healing times is clearly inadequate and likely inaccurate.

O'Connor and Cohen (1998) and Prosser *et al.* (2005) have called attention to the dearth of published information on dating of fractures specifically for children. Published juvenile staging systems and their definitions are summarized in Table 9.A.2. Although the traditional four-stage healing model (inflammation, soft callus formation, hard callus formation, remodeling) is most prominent, published schemata incorporate up to six stages. In these cases, the primary difference between staging systems is the division of the first stage into two components (induction and inflammation) by some researchers. Few scientific studies offer a specific healing timetable—those that do rely heavily on radiology as well as experience of the observer. Many simply repeat prior studies like O'Connor and Cohen's (1987, 1998) classic table, with minor adaptations or adjustments.

O'Connor and Cohen's (1987, 1998) observations of TSI are among the earliest; their system for defining fracture healing is perhaps the most often used by forensic and medical practitioners for pediatric cases. It follows the traditional four-stage healing model but recognizes (and dates) six major "categories" within these. These emphasize the initial appearance of SPNBF, loss of fracture line, and replacement of soft callus by hard and range from as early as 2–5 days for early stage 1 to 2 years for stage 4 physeal remodeling. These are partially based on broad repair rates derived from a literature summary of existing radiographic data of known pediatric fractures, data from experimentally-induced fractures in nonhuman animals, and an admitted degree of anecdotal and experiential evidence (O'Connor and Cohen, 1998; Prosser *et al.*, 2005). These healing times, although often quoted and used, have not been validated by primary research (Prosser *et al.*, 2005).

In their radiographic study of femoral shaft fractures, Yeo and Reed (1994) confine their radiographic assessment of juvenile healing stages to three aspects of callus formation. In the femoral diaphysis, stage 1 is defined as the earliest radiographically visible evidence for fracture. Stage 2 occurs when there is complete bridging of the fracture site, and stage 3 includes the mature callus. The authors present average times for patients to reach each stage (stage 1 = 11.7 days, stage 2 = 18.7 days, stage 3 = 55.3 days) and find no statistically significant correlation of fracture callus development with age or sex; however, their sample size ($n = 25$ children) is small and age range (birth to 14 years) large.

Merten *et al.* (1994) offer guidelines for healing of juvenile diaphyseal fractures based on radiographic milestones. These follow the induction–soft callus–hard callus–remodeling phase system and range from initial radiographic observations of rounding of the acute fracture margin and fat plane disruption due to soft tissue swelling during the first week to initial appearance of SPNBF and early (woven) callus formation at 7–14 days. This is followed by conversion to a hard (lamellar) callus beginning at the earliest by 14 days (peaking 21–42 days). Remodeling begins at 3 months.

Islam *et al.*'s (2000) clinical study of 707 immobilized forearm fracture radiographs of 141 children aged 1–17 years (mean age = 8 years) follows a five-stage bone repair model (induction, inflammation, soft callus, hard callus, remodeling) and evaluates the radiologic appearance of fracture margins, fracture gap, periosteal reaction, bridging and callus development, and remodeling. They find significant variability in appearance of radiological healing indicators but note trends toward the first radiological signs of healing (fracture margin blunting) at 1 week, increased sclerotic density and periosteal reaction after 2 weeks, partial bridging by 3 weeks (although their timetable (figure 6, pp. 78) lists this occurrence at 5 weeks), and remodeling seen as early as 4 weeks but lasting beyond

8 weeks in the majority of all patients. They correctly note the continuously overlapping nature of these healing signatures. However, this study is limited in that it contained a mixed sample of child ages, with only a small number ($n=23$) under the age of 4 years. In addition, few radiographs were taken in the early healing period (below 14 days) and casting preempted observation of many early healing features.

Hufnagl (2005) examines radiographic images from 62 Baton Rouge Orthopaedic Clinic male and female patients ranging in age from 2 to 93 years, with less than half of these below the age of 20 years. All show postcranial limb fractures, the majority of which have undergone internal fixation. Six stages of healing are identified. A rough radiographic timetable is approximated using the initial X-ray date as the date of injury. This date is compared to subsequent radiographs to assess relative healing time. Hufnagl (2005:51) concludes: "To suggest a strong dating timeline for fractures from radiographic observations is not advisable at this point."

Offiah and Hall (2009) do not present finite stages of healing, but instead list radiographic milestones that may or may not be visible as healing progresses. These range from initial presence of soft tissue swelling and loss of normal fat planes to first appearance of SPNBF and development of soft and hard callus. These signposts are correlated broadly with dates ranging from 7 days to 6+ weeks. They also present a mini-radiographic atlas of juvenile fractures derived from a clinical setting. These illustrate "day of presentation" as well as one to four follow-up radiographs taken from day one to a maximum of 16 months post-injury.

More recently, in a comparison of 294 radiographs of known tibial and radial fractures documented from 107 Michigan orthopedic patients below the age of 5 years, Malone *et al.* (2011) illustrate and date six stages of bone healing (modified from Hufnagl (2005)). This six-stage system focuses on evidence for granulation, bridging, and clinical union and presents healing times ranging from 3.3 days for early stage 1 to 750 days for late stage 6 (Table 9.A.2). Malone *et al.* (2011) note that forearm, arm, and upper body fractures have an accelerated healing rate compared with lower body (e.g., thigh and leg) fractures and that healing generally occurs faster in infants compared with older children; however, this differential is not quantified. The considerable overlap of mean healing times and the large standard deviations, particularly in the later stages, are remarkable. Unfortunately, this study is restricted in sample size and applies to the tibia and radius only. It is not known if other skeletal regions (e.g., ribs) exhibit comparable healing rates. It is also not known how well these radiographic healing times correlate with skeletally and histologically-derived ones.

Halliday *et al.* (2011) analyze 161 radiographs of 37 immobilized suspected non-accidental long bone fractures from 31 patients ranging in age from 0 to 44 months with known TSIs. Healing features recorded include blurring of soft tissue planes, presence of SPNBF, definition of fracture line, presence of callus, definition of callus, and presence of endosteal callus; observations of these phenomena are compared via kappa scores across three experienced radiologists. Only the appearance of SPNBF received good (high) agreement between them, generally being observed 11 days post-injury, but in one case, as early as 4 days. Agreement on the other indicators is only moderate. The authors conclude that radiographic assessment of healing time is "unreliable and poorly reproducible" (Halliday *et al.*, 2011:1054), in part due to the absence of standardized fracture terminology. It should be noted that fracture features are not explicitly defined in this study either.

Love and coworkers (2011) summarize healing rates from the radiographic literature using the four-stage system of induction–soft callus–hard callus–remodeling. Although they rely heavily upon previously published radiologically-based timetables, they identify aspects of healing specific to dry bone. For example, they note that first appearance of SPNBF has been observed as early as 4 days in dry bone post-injury. Their illustrative images of dry bone healing in abused infants provide additional observations regarding non-accidental juvenile fracture healing.

Prosser *et al.* (2012) compare digital radiographs of accidental long bone fractures of known timing from 63 children below the age of 72 months. They identify six radiologic features that consistently occur radiographically in healing fractures and can be broadly timed into acute (<1 week), recent (8–35 days), or old (≥36 days) age frames. These features include soft tissue swelling, periosteal reaction, soft callus, hard callus, bridging, and remodeling, which are scored for their presence/absence; a "time band" of percentage of radiographs showing each feature across time is derived from them. The day that each feature is first seen, peaks, and last seen is also noted in tabular form. This study's use of a fairly large number of digital radiographs of young children is its strength; however, these fracture healing stages are based, again, on radiographic visibility of immobilized fractures in a clinical (non-child abuse) setting.

Sanchez *et al.* (2013) take a unique radiological approach by focusing on measurement of callus density in non-accidental rib fractures of 16 infants below the age of 11 months to determine TSI. Callus formation and fracture line morphology (including resorption, gap widening, sclerosis, and bridging) are categorized into six stages each. The authors note that the majority of patients moved in a predictable way through these stages, spending "roughly two weeks" in each stage. Radiographic evidence for rib fracture healing completion is evident in all of the observed infants by 10–11 weeks post-injury. The authors offer radiographically-based callus density measurement guidelines that they propose are a more objective means of determining TSI.

Walters *et al.* (2014) also take a unique approach to estimating juvenile fracture healing times by analyzing radiographs of 131 cases of parturition-related clavicular fractures in infants less than 3 months of age. This study has the advantage of chronicling healing of non-immobilized fractures in very young infants. The focus is primarily on first radiographic appearance of SPNBF (seen generally within 7–10 days) and callus formation (beginning 9–15 days). They note a predictable "evolution" of healing wherein SPNBF becomes thicker and transforms from single layered to solid/multilayered, while callus thickness decreases with fracture age.

More precise estimation of fracture healing times can potentially be accomplished with histological examination of bone, particularly in the early stages (Klotzbach *et al.*, 2003). Marks and colleagues (Marks and Haden, 2002; Marks and Mileusnic-Polchan, 2007; Marks *et al.*, 2006, 2009) have employed light microscopy of histological sections from autopsy samples of non-accidentally fractured juvenile ribs to quantify the degree of SPNBF and establish preliminary estimates of healing rates. They observe SPNBF in as little as 2 days in traumatized children and state that "histological measurement of bone deposition may allow quantification of the time since injury that is not possible using radiographic or autopsy methods" (Marks *et al.*, 2009:215). However, before an actual histologically-derived TSI standard or diagnostic protocol can be established, this method requires systematic study of larger samples of known fractures from documented abuse cases (Marks *et al.*, 2009; Zumwalt and Fanizza-Orphanos, 1990).

There are no, as of yet, unique healing standards published for the elderly, but case studies provide some insight. For example, Delabarde (2008) presents observations of 27 antemortem fractures of an elderly female who died in the conflicts of Kosovo in 1999, possibly as a result of Serbian abduction and torture. The majority of fractures are from the ribs. These fractures are placed into three stages of healing based upon margin morphology and bone proliferation (i.e., callus formation). At least two (possibly three) antemortem events are identified, but no specific timetable is presented. This represents one of the few published forensic antemortem healing observations associated specifically with the elderly.

In sum, researchers have defined a variety of bone repair staging systems, which have been based primarily on radiography but rarely on histology and macroscopic dry bone. They are overwhelmingly focused on fracture healing in pediatric rather than elderly cases. Although there is broad agreement among the majority of these stage/phase systems, some significant problems and limitations are apparent when these are applied to TSI estimation in forensic cases:

1. *Inconsistency in terminology*—Although all schemes are more or less based on the anatomical stages of healing, there are discrepancies in representations of characteristic features making up healing stages. There appears to be confusion, for example, surrounding what constitutes a "soft" and "hard" callus. Many researchers (e.g., Burke, 2012; Heppenstall, 1980; Ogden, 2000; Sheikh, 2000a) define the *soft* callus as comprising the early fibrovascular scaffold that forms the initial bridge between fracture margins. Burke (2012:48) refers to the soft callus as the fibrous collagen and glycoprotein matrix composed of osteoblasts, fibroblasts, and chondroblasts that initially scaffolds the fracture margins (also see Hunt and Van Winkle, 1980). Ogden (2000:251) defines the early callus as being composed of "a thick enveloping mass of osteogenic tissue" that does not contain any bone and thus may be less visible radiographically due to its lucency. However, other researchers (e.g., Campbell and Schrader, 2006; Carter and Beaupre, 2001; Lindaman, 2001; Martin *et al.*, 1998; Merten

et al., 1994; Offiah and Hall, 2009; Ogden, 1990; Ubelaker and Montaperto, 2011) equate the soft callus with the woven, immature bone transformed from this collagen-infused fibrovascular scaffold. In addition, some researchers equate a "callus" with SPNBF (Bilo *et al.*, 2010:190; Halliday *et al.*, 2011).

These definitions significantly affect interpretations of the subsequent *hard* callus. When the soft callus is defined as non-bone or a precursor to bone, then the hard callus is identified as woven bone, which is eventually replaced by lamellar bone in the remodeling stage (Burke, 2012:48–50). But when the soft callus phase is defined as including woven bone, the hard callus becomes interpreted as solely lamellar bone (or the conversion of woven to it). This represents a significant discrepancy across healing staging systems, which has led to widespread misunderstanding and misuse of the terms "hard" and "soft" callus. However, it is only when one considers these as finite stages that these discrepancies in definition become a problem. In reality, they are simply steps along a continuous process, as Marks *et al.* (2009:213) correctly note when they differentiate "fibrous" ("temporary unmineralized scaffold") from primary (woven) and secondary (lamellar) callus formation. O'Connor and Cohen (1998:173) note that deposition of the fibrous/granulation tissue and osteoid/bone tissue is a focal event which can "coexist" and begin toward the end of the first stage of healing—induction. It is clear from this example that creation and use of standardized terminology for fracture healing is greatly needed.

2. *Reliance on radiography*—As has been seen, radiographic-based healing assessments have dominated TSI estimation efforts. Radiographic identification of fractures and assessment of radiographically-derived healing rates have been criticized on many grounds (Catteneo *et al.*, 2006; Halliday *et al.*, 2011; Johnson, 2009; Johnson and Bradshaw, 2015; Messer and Agnew, 2017), to the point that Prosser *et al.* (2005:1282) describe radiological dating of fractures as "inexact." Prosser notes that there is minimal evidence to support many of these radiologically-based staging systems. Radiography performs poorly for identification and interpretation of many antemortem pediatric fractures. Limitations of radiographic evidence for fracture identification and dating include the following:
   - Fractures in some locations (e.g., lateral curvature of ribs, metaphyses of long bones) may be difficult to detect on radiographs due to their occult position.
   - Early SPNBF may not be seen radiographically until it calcifies (by typically 7–10 days post-fracture). Standard imaging technologies may not be able to detect the very thin (<0.5 mm) SPNBF layer evident in some juvenile fractures (Brogdon, 1977, 1998, Brogdon *et al.*, 2003; Chapman, 1992; Kleinman *et al.*, 1995, 1996), although Kleinman (1998c) suggests that the early development of some pediatric SPNBF may not be visible *without* radiographs. Kleinman (1998c) notes that a minimum of 5 days is required for visibility of SPNBF radiographically, but typically more (7–10 days) (also see Brogdon *et al.*, 2013). SPNBF may never develop, depending upon the

nature, location, and treatment of the fracture. For example, as already discussed, CMLs as well as anterior costochondral rib fractures are often not accompanied by SPNBF.

- Callus development is dependent upon the treatment, location, and degree of immobilization of a fracture and thus may not develop or may be difficult to visualize radiographically.
- If a callus is visible, assessing its stage of healing from a radiograph may be challenging—increased density and sclerosis of calluses used to assess conversion of soft to hard callus status are often difficult to observe radiographically, are subjective assessments, and are dependent upon observer experience. Likewise, contouring and remodeling of lamellar bone and resorption of the hard callus are often invisible radiographically.
- Given the substantial healing that occurs quickly in pediatric fractures, healing evidence may become even more invisible to radiographic imaging if not observed during a limited window. This means that a significant number of antemortem fractures are occult on radiographs, particularly in the earlier and later stages of healing (Boyd *et al.*, 2016a; Kelloff *et al.*, 2009; McKinley and Chambliss, 2000; Prosser *et al.*, 2012; Singh *et al.*, 2012).
- In many cases, prior radiographic studies have been based on limited scientific data and have failed to consider intrinsic and extrinsic healing variables such as age and type of fracture. For example, many of them include children of wide age ranges, combining quicker infant healing times with the slower ones seen in older children and adults. And in other cases, type and anatomical location of fracture are not recorded or are combined in healing stages.

Thus, TSI estimations based on traditional radiography face significant limitations and should not be relied on as a sole methodology for fracture identification and estimation of TSI in a forensic (legal) setting. Johnson (2009) and Johnson and Bradshaw (2015) have, therefore, deemed radiographic dating of fractures "difficult" and "imprecise." The use of more sophisticated imaging (e.g., MRI, CT, ultrasound, and bone scintigraphy) has recently been incorporated into investigations of child abuse (Burke, 2012; Dedouit *et al.*, 2008; Dolinak and Matshes, 2005; Hart *et al.*, 1996; Johnson and Bache, 2008a; Kelloff *et al.*, 2009; Mandelstam *et al.*, 2003; Offiah and Hall, 2009; Thali *et al.*, 2009). These technologies offer additional potential for valuable assistance with differential diagnosis and fracture timing, but will not resolve many of these issues. In the meantime, McCormick and Love (2015) have called for revised guidelines for antemortem fracture interpretation based on macroscopic forensic bone samples rather than those based solely on radiology.

3. *Incompatibility across modalities*—Equally problematic is the realization that radiographic-based standards for TSI developed in clinical settings may not be comparable with forensic ones. Although staging systems derived across radiographic, microscopic, and macroscopic modalities have been used rather freely

and interchangeably by past researchers, this is neither ideal nor recommended. Problems with applying radiographically-based healing observations from clinical cases to forensic analysis of non-accidental antemortem fractures include the following:

- Some observations are derived from (and thus only applicable to) radiographs or other imaging modalities (e.g., CT scans or MRIs). These include notations regarding bone density, translucency, and granulation.
- The relevance of these radiological standards to forensic cases is questionable because they are typically based on immobilized fractures in otherwise living healthy children examined in a clinical setting. Per the discussion of anatomical healing, bone healing of immobilized fractures proceeds quite differently (through a different process and at a different rate) compared with mobilized ones.
- Fractures encountered in a forensic context are typically repetitive and complex and may involve forces and locations not typically encountered in an accidental setting.

The result is an array of different TSI timescales that are difficult and likely inappropriate to apply to dry bone. Boyd *et al.* (2016a; see also Garvin and Symes, 2015; McCormick and Love, 2015) have shown that accurate identification and interpretation of antemortem fractures is heavily dependent upon the modality used (gross observation, microscopy, radiology). Specific standards for healing stages should be developed for the appropriate modality used to assess and date antemortem fractures (Boyd *et al.*, 2016b).

4. *Inadequate recognition of extrinsic and intrinsic healing variables*—While most of the current fracture healing stage systems acknowledge the important roles that at least some extrinsic and intrinsic variables (particularly age) have on fracture healing and its timing, none of them allow for or accommodate these variables in their TSI estimations.
5. *Reliance on rigid classification systems*—By their very nature, current healing "stages" or "phases" rely on rigid and finite categorizations of fracture repair and do not accurately reflect the continuous, overlapping nature of the healing process. For example, it has been shown that cartilage and woven bone formation and lamellar bone remodeling can occur simultaneously, with cellular proliferation and resorption functions not limited to any one particular "stage" (Schindeler *et al.*, 2008). Direct comparison of these staging systems illustrates the somewhat arbitrary rigidity imposed upon a continuous natural process. Healing stages are neither finite nor realistic, but continuous and overlapping.

Ultimately, all of the current staging systems for TSI estimation face limitations. More precise *anatomically-based* estimates of healing ranges for infants and the elderly are greatly needed. To be used by forensic anthropologists in a legal context, these estimates should be based on not only macroscopic but also *microscopic and histological* observations of non-accidental fractures in dry bone using standardized terminology. Finally, TSI estimates should be informed by a bone repair process based more aptly on a *process-driven* rather than a temporally rigid theoretical model, one cognizant of the many extrinsic and intrinsic variables affecting bone healing.

9.6 A new model for fracture repair

Little *et al.* (2007) and Schindeler *et al.* (2008) envision bone repair as the culmination of the integrated, but often competing, physiological and cellular processes of bone deposition (anabolism) and bone resorption (catabolism). In the absence of injury, these anabolic (bone production) and catabolic (bone turnover) processes are in a homeostatic state. With fracture, the interaction of these processes is critical to both the formation of the fibrocartilaginous soft callus and its transformation into a hard callus and subsequent remodeling. The outcome of fracture repair is dictated by a "balance between anabolic (bone forming) and catabolic (bone resorbing) responses" (Schindeler *et al.*, 2008:462). Little *et al.* (2007) and Schindeler *et al.* (2008) use these concepts to explain bone repair failures, specifically focusing on inadequate callus formation through either anabolic deficiency or catabolic excess. For example, anabolic deficiency is most commonly linked not only to significant bone and tissue (and concomitant vascular) disruption but also to the influence of older age, disease, and smoking. Catabolic excess may be associated with rigid fixation of fractures through mechanical stimulation of osteoclast production. Ultimately, success of bone repair is determined by both the "magnitude and interaction" of these processes (Little *et al.*, 2007). Bone healing "speed" is determined by the efficacy of these anabolic and catabolic responses, particularly during the earliest phases of nonspecific cellular recruitment and revascularization (Schindeler *et al.*, 2008).

Boyd and Boyd (2017) have integrated these concepts into a new fracture healing model that is applicable to dry bone and reflects the continuous nature of bone repair. This model relies on documenting the anabolic and catabolic-driven fracture healing process with the aid of a digital light microscope ranging in magnification from 5 to 200×. Although all healing features are described with the aid of a light microscope, they are visible macroscopically or through a simple handheld magnifier as well. From these images, skeletal manifestations of anatomical milestones of the fracture healing continuum can be visualized, summarized, and ordinally scored. Healing progression is characterized by the sometimes overlapping appearance of skeletal manifestations of these processual milestones (Table 9.A.3) associated with bone deposition and resorption.

"Nonspecific" anabolic osteoblastic activity predominates in the earliest stages of repair, named as such because it is driven by a generalized tissue injury cellular response not necessarily specific to the bone. This includes the inflammatory recruitment of a variety of cells (e.g., cytokines, growth hormones) involved in tissue injury (Schindeler *et al.*, 2008). Although the accompanying initial signs of bone injury repair (including embedded blood, staining from hemorrhage, and bone necrosis) may be visible quite early microscopically in some samples, the effects of inflammation do not always leave clear markers on the bone that can consistently be used to infer the temporal progression of healing. For this reason, these observations are not included here.

Anabolic osteoblastic activity that *is* observable macroscopically and microscopically on forensic samples includes aspects of bone deposition ranging from initial SPNBF, fibrocartilage, woven, and lamellar bone development and bridging. These can be assessed (i.e., scored ordinally) based on the degree of development of each process:

- *SPNBF* is often an early histological, macroscopic/microscopic, and radiological sign of healing, seen as early as 2 days, 4 days, and 7–10 days, respectively. This variable is scored in terms of the percent of SPNBF development observed both at and peripheral to the fracture site (Figure 9.1). However, it is cautioned that depending upon the fracture type and location, classic SPNBF may not form. As previously discussed, CMLs and other regions may manifest inhibited SPNBF due to the absence of a periosteal cambium layer in the metaphysis.
- *Fibrocartilage and woven and lamellar bone development* is typically broadly associated with "callus" development. Microscopically, this process is first observed as early fibrocartilage initiation and formation (Figure 9.2); it then proceeds with woven bone formation through mineralization of this fibrous matrix (Figure 9.3), followed by replacement of the disorganized and immature woven bone by more mature and organized lamellar bone (Figure 9.4). (Note: Due to the aforementioned confusion in the literature regarding definition of soft and hard callus, "callus" terminology is avoided altogether here).
- Within this fracture healing matrix, *bridging* is initially seen as a fibrocartilaginous scaffolding derived from the subperiosteum (Figure 9.2). This fibrocartilage initially stabilizes (bridges) the fracture but often comes apart and/or disintegrates upon maceration. This necessitates close scrutiny and careful monitoring on the part of forensic anthropologists at autopsy and during processing. With careful (and limited) processing, it can still be observed microscopically. This fibrous scaffold eventually is replaced (through mineralization) with a woven-based and then permanent lamellar bone bridge.

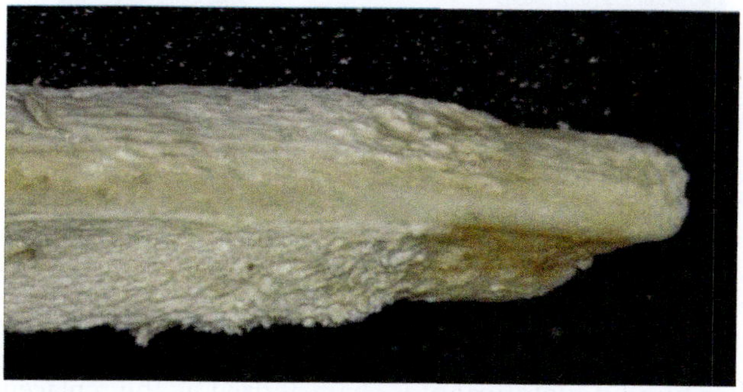

Figure 9.1 Subperiosteal new bone formation (SPNBF): early osteoblastic-driven bone deposition may be seen microscopically or macroscopically as early as 4 days, or may not be seen at all (rib fracture, 27-day old male, 30×).

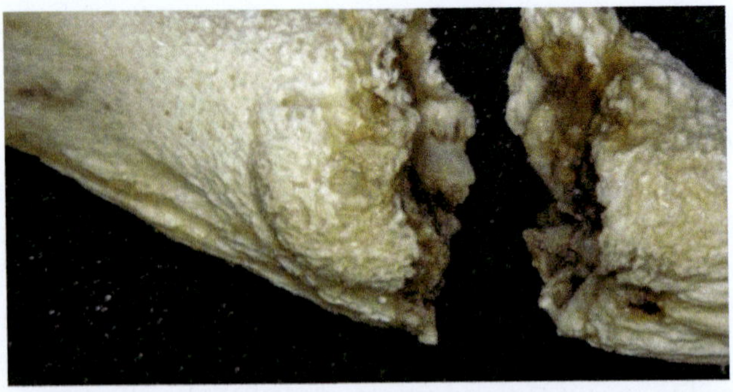

Figure 9.2 Fibrocartilage formation and bridging are seen as a fibrocartilaginous scaffolding derived from the subperiosteum that initially stabilizes the fracture, but may disintegrate upon maceration (rib fracture, 27-day old male, 30×).

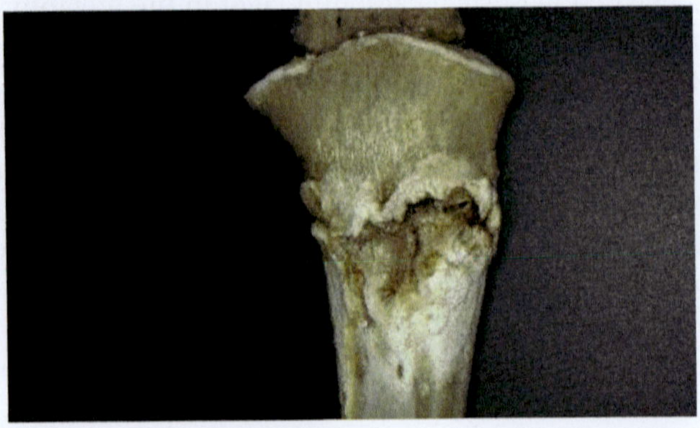

Figure 9.3 Woven bone development is characterized by the mineralization of the fibrocartilaginous scaffold to form woven bone (tibial fracture in a 13-month-old female, 20×).

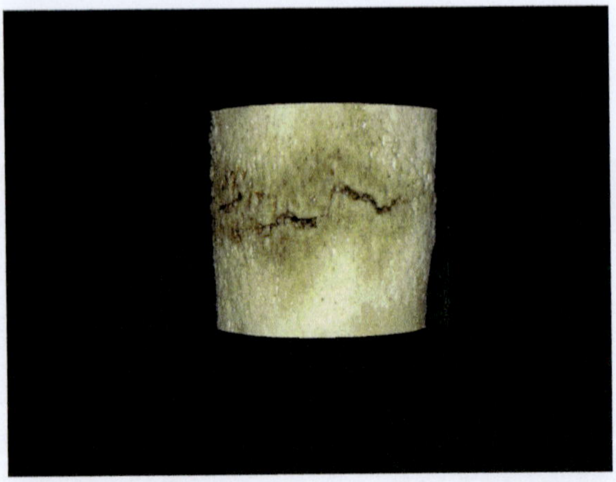

Figure 9.4 Lamellar bone development is characterized by the replacement of immature and disorganized woven bone with mature, organized lamellar bone (radius fracture in a 13-month old female, 30×).

Again, it must be cautioned that "callus" development (and, thus, overt fibrocartilaginous bridging) may not be visible in incomplete fractures or those minimally displaced or immobilized, where bone healing may occur through a primarily intramembranous rather than endochondral process. It is also not likely to be observed at the physis and in the cranium. Extreme displacement of some fractures may preclude the bridging process altogether.

Catabolic processes focusing on bone resorption are, by definition, largely osteoclastic. Although removal of inflammatory tissue is important during the early bone repair stages, many researchers (e.g., Schindeler *et al.*, 2008) have noted that this may not be dependent upon osteoclastic activity but instead a generalized cellular response. Thus, this earliest catabolic response is termed "nonspecific" and is likely to result in one of the earliest observable signs of fracture healing—fracture margin resorption/rounding (see preceding text). True osteoclast-driven catabolic bone and tissue resorption and remodeling are typically seen in middle and later stages of bone repair, namely, woven and lamellar bone remodeling (Schindeler *et al.*, 2008). These processes are influenced by local mechanical forces and play the greatest role in the *strength* of bone repair rather than its speed. Catabolic processes of bone resorption include fracture margin resorption/rounding, fibrocartilage resorption, woven to lamellar bone conversion, and remodeling/callus resorption:

- A healing signature visible quite early microscopically (by day 4 post-injury) is *fracture margin resorption/rounding*, which is assessed here on an ordinal scale based on the percentage of rounding of fracture edges and degree of visibility/obliteration of fracture line (Figure 9.5). Presence of a hematoma early in the inflammation phase stimulates osteoclasts to actively remove (absorb) necrotic

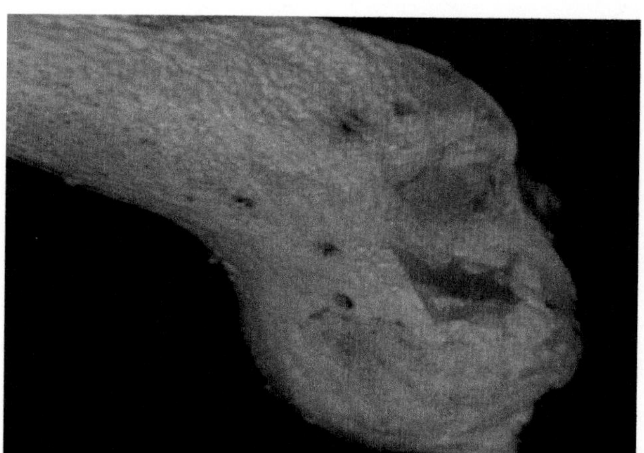

Figure 9.5 Fracture margin rounding/resorption reflects the osteoclastic resorption of necrotic fracture margins, leading to potential obliteration of the original fracture line (rib fracture, 27-day old male, 30×).

bone at the fracture margin. Osteoclastic resorption of necrotic fracture margins may be manifest by a *widening* of the fracture gap during the first week or two post-injury. This resorption process eventually promotes a gradual rounding of the initial sharp, well-defined fracture boundaries. Given more time, fracture line evidence may obliterate; thus, this process may span across the entire healing continuum, from early to late healing.

- *Fibrocartilage to woven bone conversion* reflects the process of fibrocartilage resorption in favor of irregular immature woven bone deposition at the fracture site and is evaluated by the percent conversion of fibrocartilage to woven bone (Figure 9.6).
- *Woven to lamellar bone conversion* reflects the process of woven bone resorption in favor of lamellar bone deposition at the fracture site and is evaluated by the percent conversion of woven to lamellar bone (Figure 9.7).
- *Remodeling/lamellar resorption* (contouring) involves larger-scale regional resorption of lamellar bone following Wolff's Law and other biomechanical principles and can be visualized along a scale of increasing percentages of osteoclast-driven remodeling of mature lamellar bone (although, undoubtedly, osteoblastic bone deposition plays a role here also). Clearly, this is the most temporally broad and unpredictable aspect of bone healing (Figure 9.8).

Figure 9.9a depicts the continuous progression of these anabolic and catabolic processes in bone fracture healing. As can be seen, there is considerable overlap in the features discussed due to the fact that the anabolic and catabolic processes of bone deposition and resorption are *coupled* through much of the healing process. Thus, this coupling process is one that does not lend itself to assigning discrete

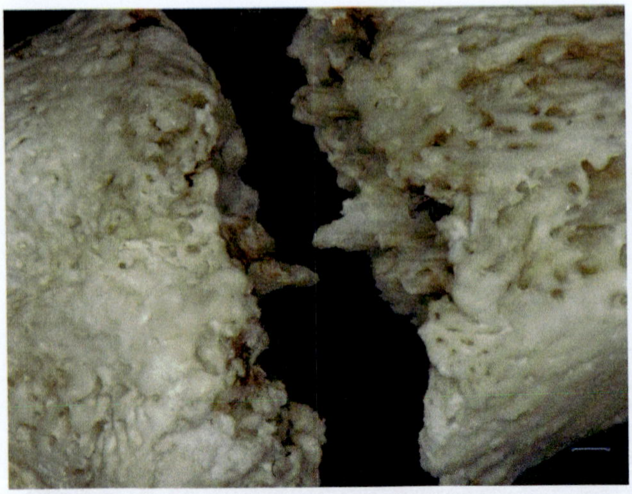

Figure 9.6 Fibrocartilage to woven bone conversion reflects resorption of the fibrocartilage in favor of woven bone deposition (mineralization) (rib fracture in a 10-month-old male, 40×).

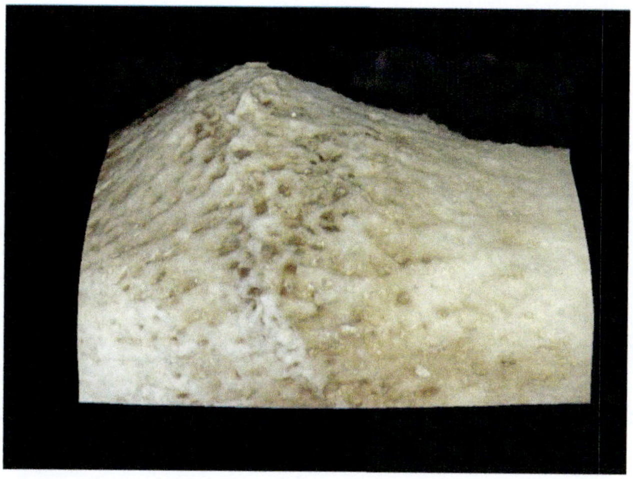

Figure 9.7 Woven to lamellar bone conversion reflects the conversion of woven to lamellar bone at the fracture site (rib fracture, 10-month old male, 40×).

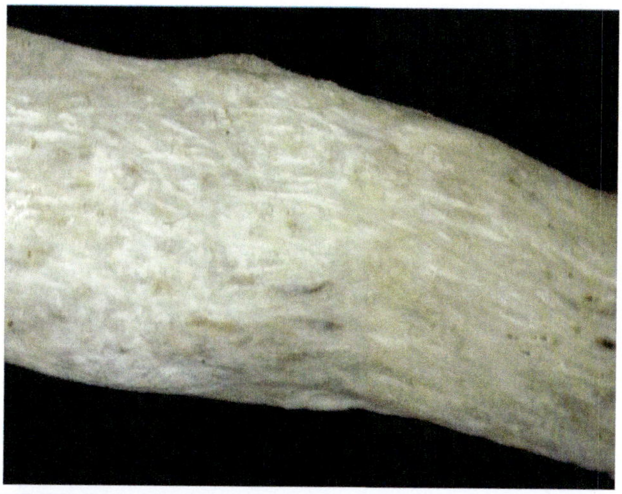

Figure 9.8 Remodeling/lamellar resorption (contouring) involves larger-scale regional resorption of mature lamellar bone (rib fracture, 4-year old male, 20×).

stages or phases. This model has the ability to illustrate the potential effect of extrinsic and intrinsic variables upon the healing process. Figure 9.10, for example, illustrates a projected scenario of reduced anabolic bone healing response that might be modeled in fractures affecting the elderly.

The key to TSI estimation is to assess where an unknown fracture lies along this healing continuum. This is achieved first through accurate knowledge and identification of the skeletal manifestations of the anatomical healing process and then through comparison of these manifestations from unknowns to those

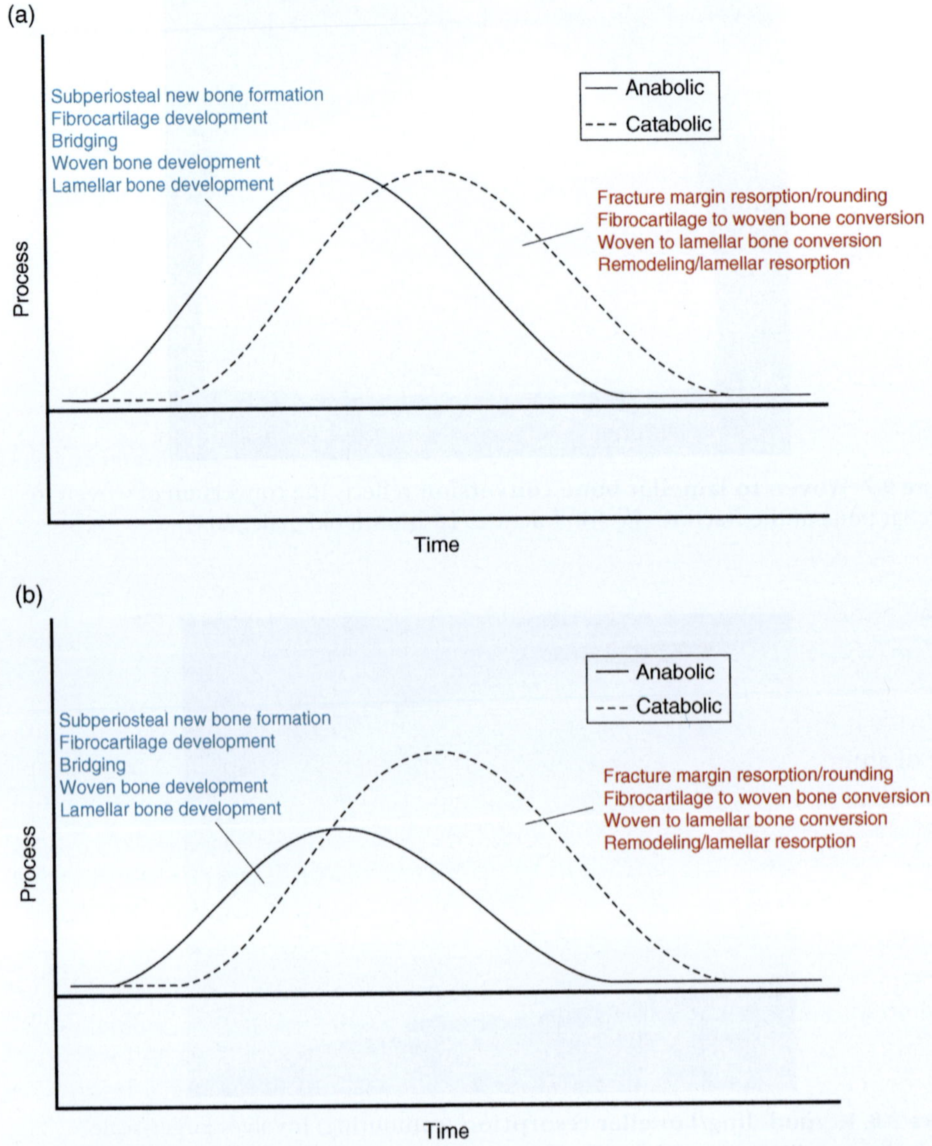

Figure 9.9 (a) Model of anabolic (solid line)/catabolic (dotted line) bone healing response in a normal fracture (Source: Adapted from Little *et al.*, 2007). (b) Model of deficient anabolic bone healing response resulting in lower than normal bone production (Source: Adapted from Little *et al.*, 2007).

from reference fractures—non-accidental antemortem fractures with known TSI dates. However, these samples are currently woefully inadequate for fairly obvious reasons—knowledge of specific TSI for fractures in forensic settings is not common. A definitive and complete TSI timetable for dry bone is, thus, not possible until a comparative fracture database is assimilated. The Antemortem Fracture Archive (AFA) is an important tool for the development of such a database.

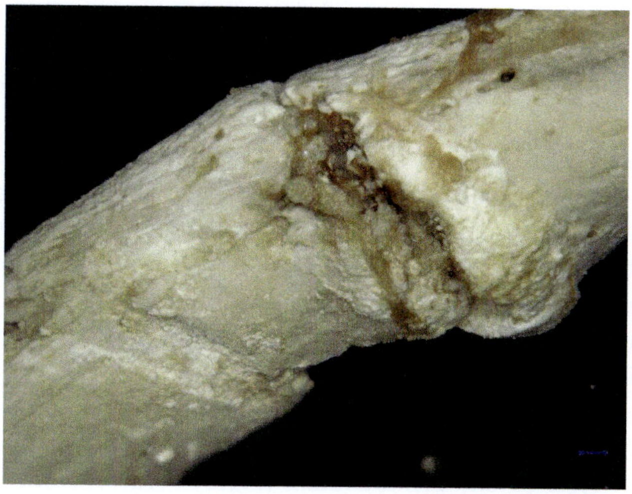

Figure 9.10 Moderate fracture margin resorption and rounding in day 15 individual (rib fracture, 3-month old male, 30×).

9.7 Expanding and refining TSI estimation through the Antemortem Fracture Archive

The AFA is a digital archive consisting of a searchable online (web-based) database of antemortem fracture imagery incorporating macroscopic and microscopic modalities. The database is implemented as a web app, developed in python using a Flask micro-framework and a MySQL database; both the database and website are hosted on a single Linux platform (located at http://bone-trauma.aciwebs.com).

Currently, the archive contains over 2000 digital micrographs of 147 antemortem fractures from 15 individuals (6 females, 9 males) exhibiting non-accidental fatal pediatric, domestic, or elderly traumatic injury. These individuals range in age-at-death from 27 days to 79 years; over half (57%) of the fractures are from juveniles below the age of 4 years. Fracture location is primarily focused on ribs but also includes long bone diaphyses, the clavicle, and the cranium. Each fracture is represented macroscopically and microscopically at magnifications of 5–200×. Forensic practitioners have the ability to add to this database through submission of de-identified antemortem fracture casework to the archive in a variety of modalities (macroscopic, microscopic, radiographic, and histological).

Although the majority of fractures in the database have unknown TSIs, there are currently three individuals within the AFA with known or limited TSI estimates. These include:

- An 8-week-old male who lived 4 days post-fracture (hereafter referred to as "day 4 individual")
- A 3-month-old male who lived 15 days post-fracture ("day 15 individual")

- A 27-day-old male whose fractures are no older than 27 days ("<day 27 individual").

Although limited in scope, the continuous nature of this healing process becomes apparent upon comparison of fractures from these individuals and a broad timetable of TSI estimates can begin to be formed.

For example, a very slight degree of rounding of the fracture margin is observed in the day 4 individual, while the day 15 individual manifests significantly greater rounding and beginning resorption (Figure 9.10). Partial resorption (defined as 25–75% resorption) and full margin resorption (defined as >75%) can proceed fairly quickly in juvenile fractures and can vary within the same individual, as witnessed in multiple right rib fractures from the <27-day-old individual. Beginning obliteration of fracture lines is seen by day 27 for some of the rib fractures (Figure 9.11). No SPNBF was observable in the day 4 individual but fully enveloped ribs from the day 15 and <day 27 individuals (Figure 9.12). Advanced woven bone development and bridging are observed in both the older fractures as well (Figure 9.13). Lamellar bone conversion is moderately seen in the <day 27 individual, coded as 2 (25–75%) (Figure 9.14), but only slightly in the day 15 individual.

Overall, ordinal healing score totals generally correlate with increased TSI. However, there is appreciable overlap in healing features that a finite staging system would not accommodate or explain. The current model of continuous healing based on anabolic (bone deposition) and catabolic (bone resorption) responses allows for a more realistic interpretation of healing as a process (not a finite stage) and, ultimately, has the potential to provide more accurate TSI estimations. It is recommended that light microscopy be utilized in antemortem healing assessments to more readily assess the subtle physiological changes accompanying the healing continuum, which may not be evident radiographically or macroscopically.

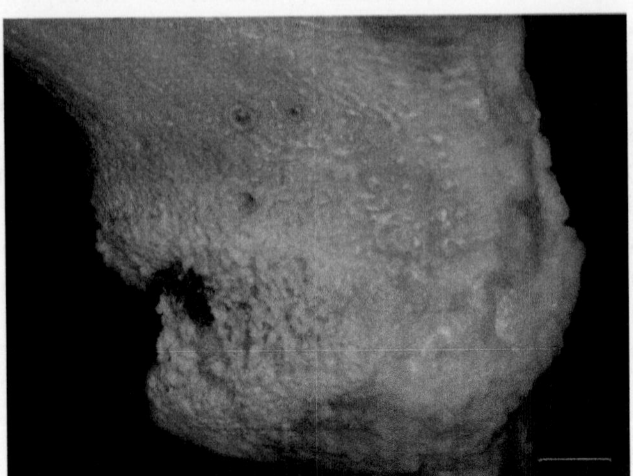

Figure 9.11 Fracture line obliteration in 27-day old male (rib fracture, 40×).

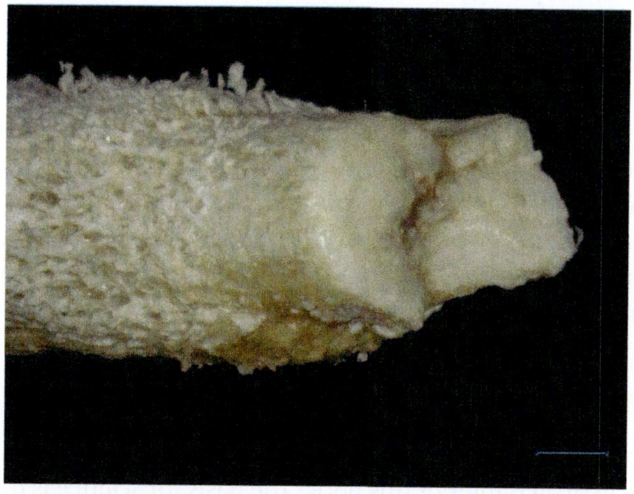

Figure 9.12 SPNBF development in 27-day old male (rib fracture, 30×).

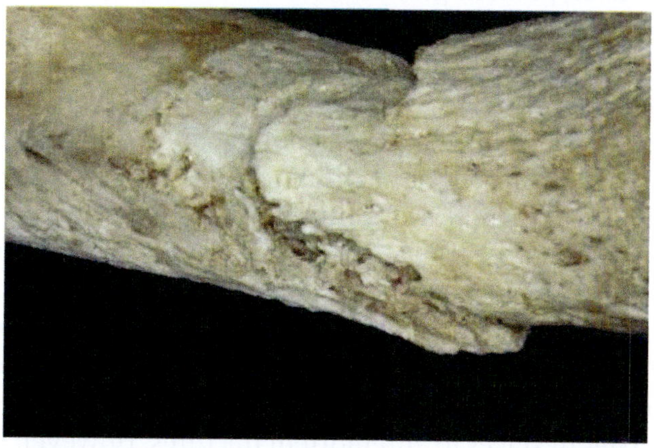

Figure 9.13 Advanced woven bone development in day 15 individual (rib fracture, 3-month old male, 30×).

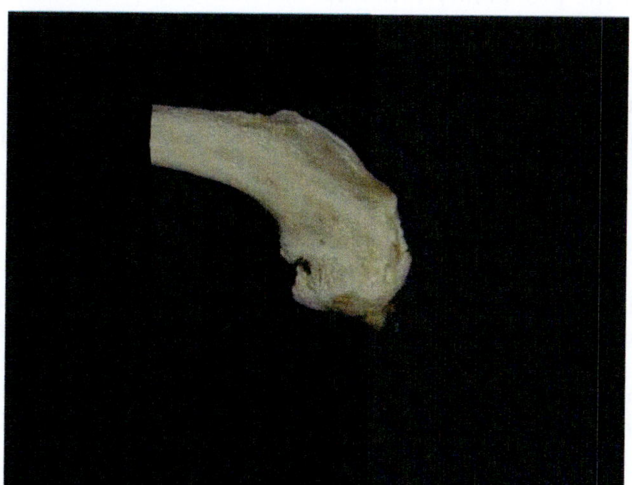

Figure 9.14 Lamellar Conversion in 27-day old male (rib fracture, 20×).

Currently, we do not possess enough samples with known TSI to fit a statistical model capable of predicting TSI from score values. However, with the collection of additional samples of known or limited TSI ranges, the generation of such predictive statistics will be possible. Anatomical indicators reflecting the visual progression of the healing process can be used as dependent variables to predict the independent variable of TSI. With future larger samples in the AFA for comparison, it is expected that this more objective assessment of healing will become possible.

9.8 Theory and the future of TSI estimation

As discussed in the first chapter of this book, the basis for science is theory building, which is dependent upon a cyclical feedback of abductive, deductive, and inductive logical processes. Hypothesis generation is followed by an often arduous period of inductive data collection—this is where the science of TSI fracture determination currently lies. While the theoretical basis for TSI estimation has been described through an anatomical model of the healing continuum, testing of hypotheses regarding TSI estimation awaits the assimilation of larger comparative samples.

Most important is the realization that the choice of theoretical models for interpreting fracturing repair significantly influences TSI estimations: these choices will ultimately affect adjudication of pediatric and elderly death investigations. Use of finite staging systems for understanding and interpreting bone repair results in arbitrary (at best) and inaccurate (at worst) TSI estimations and leads to unrealistic legal expectations of exact TSI dates. Given the continuous and overlapping nature of the fracture healing process, it may never be possible to assign rigorous specific dates or stages to antemortem fractures. However, with additions of forensically-based samples of known TSI to the AFA database, realistic time *ranges* for the skeletal signatures of fracture healing can be tightened, increasing the reliability of the probability estimates for TSI. Thus, while it is true that we face limitations in TSI estimation because of the "unknowable" nature of the timing of many of these fracture events, anatomically-informed microscopically based chronicling of the healing process can lead to more realistic and accurate TSI estimates and adjudication of fatal pediatric and elderly death investigations.

References

Abel, S. M. (2011) Nonaccidental skeletal trauma. In: *The Juvenile Skeleton in Forensic Abuse Investigations* (eds. A. H. Ross and S. M. Abel). Springer/Humana Press, New York, pp. 61–77.

Agnew, A. M. and Bolte, J. H., IV (2012) Bone fracture: biomechanics and risk. In: *Bone Histology: An Anthropological Perspective* (eds. C. Crowder and S. Stout). CRC Press, Boca Raton, FL, pp. 221–240.

AMA Council on Scientific Affairs. (1987) American Medical Association: Council on Scientific Affairs Report: Elder abuse and neglect. *JAMA*, **257**, 966–971.

American Academy of Pediatrics Policy Statement: diagnostic imaging of pediatric child abuse. (2009) *Pediatrics*, **123**, 1430–1435.

Arkader, A. and Skaggs, D. L. (2015) Physeal injuries. In: *Green's Skeletal Trauma in Children*, 5th ed. (eds. G. A. Mencio and M. F. Swiontkowski). Elsevier, Saunders, Philadelphia, PA, pp. 16–35.

Ashraf, N., Meyer, M. H., Frick, S., and Meyer, R. A., Jr. (2007) Evidence for overgrowth after midfemoral fracture via increased RNA for mitosis. *Clinical Orthopaedics and Related Research*, **454**, 214–222.

Baker, A. M., Fulginitti, L. C., Brogdon, B. G., Symes, S., *et al.* (2011) Bones and children: an interdisciplinary approach to forensic issues. *Proceedings of the American Academy of Forensic Sciences*, **XVII**, 12.

Barbian, L. T. and Sledzik, P. S. (2008) Healing following cranial trauma. *Journal of Forensic Sciences*, **53** (2), 263–268.

Barsness, K. A., Cha, E. S., Bensard, D. D., Calkins, C. M., *et al.* (2003) Positive predictive value of rib fractures as an indicator of non-accidental trauma in children. *Journal of Trauma*, **56**, 1107–1110.

Bilkay, U., Tokat, C., Helvaci, E., Ozek, C., *et al.* (2008) Osteogenic capacities of tibial and cranial periosteum: a biochemical and histologic study. *The Journal of Craniofacial Surgery*, **19** (2), 453–458.

Bilo, R. A. C., Robben, S. G. F., and van Rijn, R. R. (2010) *Forensic Aspects of Paediatric Fractures: Differentiating Accidental Trauma from Child Abuse*. Springer, Heidelberg.

Boyd, D. and Boyd, C. (2017) Documenting antemortem time since injury for use in forensic abuse cases through an archival bone database of antemortem fracture healing. *Proceedings of the 69th American Academy of Forensic Sciences*, **XXIII**, 223–224.

Boyd, C., Boyd, D., Roller, S., and Foley, D. (2016a) Comparability of macroscopic, microscopic, and radiologically defined pediatric antemortem healing stages. *Proceedings of the 68th American Academy of Forensic Sciences*, **XXII**, 68.

Boyd, D., Boyd, C., and Roller, S. (2016b) Pediatric antemortem healing standards based on microscopic analysis of fractures in known forensic child abuse cases. *Proceedings of the 68th American Academy of Forensic Sciences*, **XXII**, 130.

Brighton, C. T. (1980) Biophysics of fracture healing. In: *Fracture Treatment and Healing* (ed. R. B. Heppenstall). W. B. Saunders, Philadelphia, PA, pp. 65–79.

Brogdon, B. G. (1977) Child abuse: the radiologists' role. *College of American Pathologists*, **31**, 134–136.

Brogdon, B. G. (1998) *Forensic Radiology*. CRC Press, Boca Raton, FL.

Brogdon, B. G. and McDowell, J. D. (2003) Abuse of the aged. In: *A Radiologic Atlas of Abuse, Torture, Terrorism, and Inflicted Trauma* (eds. B. G. Brogdon, H. Vogel, and J. D. McDowell). CRC Press, Boca Raton, FL, pp. 61–67.

Brogdon, B. G. and McDowell, J. D. (2011) Abuse of intimate partners and of the elderly: an overview. In: *Brogdon's Forensic Radiology*, 2nd ed. (eds. M. J. Thali, M. D. Viner, and D. G. Brogdon). CRC Press, Boca Raton, FL, pp. 279–293.

Brogdon, B. G., Vogel, H., and McDowell, J. D. (2003) *A Radiologic Atlas of Abuse, Torture, Terrorism, and Inflicted Trauma*. CRC Press, Boca Raton, FL.

Brogdon, B. G., Shwayder, T., and Elifritz, J. (2013) *Child Abuse and Its Mimics in Skin and Bone*. CRC Press, Boca Raton, FL.

Burke, M. P. (2012) *Forensic Pathology of Fractures and Mechanisms of Injury*. CRC Press, Boca Raton, FL.

Caffey, J. (1946) Multiple fractures in the long bones of infants suffering from chronic subdural hematoma. *American Journal of Roentgenology*, **56** (2), 163–173.

Cameron, J. M. (1978) Radiological pathological aspects of the battered child syndrome. In: *The Maltreatment of Children* (ed. S. M. Smith). University Park Press, Lancaster, England, pp. 69–81.

Campbell, R. M. and Schrader, T. (2006) Child abuse. In: *Rockwood and Wilkin's Fractures in Children*, 6th ed. (eds. J. H. Beaty and J. R. Kasser). Lippincott Williams & Wilkins, Philadelphia, PA, pp. 223–253.

Carter, D. R. and Beaupre, G. S. (2001) *Skeletal Form and Function—Mechanobiology of Skeletal Development, Aging, and Regeneration*. Cambridge University Press, Cambridge.

Carter, K. W. and Moulton, S. L. (2016) Pediatric abdominal injury patterns caused by "falls": a comparison between nonaccidental and accidental trauma. *Journal of Pediatric Surgery*, **51** (2), 326–328.

Case, M. E. (2008a) Forensic pathology of child brain trauma. *Brain Pathology*, **18**, 562–564.

Case, M. E. (2008b) Inflicted traumatic brain injury in infants and young children. *Brain Pathology*, **18**, 571–582.

Catteneo, C. E., Marinelli, A., DiGiancamillo, M., DiGiancamillo, O., *et al.* (2006) Sensitivity of autopsy and radiological examination in detecting bone fractures in an animal model: implications for the assessment of fatal child physical abuse. *Forensic Science International*, **164**, 131–137.

Chapman, S. (1992) The radiological dating of injuries. *Archives of Disease in Childhood*, **67**, 1063–1065.

Chen, L., Yang, L., Yao, M., Cui, X.-J., Xue, C.-C., Wang, Y.-J., and Shu, B. (2016) Biomechanical characteristics of osteoporotic fracture healing in ovariectomized rats: a systematic review. *PLoS One*, **11** (4), e0153120.

Collins, K. A. (2006) Elder maltreatment. *Archives of Pathology & Laboratory Medicine*, **130**, 1290–1296.

Cooper, C., Selwood, A., and Livingston, G. (2008) The prevalence of elder abuse and neglect: a systematic review. *Age and Ageing*, **37**, 151–160.

Cramer, K. E. (1996) Orthopedic aspects of child abuse. *Pediatric Clinics of North America*, **43** (5), 1035–1051.

Crowder, C. and Stout, S. (eds.) (2012) *Bone Histology: An Anthropological Perspective*. CRC Press, Boca Raton, FL.

Cruess, R. L. (1984) Healing of bone, tendon, and ligament. In: *Fractures in Adults*, Vol. 1 (eds. C. A. Rockwood and D. P. Green). J. B. Lippincott, Philadelphia, PA, pp. 147–167.

Cruess, R. L. and Dumont, J. (1975) Healing of bone, tendon, and ligament. In: *Fractures* (eds. C. A. Rockwood and D. P. Green). J. B. Lippincott, Philadelphia, PA, pp. 97–118.

Cumming, W. (1979) Neonatal skeletal fractures: birth trauma or child abuse? *Journal of the Canadian Association of Radiologists*, **30**, 30–33.

Cunha, E. and Pinheiro, J. (2009) Antemortem trauma. In: *Handbook of Forensic Anthropology and Archaeology* (eds. S. Blau and D. Ubelaker). Left Coast Press, Walnut Creek, CA, pp. 246–262.

Dedouit, F., Guilbeau-Frugier, C., Capuani, C., Sévely, A., *et al.* (2008) Child abuse: practical application of autopsy, radiological, and microscopic studies. *Journal of Forensic Sciences*, **5** (6), 1424–1429.

Delabarde, T. (2008) Case study 5.2: multiple healed rib fractures—timing of injuries in regard to death. In: *Skeletal Trauma: Identification of Injuries Resulting from Human Rights Abuse and Armed Conflict* (eds. E. H. Kimmerle and J. P. Baraybar). CRC Press, Boca Raton, FL, pp. 236–244.

DiMaio V. J. M. and Dana, S. E. (2007) *Handbook of Forensic Pathology*, 2nd ed. Taylor & Frances, Boca Raton, FL.

Dolinak, D. and Matshes, E. (2005) Child abuse. In: *Forensic Pathology: Principles and Practice* (eds. D. Dolinak, E. Matshes, and E. Lew). Elsevier, Amsterdam, pp. 369–412.

Duffy, S. O., Squires, J., Fromkin, J. B., and Berger, R. P. (2011) Use of skeletal surveys to evaluate for physical abuse: analysis of 703 consecutive skeletal surveys. *Pediatrics*, **127** (1), e47–e52.

Dwek, J. R. (2010) The periosteum, what is it, where is it, and what mimics it in its absence? *Skeletal Radiology*, **39** (4), 319–323.

Ferguson, C., Alpern, E., Miclau, T., and Helms, J. A. (1999) Does adult fracture repair recapitulate embryonic skeletal formation? *Mechanisms of Development*, **87** (1–2), 57–66.

Flaherty, E. G., Perez-Rossello, J. M., Levine, M. A., Hennrikus, W. L. *et al.* (2014) Evaluating children with fractures for child physical abuse. *Pediatrics*, **133** (2), 477–489.

Frick, S. L. (2015) Skeletal growth, development, and healing as related to pediatric trauma. In: *Green's Skeletal Trauma in Children*, 5th ed. (eds. G. A. Mencio and M. F. Swiontkowski). Elsevier, Saunders, Philadelphia, PA, pp. 1–15.

Frick, S. L. and Jones, E. T. (2009) Skeletal growth, development, and healing as related to pediatric trauma. In: *Skeletal Trauma in Children*, 4th ed. (eds. N. E. Green and M. F. Swiontkowski). W. B. Saunders, Philadelphia, PA, pp. 1–18.

Frost, H. M. (1989a) The biology of fracture healing: an overview for clinicians, Part I. *Clinical Orthopaedics and Related Research*, **248**, 283–293.

Frost, H. M. (1989b) The biology of fracture healing: an overview for clinicians, Part II. *Clinical Orthopaedics and Related Research*, **248**, 294–309.

Galloway, A. (1999) *Broken Bones*. Charles C. Thomas, Springfield, IL.

Garvin, H. M. and Symes, S. A. (2015) A comparison of radiographic and osteological findings in suspected infant abuse cases. *Proceedings of the 67th American Academy of Forensic Sciences*, **XXI**, 177.

Gerstenfeld, L. C., Cullinane, D. M., Barnes, G. L., Graves, D. T., *et al.* (2003) Fracture healing as a post-natal developmental process: molecular spatial, and temporal aspects of its regulation. *Journal of Cellular Biochemistry*, **88**, 873–884.

Giannoudis, P., Tzioupis, C., Almalki, T., and Buckley, R. (2007) Fracture healing in osteoporotic fractures: is it really different? A basic science perspective. *Injury*, **38** (1), S90–S99.

Gill, J. R., Andrew, T., Gilliland, M. G. F., Love, J., Matshes, E., and Reichard, R. R. (2013) National Association of Medical Examiners position paper: recommendations for the postmortem assessment of suspected head trauma in infant and young children. *Academic Forensic Pathology*, **4** (2), 206–213.

Gironda, M. W., Nguyen, A. L., and Mosqueda, L. M. (2016) Is this broken bone because of abuse? Characteristics and comorbid diagnoses in older adults with fractures. *Journal of the American Geriatrics Society*, **64** (8), 1651–1655.

Gonza, E. R. (1982) *Biomechanics of Musculoskeletal Injury*. Williams & Wilkins, Baltimore, MD.

Green, N. E. and Swiontkowski, M. F. (2009) *Skeletal Trauma in Children*, 4th ed. W. B. Saunders, Philadelphia, PA.

Greenwald, J. A., Mehrara, B. J., Spector, J. A., *et al.* (2000a) Biomolecular mechanisms of calvarial bone induction: immature versus mature dura matter. *Plastic and Reconstructive Surgery*, **105** (4), 1382–1392.

Greenwald, J. A., Mehrara, B. J., Spector, J. A., *et al.* (2000b) Immature versus mature dura matter: II. Differential expression of genes important to calvarial reossification. *Plastic and Reconstructive Surgery*, **106** (3), 630–638.

Griest, K. (ed.) (2010) *Pediatric Homicide: Medical Investigation*. CRC Press, Boca Raton, FL.

Gunther, W. M., Symes, S. A., and Berryman, H. E. (2000) Characteristics of child abuse by anteroposterior manual compression versus cardiopulmonary resuscitation: case reports. *American Journal of Forensic Medicine and Pathology*, **21** (1), 5–10.

Halliday, K. E., Broderick, N. J., Somers, J. M., *et al.* (2011) Dating fractures in infants. *Clinical Radiology*, **66**, 1049–1054.

Harper, N. S., Lewis, T., Eddleman, S., Lindberg, D. M., *et al.* (2016) Follow-up skeletal survey use by child abuse pediatricians. *Child Abuse & Neglect*, **51**, 336–342.

Hart, B. L., Dudley, M. H., and Zumwalt, R. E. (1996) Postmortem cranial MRI and autopsy correlation in suspected child abuse. *The American Journal of Forensic Medicine and Pathology*, **17** (3), 217–224.

Hassler, W. and Zentner, J. (1990) Radical osteoclastic craniectomy in sagittal synostosis. *Neurosurgery*, **27**, 539–543.

Hendrix, R. W. (2002) Fracture healing. In: *Radiology of Skeletal Trauma*, Vol. 2, 3rd ed. (ed. L. F. Rogers). Churchill Livingstone, Philadelphia, PA, pp. 302–230.

Heppenstall, R. B. (1980) Fracture healing. In: *Fracture Treatment and Healing* (ed. R. B. Heppenstall). W. B. Saunders, Philadelphia, PA, pp. 35–64.

Hilton, S. V. W. (1994) Differentiating the accidentally injured from the physically abused child. In: *Practical Pediatric Radiology* (eds. S. V. W. Hilton and D. K. Edwards, III). W. B. Saunders, Philadelphia, PA, pp. 389–436.

Hipp, J. A., Cheal, E. J., and Hayes, W. C. (1992) Biomechanics of fractures. In: *Skeletal Trauma, Fractures, Dislocations, Ligamentous Injuries* (eds. B. Browner, J. B. Jupiter, A. M. Levine, and P. G. Trafton). W. B. Saunders, Philadelphia, PA, pp. 95–125.

Hirsch, F. W., Sorge, I., Roth, C., and Gosemann, J. H. (2016) Accident or maltreatment? Radiographic X-ray patterns in non-accidental trauma: the concept of sentinel injuries. *Radiologe*, **56** (5), 414–423.

Hufnagl, K. B. D. P. (2005) *An Investigation of Time Since Injury: A Radiographic Study of Fracture Healing*. M.A. Thesis, Department of Geography and Anthropology, Louisiana State University, Baton Rouge.

Humphries, A. L. (2011) Basic juvenile skeletal anatomy and growth and development. In: *The Juvenile Skeleton in Forensic Abuse Investigations* (eds. A. H. Ross and S. M. Abel). Springer/Humana Press, New York, pp. 19–31.

Hunt, T. K. and Van Winkle, W. (1980) Wound healing. In: *Fracture Treatment and Healing* (ed. R. B. Heppenstall). W. B. Saunders, Philadelphia, PA, pp. 1–34.

Islam, O., Soboleski, D., Symons, S., Davidson, L., *et al.* (2000) Development and duration of radiographic signs of bone healing in children. *American Journal of Roentgenology*, **175**, 75–78.

Jayawardena, K. M. and Liao, S. (2006) Elder abuse at end of life. *Journal of Palliative Medicine*, **9** (1), 127–136.

Jenny, C. (1994) The state of child abuse medical research—1993. In: *Child Abuse: Medical Diagnosis and Management* (ed. R. M. Reece). Lea and Febiger, Philadelphia, PA, pp. 447–451.

Johnson, K. (2009) Skeletal aspects of non-accidental injury. In: *Calcium and Bone Disorders in Children and Adolescents* (eds. J. Allgrove and N. J. Shaw). Endocrine Development, **16**. Karger, Basel, pp. 233–245.

Johnson, K. J. and Bache, E. (eds.) (2008a) *Imaging in Pediatric Trauma*. Springer, Berlin.

Johnson, K. J. and Bache, E. (2008b) Basic science of pediatric fractures. In: *Imaging in Pediatric Trauma* (eds. K. J. Johnson and E. Bache). Springer, Berlin.

Johnson, K. and Bradshaw, K. (2015) Skeletal aspects of non-accidental injury. *Endocrine Development*, **28**, 247–258.

Kalaitzoglou, E., Popescu, I., Bunn, R. C., Fowlkes, J. L., and Thraillkill, K. M. (2016) Effects of type 1 diabetes on osteoblasts, osteocytes, and osteoclasts. *Current Osteoporosis Reports*, **14** (6), 310–319.

Kelloff, J., Hulett, R., and Spivey, M. (2009) Acute rib fracture diagnosis in an infant by US: a matter of child protection. *Pediatric Radiology*, **39** (1), 70–72.

Kemp, A. M., Dunstan, F., Harrison, S., Morris, S., *et al.* (2008) Patterns of skeletal fractures in child abuse: systematic review. *BMJ*, **337**, a1518.

Kempe, C. H., Silverman, F. H., Steele, B. F., Droegemueller, W. *et al.* (1962) The battered child syndrome. *JAMA*, **181**, 17–24.

Kerley, E. R. (1976) Forensic anthropology and crimes involving children. *Journal of Forensic Sciences*, **21**, 333–339.

King, J., Diefendorf, D., Apthorp, J., Negrette, V. F., *et al.* (1988) Analysis of 429 fractures in 189 battered children. *Journal of Pediatric Orthopaedics*, **8**, 585–589.

Kirschner, R. H. and Wilson, H. L. (1994) Fatal child abuse: the pathologist's perspective. In: *Child Abuse: Medical Diagnosis and Management*. Lea & Febiger, Philadephia, PA, pp. 325–357.

Kleinman, P. K. (1998a) *Diagnostic Imaging of Child Abuse*, 2nd ed. Mosby, St. Louis, MO.

Kleinman, P. K. (1998b) The radiologist's response to child abuse. In: *Diagnostic Imaging of Child Abuse*, 2nd ed. (ed. P. K. Kleinman). Mosby, St. Louis, MO, pp. 383–389.

Kleinman, P. K. (1998c) Skeletal trauma: general considerations. In: *Diagnostic Imaging of Child Abuse*, 2nd ed. (ed. P. K. Kleinman). Mosby, St. Louis, MO, pp. 8–25.

Kleinman, P. K. (2015) *Diagnostic Imaging of Child Abuse*, 3rd ed. Cambridge University Press, Cambridge.

Kleinman, P. K. and Barnes, P. D. (1998) Head trauma. In: *Diagnostic Imaging of Child Abuse*, 2nd ed. (ed. P. K. Kleinman). Mosby, St. Louis, MO, pp. 285–342.

Kleinman, P. K. and Marks, S. C., Jr. (1996a) A regional approach to the classic metaphyseal lesion in abused infants: the proximal tibia. *American Journal of Roentgenology*, **166**, 421–426.

Kleinman, P. K. and Marks, S. C., Jr. (1996b) A regional approach to the classic metaphyseal lesion in abused infants: the distal tibia. *American Journal of Roentgenology*, **166**, 1207–1212.

Kleinman, P. K. and Marks, S. C., Jr. (1996c) A regional approach to the classic metaphyseal lesion in abused infants: the proximal humerus. *American Journal of Roentgenology*, **167**, 1399–1403.

Kleinman, P. K. and Marks, S. C., Jr. (1998) A regional approach to the classic metaphyseal lesion in abused infants: the distal femur. *American Journal of Roentgenology*, **170**, 43–47.

Kleinman, P. K. and Schlesinger, A. E. (1997) Mechanical factors associated with posterior rib fractures: laboratory and case studies. *Pediatric Radiology*, **27**, 87–91.

Kleinman, P. K. and Walters, M. M. (2015) Dating fractures. In: *Diagnostic Imaging of Child Abuse*, 3rd ed. (ed. P. K. Kleinman). Cambridge University Press, Cambridge, pp. 208–216.

Kleinman, P. K., Marks, S. C., and Blackbourne, B. (1986) The metaphyseal lesion in abused infants: a radiologic-histopathologic study. *American Journal of Roentgenology*, **146**, 895–905.

Kleinman, P. K., Blackbourne, B. D., Marks, S. C., Karellas, A., *et al.* (1989) Radiologic contributions to the investigation and prosecution of cases of fatal infant abuse. *The New England Journal of Medicine*, **320**, 507–511.

Kleinman, P. K., Marks, S. C., Spevak, M. R., Belanger, P. L., *et al.* (1991) Extension of growth-plate cartilage into the metaphysis: a sign of healing fracture in abused infants. *American Journal of Roentgenology*, **156**, 775–779.

Kleinman, P. K., Marks, S. C., Spevak, M. R., and Richmond, J. M. (1992) Fractures of the rib head in abused infants. *Radiology*, **185**, 119–123.

Kleinman, P. K., Marks, S. C., and Richmond, J. M., Blackbourne, B. D. (1995) Inflicted skeletal injury: a postmortem radiologic-histopathologic study in 31 infants. *American Journal of Roentgenology*, **165**, 647–650.

Kleinman, P. K., Nimkin, K., Spevak, M. R., Rayder, S. M., *et al.* (1996) Follow-up skeletal surveys in suspected child abuse. *American Journal of Roentgenology*, **167**, 893–896.

Klepinger, L. L. (2006) *Fundamentals of Forensic Anthropology*. John Wiley & Sons, Inc., Hoboken, NJ.

Klotzbach, H., Delling, G., Richter, E., Sperhake, J. P., *et al.* (2003) Post-mortem diagnosis and age estimation of infants' fractures. *International Journal of Legal Medicine*, **117**, 82–89.

Kogutt, M. S., Swischuk, L. E., and Fagan, C. J. (1974) Patterns of injury and significance of uncommon fractures in the battered child syndrome. *American Journal of Roentgenology*, **121** (1), 143–149.

Kovaks, E. J. (2005) Aging, traumatic injury, and estrogen treatment. *Experimental Gerontology*, **40** (7), 549–555.

Kroman, A. M., Symes, S. A., Smith, O. C. B., Love, J. C., *et al.* (2002) The hidden truth: mandibular condylar fractures in child abuse. *Proceedings of the 54th American Academy of Forensic Sciences*, **VIII**, 250.

Kwon, D. S., Spevak, M. R., Fletcher, K., and Kleinman, P. K. (2002) Physiologic subperiosteal new bone formation: prevalence, distribution, and thickness in neonates and infants. *American Journal of Roentgenology*, **179**, 985–988.

Lantz, P. E. and Couture, D. E. (2011) Fatal acute intracranial injury, subdural hematoma, and retinal hemorrhages caused by stairway fall. *Journal of Forensic Sciences*, **56** (6), 1648–1653.

Lee, C. K. and Lathrop, S. L. (2010) Child abuse-related homicides in New Mexico: a 6-year retrospective review. *Journal of Forensic Sciences*, **55** (1), 100–103.

Lett, J. E. (1995) Abuse of the elderly. *Journal of the Florida Medical Association*, **82**, 675–678.

Leventhal, J., Thomas, S., Rosenfield, N., and Markowitz, R. (1993) Fractures in young children. Distinguishing child abuse from unintentional injuries. *American Journal of Diseases of Children*, **147**, 87–92.

Levy, A. D. and Harcke, H. T. (2011) *Essentials of Forensic Imaging: A Text Atlas*. CRC Press, Boca Raton, FL.

Lindaman, L. M. (2001) Bone healing in children. *Clinics in Podiatric Medicine and Surgery*, **18** (1), 97–108.

Little, D. G., Ramachandran, M., and Schindeler, A. (2007) The anabolic and catabolic responses in bone repair. *The Journal of Bone and Joint Surgery*, **89-B**, 425–433.

Loder, R. and Bookout, C. (1991) Fracture patterns in battered children. *Journal of Orthopaedic Trauma*, **5**, 428–433.

Lonergan, G. J., Baker, A. M., Morey, M. K., and Boos, S. C. (2003) Child abuse: radiologic-pathologic correlation. *RadioGraphics*, **23**, 811–845.

Love, J. C. (2016) The value of anthropology in medicolegal death investigation of pediatric non-accidental injury. *Academic Forensic Pathology*, **6** (3), 478–485.

Love, J. C. and Sanchez, L. (2009) Recognition of skeletal fractures in infants: an autopsy technique. *Journal of Forensic Sciences*, **54** (6), 1443–1446.

Love, J. C., Derrick, S. M., and Wiersema, J. M. (2011) *Skeletal Atlas of Child Abuse*. Springer/Humana Press, New York.

Love, J. C., Derrick, S. M., Wiersema, J. M., *et al.* (2013) Novel classification system of rib fractures observed in infants. *Journal of Forensic Sciences*, **58** (2), 330–335.

Love, J. C., Wiersema, J. M., Derrick, S. M., and Haden-Pinneri, K. (2014) The value of the pediatric skeletal examination in the autopsy of children. *Academic Forensic Pathology*, **4** (1), 100–108.

Maat, G. J. R. (2008) Case study 5.3: dating of fractures in human dry bone tissue—the Berisha case. In: *Skeletal Trauma: Identification of Injuries Resulting from Human Rights Abuse and Armed Conflict* (eds. E. H. Kimmerle and J. P. Baraybar). CRC Press, Boca Raton, FL, pp. 245–254.

Maat, G. J. R. and Huls, N. (2010) Histological fracture dating of fresh and dried bone tissue. In: *Forensic Aspects of Paediatric Fractures: Differentiating Accidental Trauma from Child Abuse.* (eds. R. A. C. Bilo, S. G. F. Robben, and R. R. van Rijn). Springer, Heidelberg, pp. 194–201.

Malinin, T. I. and Temple, T. (2016) Fracture healing: an overview of existing concepts. *Current Orthopaedic Practice,* **27** (2), 192–197.

Malone, C. A., Sauer, N. J., and Fenton, T. W. (2011) A radiographic assessment of pediatric fracture healing and time since injury. *Journal of Forensic Sciences,* **56** (5), 1123–1130.

Mandelstam, S. A., Cook, D., Fitzgerald, M., and Ditchfield, M. R. (2003) Complementary use of radiological skeletal survey and bone scintigraphy in detection of bony injuries in suspected child abuse. *Archives of Disease in Childhood,* **88**, 387–390.

Mann, R. W. and Hunt, D. R. (2005) *Photographic Regional Atlas of Bone Disease,* 2nd ed. Charles C. Thomas, Springfield, IL.

Maples, W. R. (1986) Trauma analysis by the forensic anthropologist. In: *Forensic Osteology: Advances in the Identification of Human Remains,* 1st ed. (ed. K. J. Reichs). Charles C. Thomas, Springfield, IL, pp. 218–228.

Marks, S. C., Jr. (1998) The structural and developmental contexts of skeletal injury. In: *Diagnostic Imaging of Child Abuse,* 2nd ed. (ed. P. K. Kleinman). Mosby, St. Louis, MO, pp. 2–7.

Marks, M. K. and Haden, K. H. (2002) Child abuse case: multiple forensic issues. *Proceedings of the American Academy of Forensic Sciences,* **VIII**, 250.

Marks, M. K. and Mileusnic-Polchan, P. (2007) Histopathology of antemortem infant bone fractures: estimation of time since insult. *Proceedings of the 59th American Academy of Forensic Sciences,* **XIII**, 315.

Marks, M. K., Tersigni, M. A., and Mileusnic-Polchan, D. (2006) Antemortem infant rib fracture: the histological evidence. *Proceedings of the 58th American Academy of Forensic Sciences,* **XII**, 307.

Marks, M. K., Marden, K., and Mileusnic-Polchan, D. (2009) Forensic osteology of child abuse. In: *Hard Evidence: Case Studies in Forensic Anthropology,* 2nd ed. (ed. D. W. Steadman). Prentice-Hall, Upper Saddle River, NJ, pp. 205–220.

Martin, R. B., Burr, D. B., and Sharkey, N. A. (1998) *Skeletal Tissue Mechanics.* Springer, New York.

McCormick, L. E. and Love, J. C. (2015) Healing rates of antemortem injuries to bone. *Proceedings of the 67th American Academy of Forensic Sciences,* **XXI**, 184.

McGraw, E. P., Pless, J. E., Pennington, D. J., and White, S. J. (2002) Postmortem radiography after unexpected death in neonates, infants, and children: should imaging be routine? *American Journal of Roentgenology,* **178**, 1517–1521.

McKibbin, B. (1978) The biology of fracture healing in long bones. *The Journal of Bone and Joint Surgery,* **60B** (2), 150–162.

McKinley, D. W. and Chambliss, M. L. (2000) Follow-up radiographs to detect callus formation after fractures. *Archives of Family Medicine,* **9**, 373–374.

Merten, D., Kirks, D., and Ruderman, R. (1981) Occult humeral epiphyseal fractures in battered infants. *Pediatric Radiology,* **10**, 151–154.

Merten, D., Radlowski, M., and Leonidas, J. (1983) The abused child: a radiological reappraisal. *Radiology,* **146**, 377–381.

Merten, D. F., Cooperman, D. R., and Thompson, G. H. (1994) Skeletal manifestations of child abuse. In: *Child Abuse: Medical Diagnosis and Management* (ed. R. M. Reece). Lea and Febiger, Philadelphia, PA, pp. 23–53.

Messer, D. L. and Agnew, A. M. (2017) Exploring the gap between anthropological and clinical literature on pediatric fracture healing. *Proceedings of the 69th American Academy of Forensic Sciences,* **XXIII**, 182–183.

Meyer, R. A., Meyer, M. H., Phieffer, L. S., and Banks, D. M. (2001) Delayed union of femoral fractures in older rats: decreased gene expression. *BMC Musculoskeletal Disorders*, **2**, 2.

Namkung-Matthai, H., Appleyard, R., Jansen, J., Hao, L., *et al.* (2001) Osteoporosis influences the early period of fracture healing in a rat osteoporotic model. *Bone*, **28** (1), 80–86.

Ng, C. S. and Hall, C. M. (1998) Costochondral junction fractures and intra-abdominal trauma in non-accidental injury (child abuse). *Pediatric Radiology*, **28**, 671–676.

Nightengale, J. (2005) Anatomy, physiology, and pathology of the skeletal system. In: *Interpreting Trauma Radiographs* (eds. J. McConnell, R. Eyres, and J. Nightengale). Blackwell, Oxford, pp. 63–105.

O'Connor, J. F. and Cohen, J. (1987) Dating fractures. In: *Diagnostic Imaging of Child Abuse*, 1st ed. (ed. P. K. Kleinman). Williams & Wilkins, Baltimore, MD.

O'Connor, J. F. and Cohen, J. (1998) Dating fractures. In: *Diagnostic Imaging of Child Abuse*, 2nd ed (ed. P. K. Kleinman). Williams & Wilkins, Baltimore, MD, pp. 168–177.

Offiah, A. C. and Hall, C. M. (2009) *Radiological Atlas of Child Abuse*. Radcliffe Publishing, Oxford.

Ogden, J. A. (1990) Biology of chondro-osseous repair. In: *Skeletal Injury in the Child*, 2nd ed. (ed. J. A. Ogden). W. B. Saunders, Philadelphia, PA, pp. 175–198.

Ogden, J. A. (2000) Biology of repair of the immature skeleton. In: *Skeletal Injury in the Child*, 3rd ed (ed. J. A. Ogden). Springer, New York, pp. 243–268.

Oliver, R. A., Yu, Y., Yee, G., Low, A. K., Diwan, A. D., and Walsh, W. R. (2013) Poor histological healing of a femoral fracture following 12 months of oestrogen deficiency in rats. *Osteoporosis International*, **24** (10), 2581–2589.

Ortner, D. J. (2003) *Identification of Pathological Conditions of Human Skeletal Remains*, 2nd ed. Academic Press, Amsterdam.

Paige, K. T., Vega, S. J., Kelly, C. P., *et al.* (2006) Age-dependent closure of bony defects after frontal orbital advancement. *Plastic and Reconstructive Surgery*, **118**, 977–984.

Pergolizzi, R. J. and Oestreich, A. (1995) Child abuse fracture through physiological periosteal reaction. *Pediatric Radiology*, **25**, 566–567.

Perkins, R. and Skirving, A. (1987) Callus formation and the rate of healing of femoral fractures in patients with head injuries. *Journal of Bone and Joint Surgery (British)*, **69**, 521–524.

Pillemer, K. and Finkelhor, D. (1988) The prevalence of elder abuse: a random sample survey. *Gerontologist*, **28**, 51–57.

Pinto, D. C., Love, J. C., Derrick, S. M., *et al.* (2015) A proposed scheme for classifying pediatric rib head fractures using case examples. *Journal of Forensic Sciences*, **60** (1), 112–117.

Prosser, I., Maguire, S., Harrison, S. K., Mann, M., *et al.* (2005) How old is this fracture? Radiologic dating of fractures in children: a systematic review. *American Journal of Roentgenology*, **184**, 1282–1286.

Prosser, I., Lawson, Z., Evans, A., Harrison, S., *et al.* (2012) A timetable for the radiologic features of fracture healing in young children. *American Journal of Roentgenology*, **198**, 1014–1020.

Ragan, K. L. (2011) Fatal child maltreatment: the challenges of identifying the causes and incidence of deaths from abuse and neglect. In: *The Juvenile Skeleton in Forensic Abuse Investigations* (eds. A. H. Ross and S. M. Abel). Springer/Humana Press, New York, pp. 7–17.

Rang, M. (1983) *Children's Fractures*, 2nd ed. J. B. Lippincott, Philadelphia, PA.

Reece, R. M. (1994) *Child Abuse: Medical Diagnosis and Management*. Lea and Febiger, Philadelphia, PA.

Resnick, D., Manolagas, S., and Fallon, M. (2002) Histogenesis, anatomy and physiology of bone. In: *Diagnosis of Bone and Joint Disorders*, Vol. **4** (ed. D. Resnick). W. B. Saunders, Philadelphia, PA, pp. 647–687.

Riezzo, I. (2010) Pediatric and fetal autopsies. In: *Forensic Autopsy: A Handbook and Atlas* (eds. C. Pomara, S. B. Karch, and V. Fineschi). CRC Press, Boca Raton, FL, pp. 79–98.

Rodriguez-Martin, C. (2006) Identification and differential diagnosis of traumatic lesions of the skeleton. In: *Forensic Anthropology and Medicine: Complementary Sciences from Recovery to Cause of Death* (eds. A. Schmitt, E. Cunha, and J. Pinheiro). Humana Press, Totowa, NJ, pp. 197–221.

Rodriguez-Merchan, E. C. (2005) Pediatric skeletal trauma: a review and historical perspective. *Clinical Orthopaedics and Related Research*, **432**, 8–13.

Rosenberg, A. E. (2015) The skeleton: structure, growth and development, and basis of skeletal injury. In: *Diagnostic Imaging of Child Abuse*, 3rd ed. (ed. P. K. Kleinman). Cambridge University Press, Cambridge, pp. 9–22.

Ross, A. H. and Abel, S. M. (eds.) (2011) *The Juvenile Skeleton in Forensic Abuse Investigations*. Springer/Humana Press, New York.

Salter, R. B. (1980) Birth and pediatric fractures. In: *Fracture Treatment and Healing* (ed. R. B. Heppenstall). W. B. Saunders, Philadelphia, PA, pp. 189–234.

Sanchez, T. R., Nguyen, H., Palacios, W., Doherty, M., and Coulter, K. (2013) Retrospective evaluation and dating of non-accidental rib fractures in infants. *Clinical Radiology*, **68** (8), e467–e471.

Sauer, N. J. (1998) The timing of injuries and manner of death: distinguishing among antemortem, perimortem, and postmortem trauma. In: *Forensic Osteology: Advances in the Identification of Human Remains*, 1st ed. (ed. K. J. Reichs). Charles C. Thomas, Springfield, IL, pp. 321–332.

Sauer, N. J. and Dunlap, S. S. (1985) The asymmetrical remodeling of two neurosurgical burr holes: a case study. *Journal of Forensic Sciences*, **30**, 953–957.

Scheuer, L. and Black, S. (2000) *Developmental Juvenile Osteology*. Elsevier, Amsterdam.

Scheuer, L. and Black, S. (2004) *The Juvenile Skeleton*. Elsevier, London.

Schiller, A. L. and Teitelbaum, S. L. (1999) Bones and joints. In: *Pathology*, 3rd ed. (eds. E. Rubin and J. L. Farber). Lippincott-Raven, Philadephia, PA, pp. 1354–1356.

Schindeler, A., McDonald, M. M., Bokko, P., and Little, D. G. (2008) Bone remodeling during fracture repair: the cellular picture. *Seminars in Cell and Developmental Biology*, **19** (5), 459–466.

Sevitt, S. (1981) *Bone Repair and Fracture Healing in Man*. Churchill Livingstone, Edinburgh.

Shapiro, F. (2008) Bone development and its relation to fracture repair: the role of mesenchymal osteoblasts and surface osteoblasts. *European Cells & Materials*, **15**, 53–76.

Sheikh, B. (2000a) Bone healing. In: *Treatment and Rehabilitation of Fractures*, 1st ed. (eds. S. Hoppenfield and V. L. Murthy). Lippincott Williams & Wilkins, Philadelphia, PA, pp. 1–6.

Sheikh, B. (2000b) Determining when a bone fracture has healed. In: *Treatment and Rehabilitation of Fractures*, 1st ed. (eds. S. Hoppenfield and V. L. Murthy). Lippincott Williams & Wilkins, Philadelphia, PA, pp. 7–10.

Shilt, J. and McPherson, P. (2015) Nonaccidental trauma. In: *Green's Skeletal Trauma in Children*, 5th ed. (eds. G. A. Mencio and M. F. Swiontkowski). Elsevier, Saunders, Philadelphia, PA, pp. 543–563.

Shipman, P., Walker, A., and Bichell, D. (1985) *The Human Skeleton*. Harvard University Press, Cambridge, MA.

Shopfner, C. E. (1966) Periosteal bone growth in normal infants. A preliminary report. *The American Journal of Roentgenology, Radium Therapy, and Nuclear Medicine*, **97**, 154–163.

Silverman, F. N. (1953). The roentgen manifestations of unrecognized skeletal trauma in infants. *American Journal of Roentgenology*, **69** (3), 413–427.

Singh, R., Squires, J., Fromkin, J. B., and Berger, R. P. (2012) Assessing the use of follow-up skeletal surveys in children with suspected physical abuse. *Journal of Trauma and Acute Care Surgery*, **73** (4), 972–976.

Skak, S. V. and Jensen, T. T. (1988) Femoral shaft fractures in 265 children: log-normal correlation with ages of speed of healing. *Acta Orthopaedica Scandinavica*, **59**, 704–707.

Smith, R. (1987) Head injury, fracture healing and callus. *The Journal of Bone and Joint Surgery*, **69**, 518–520.

Soto Martinez, M. E. and Love, J. C. (2016) Infant bone health: an evaluation of quantitative ultrasound. *Proceedings of the 68th American Academy of Forensic Sciences*, **XXII**, 160.

Spencer, R. (1987) The effect of head injury on fracture healing: a quantitative assessment. *Journal of Bone and Joint Surgery (British)*, **69**, 525–528.

Steyn, M., DeBoer, H., and Van der Merwe, A. E. (2014) Cranial trauma and the assessment of posttraumatic survival time. *Forensic Science International*, **244**, e25–e29.

Strouse, P. J. and Owings, C. L. (1995) Fractures of the first rib in child abuse. *Radiology*, **197** (3), 763–765.

Thali, M. J., Dirnhofer, R. and Vock, P. (2009) *The Virtopsy Approach: 3D Optical and Radiological Scanning and Reconstruction in Forensic Medicine*. CRC Press, Boca Raton, FL.

Thali, M. J., Viner, M. D., and Brogdon, B. G. (2011) *Brogdon's Forensic Radiology*, 2nd ed. CRC Press, Boca Raton, FL.

Thomsen, T. K., Elle, B., and Thomsen, J. L. (1997) Post-mortem radiological examination in infants: evidence of child abuse? *Forensic Science International*, **90**, 223–230.

Thorpe, E. L., Zuckerbraun, N. S., Wolford, J. E., and Berger, R. P. (2014) Missed opportunities to diagnose child physical abuse. *Pediatric Emergency Care*, **30** (11), 771–776.

Ubelaker, D. H. and Montaperto, K. M. (2011) Biomechanical and remodeling factors in the interpretation of fractures of juveniles. In: *The Juvenile Skeleton in Forensic Abuse Investigations* (eds. A. H. Ross and S. M. Abel). Springer/Humana Press, New York, pp. 33–48.

Volberg, F. M., Whalen, J. P., Krook, L., and Winchester, P. (1977) Lamellated periosteal reactions: a radiologic and histologic investigation. *American Journal of Roentgenology*, **128**, 85–87.

Walker, P. L., Cook, D. C., and Lambert, P. M. (1997) Skeletal evidence for child abuse: a physical anthropological perspective. *Journal of Forensic Sciences*, **42**, 196–207.

Walters, M. M., Forbes, P. W., Buonoma, C., and Kleinman, P. K. (2014) Healing patterns of clavicular birth injuries as a guide to fracture dating in cases of possible infant abuse. *Pediatric Radiology*, **44** (10), 1224–1229.

Wedell, V. and Galloway, A. (2014) *Broken Bones*, 2nd ed. Charles C. Thomas, Springfield, IL.

Wiersema, J. M. and Love, J. C. (2015) Skeletal injuries in cases of child abuse: two case studies from the Harris County Institute of Forensic Science. In: *Skeletal Trauma Analysis: Case Studies in Context* (eds. N. V. Passalacqua and C. W. Rainwater). John Wiley & Sons, Ltd, Chichester, UK, pp. 42–55.

Wiersema, J. M., Love, J. C., Derrick, S. M., *et al.* (2014) Standardized descriptive method for the anthropological evaluation of pediatric skull fractures. *Journal of Forensic Sciences*, **59** (6), 1487–1492.

Wilkins, K. E. (2005) Principles of fracture remodeling in children. *Injury—International Journal of the Care of the Injured*, **36**, S-A3–S-A11.

Wolf, R. S. (1988) Elder abuse: ten years later. *Journal of the American Geriatrics Society*, **36**, 758–762.

Worlock, P., Stower, M., and Barbor, P. (1986) Patterns of fractures in accidental and non-accidental injury in children: a comparative study. *BMJ*, **293**, 100–102.

Yeo, L. and Reed, M. (1994) Staging of healing of femoral fractures in children. *Canadian Association of Radiologists Journal*, **45**, 16–19.

Zumwalt, R. and Fanizza-Orphanos, A. (1990) Dating of healing rib fractures in fatal child abuse. In: *Advances in Pathology*, Vol. 3 (eds. C. Fenoglio-Presier and R. Weinstein). Wolf Publishing, London, pp. 193–205.

Appendix A

Major fracture repair stages and TSI estimations

Table 9.A.1 Major fracture repair stages for adults

Heppenstall (1980:41–45) (radiography)
Stage 1—Inflammation
• Disruption of vascular supply, hemorrhage, hematoma formation
• Hypoxic, acidic environment
• Necrosis of bone at fx margin (endosteal and periosteal)
• Disruption of osteons and lacunae, leading to release of enzymes
• Removal of dead tissue and by-products by macrophages
• Activation of fibroblasts to initiate fx repair
• Osteoclast activation leads to osteolytic activity at cell borders
Stage 2—Soft callus
• Proliferation of osteoblasts in periosteal layer forms external callus and soft tissue collar
• Development of internal callus
Stage 3—Hard callus
• Conversion of external and internal callus to fiber (immature) bone
• Increased vascularity and cellularity
• Firm union w/ new bone
Stage 4—Remodeling
• Gradual conversion of fiber (woven) bone to lamellar bone by osteoclasts (external surface and medullary cavity)

Source: Adapted from Heppenstall, 1980.

Table 9.A.2 Major fracture repair staging systems for juveniles

O'Connor and Cohen (1987, 1998) (radiography)
Stage 1—Induction (early = 2–5 days; peak = 4–10 days; late = 10–21 days)
• Resolution of soft tissues
• Deposition of fibrous/granulation tissue and osteoid/bone tissue
Stage 2—Soft callus
• SPNBF visible **(early = 4–10 days, peak = 10–14 days; late = 14–21 days)**
• Loss of fx line definition **(early = 10–14 days; peak = 14–21 days)**
• Soft callus formation **(early = 10–14 days; peak = 14–21 days)**
Stage 3—Hard callus (early = 14–21 days; peak = 21–42 days; late = 42–90 days)
Stage 4—Remodeling (early = 3 months; peak = 1 year; late = 2 years to physeal closure)

(Continued)

Table 9.A.2 (Continued)

Yeo and Reed (1994) (radiography; femoral diaphysis)

Stage 1—Earliest radiographically visible evidence for fracture **(*x* = 11.7 days)**
Stage 2—Complete bridging of the fracture site **(*x* = 18.7 days)**
Stage 3—Mature callus **(*x* = 55.3 days)**

Merten *et al.* (1994) (radiography; diaphyseal)

Phase I—Induction (0–7 days)
- Soft tissue swelling
- Displacement/obliteration of normal fat and fascial planes
- Reducing definition of sharp acute fx line

Phase II—Soft callus (beginning 7–10 days in young children; 10–14 in older children)
- Appearance of SPNBF
- Callus formation at fx site

Phase III—Hard callus (begins 14–21 days; peaks 21–42 days)
- Conversion of periosteal and endosteal bone to lamellar bone
- Radiological solid union at fx site

Phase IV—Remodeling (begins at 3 months; peaks 1–2 years)
- Restoration of bony configuration
- Correction of deformity

Islam *et al.* (2000) (radiography; 1–17 years; forearm diaphysis)

Stages 1—Induction (0–3 week range)
Stage 2—Inflammation
- Loss of fx line definition (peaks 2–3 weeks post-injury)
- Fracture gap widening (peak = 4–6 weeks; range = 3–7 weeks)

Stage 3—Soft callus
- Sclerosis at fx margin (peak = 4–6 weeks; range 3–11 weeks)
- Periosteal reaction presence (peak = 4–7 weeks; range = 2–14 weeks)
- Callus presence (peak = 4–7 weeks; range = 2–14 weeks)

Stage 4—Hard callus (2–13 weeks)
- Callus density greater than cortex (peak = 13 weeks; range = 5–14 weeks)
- Bridging (peak = 13 weeks; range = 5–14 weeks)
- Periosteal reaction incorporation (peak = 14 weeks; range = 7–14 weeks)

Stage 5—Remodeling (3 months–2 years)

Hufnagl (2005) (adapted from Hendrix, 2002) (radiography; adults and juveniles combined)

Stage 1—Fracture event
- No fx healing
- Sharp fragment edges

Stage 2—Granulation
- Beginning resorption along fx margins leading to widening fx gap and blurring of fx edges
- Initial callus formation

Table 9.A.2 (Continued)

Stage 3—Mature callus
• Radiopaque mature callus bulging out and over fx gap
• Fx line still visible
Stage 4—Partial bridging
• Partial connection of callus across fx gap
• Blurring of fx line
Stage 5—Almost complete bridging
• Clinical union
• Fx line almost completely obscured
Stage 6—Complete bridging
• Eradication of fx line
Offiah and Hall (2009) (radiography)
Soft tissue swelling, loss of normal fat planes (within 7–10 days)
SPNBF first visibility (7–10 days+)
Fracture margin
• Acute/sharp **(<7–10 days)**
• Loss of definition **(7+ days)**
Fracture gap widening (7+ days)
Soft callus (osteoid) formation (1–6 weeks)
• Subtle increased density around fx site
• Fx line still visible
Hard callus formation (ends 6–8 weeks)
• Conversion of woven to lamellar bridging bone
• Observed as definite sclerosis around fx
• Consolidation of callus
• Fx line may or may not be visible, but disappears by 6–8 weeks
Remodeling
• Not reliable radiographically for dating of fxs
Malone *et al.* (2011) (adapted from Hufnagl, 2005) (radiography; tibial and radial diaphysis)
Stage 1—No healing (*x*=3.3 days; range=0–14 days)
• Sharp fx lines
• Absence of bridging and callus formation
Stage 2—Granulation (*x*=21 days; range=4–50 days)
• Beginning of resorption along fx line leading to blurring of fx line
• "Fluffy" callus formation but absence of a complete mature callus
Stage 3—Callus (*x*=38.4 days; range=15–75 days)
• Mature callus formation around fx site
• Radiopaque callus bulging over site
• Fx line visible but may be blurred

(Continued)

Table 9.A.2 (Continued)

Stage 4—Bridging (*x*=43.9 days; range=24–93 days)
- Fx gap connected across fx in some but not all areas (<50%)
- Blurring of fx line
- Callus may still be present

Stage 5—Clinical union (*x*=65.2 days; range=24–156 days)
- Fx line significantly blurred
- Fx line connected in most areas (>50%)
- Callus presence minimal

Stage 6—Completion (*x*=313.3 days; range=42–750 days)
- No fx line visible
- Minimal or no callus visibility

Halliday *et al.* (2011) (radiography; diaphyseal; 0–44 months)

Blurring of soft tissue (soft tissue swelling) ≤ 10 days
SPNBF = seen 11 days+, except for one case at 4 days and another at 8 days
Loss of fx line definition = 1–4 weeks
Presence of callus = not differentiated from SPNBF
Definition of callus: Ill-defined = 8–29 days; well-defined = 20–106 days
Endosteal callus = 3 weeks+, except for one case at 8 days

Love *et al.* (2011) (radiography and dry bone) (summarizing and citing Chapman, 1992; Lindaman, 2001; McKibbin, 1978; O'Connor and Cohen, 1998; Ogden, 1990; Salter, 1980)

Phase I—Inflammation
- Bleeding leads to hematoma development
- Vascular disruption, leading to bone, cartilage, and soft tissue necrosis
- Migration of inflammatory cells into injury site; fx hematoma organization
- Resorption of necrotic tissue
- Replacement of clot with fibrovascular tissue
- Mineralization of collagen fibers to form woven bone of primary callus

Phase II—Soft callus (first observed possibly as early as 4 days)
- Gross recognition of SPNBF
- Initial fx line bridging (fibrous matrix, then primary woven bone)
- Disorganized callus

Phase III—Hard callus
- Full bridging of fx callus
- Obliteration of fx line
- Replacement of woven with lamellar bone (consolidation)
- Resorption of hematoma and inflammatory tissue

Phase IV—Remodeling
- Late conversion of woven to lamellar bone to reforming of normal bone contour and medullary cavity

Table 9.A.2 (Continued)

Prosser *et al.* (2012) (digital radiography; diaphyseal)
1. Soft tissue swelling (first seen = 1 day; peak = 1–2 days; last seen = 31 days)
2. Periosteal reaction (first seen = 5 days; peak = 15–35 days; last seen = 96 days)
3. Soft callus (first seen = 12 days; peak = 22–35 days; last seen = 66 days)
4. Hard callus (first seen = 19 days; peak ≥ 22 days; last seen = 96 days)
5. Bridging (first seen = 19 days; peak ≥ 36 days; last seen = 300 days)
6. Remodeling (first seen = 45 days; peak ≥ 36 days; last seen = 421 days)
Sanchez *et al.* (2013) (radiography; ribs)
Stage 1—No periosteal rxn; barely visible fx line (0–1 week)
Stage 2—Periosteal rxn < 2 mm thick; Some fx line resorption (1–3 weeks)
Stage 3—Early callus formation <4 mm thick; fx line clearly visible (3–5 weeks)
Stage 4—Callus thickest (4 mm+) (5–7 weeks)
Stage 5—Callus remodeling (<4 mm); near-complete bridging (7–9 weeks)
Stage 6—Focal sclerosis, cortical thickening (9–11 weeks)
Walters *et al.* (2014) (radiography; clavicle birth fxs)
SPNBF—Highly unlikely before 7 days; often present by 10 days
Callus formation—Unlikely before 9 days; often present by 15 days

Table 9.A.3 Fracture repair processual observations

Anabolic/osteoblastic activity
I. SPNBF development
1. None
2 Slight (<25%)
3. Moderate (25–75%)
4. Advanced (>75%)
5. Resorption/obliteration
II. Fibrocartilage development
1. None
2. Initial (<25%)
3. Moderate (25–75%)
4. Advanced (>75%)
5. Completed
III. Woven bone development
1. None
2. Initial (<25%)
3. Moderate (25–75%)
4. Advanced (>75%)
5. Completed

(Continued)

Table 9.A.3 (Continued)

IV. Lamellar bone development
1. None
2. Initial (<25%)
3. Moderate (25–75%)
4. Advanced (>75%)
5. Completed
V. Bridging
1. None
2. Slight (<25%; mostly fibrous)
3. Moderate (25–50%; fibrous and woven)
4. Advanced (50–75%; woven and fibrous)
5. Complete (<75%; woven and lamellar)
Catabolic/osteoclastic activity
I. Fx margin morphology
1. Sharp—fx margin/line clearly visible
2. Initial rounding (<25%)
3. Moderate rounding and visibility (25–75%)
4. Fx line poorly visible (>75%)
5. Fx line no longer visible
II. Fibrocartilage to woven bone conversion
1. None
2. Slight (<25%)
3. Moderate (25–75%)
4. Advanced (>75%)
5. Completed
III. Woven to lamellar bone conversion
1. None
2. Slight (<25%)
3. Moderate (25–75%)
4. Advanced (>75%)
5. Completed
IV. Remodeling/lamellar bone resorption
1. None
2. Slight (<25%)
3. Moderate (25–75%)
4. Advanced (>75%)
5. Completed—full "callus" resorption

CHAPTER 10

Theoretical foundation of child abuse

Jennifer C. Love[1] and Miriam E. Soto Martinez[2]

[1] *Office of the Chief Medical Examiner, Washington, DC, USA*

[2] *Forensic Anthropology Division, Harris County Institute of Forensic Sciences, Houston, TX, USA*

10.1 Introduction

Recognizing non-accidental injury in children is a difficult task that requires a multidisciplinary team approach including pediatricians, child protective services, and law enforcement. When the child is deceased, the team expands to include medicolegal death investigators, forensic pathologists, and forensic anthropologists. During the medicolegal death investigation of a child, the roles of the forensic anthropologist are threefold: identify skeletal injury, assess the probability that the injury resulted from non-accidental injury, and estimate the timing of the injury. The body of knowledge called upon by the anthropologist to perform these roles is soundly grounded in foundational, interpretive, and methodological theories. In this chapter, the theoretical foundation of skeletal injury examination and interpretation is framed by a case study to add context for the reader.

10.2 Case study

A 2-month-old infant was discovered unresponsive in her crib by her mother after an afternoon nap. Reportedly, the child's mother fed the infant 5 oz. of formula milk prior to putting her down for a nap at 1:00 in the afternoon. The mother checked on the infant around 2:00 p.m. and found her unresponsive, at which point she called 911 and initiated CPR. Paramedics arrived at the home, continued CPR, and transported the decedent to the local children's hospital. Resuscitation efforts continued at the hospital to no avail, and the infant was pronounced dead soon after arrival. According to the police record, the mother reported that the

Forensic Anthropology: Theoretical Framework and Scientific Basis, First Edition.
Edited by C. Clifford Boyd Jr and Donna C. Boyd.

decedent had been fussy prior to the nap and had rolled off the changing table earlier in the morning; otherwise, the infant was in normal health. The pediatrician's records indicated that the infant was observed to be healthy at her 2-month-old well-child examination and had received all standard vaccinations.

During the autopsy, the infant was found to be well-nourished and well-developed. Upon external examination, a few small contusions were noted on the decedent's forehead, right shoulder, and left knee. Internal examination revealed a subdural hematoma, optic nerve sheath hemorrhage, retinal hemorrhages, several acute posterior rib fractures, a right distal femoral metaphyseal fracture, and a complex skull fracture. The cause and manner of death were classified as multiple blunt force trauma and homicide.

10.3 Anthropologists and child abuse

Historically, the anthropologists' role in medicolegal death investigation of child abuse was limited to pediatric skeletal remains (Walker *et al.*, 1997; Lewis, 2007). As anthropologists have become embedded in medical examiner offices, their role in the recognition of child abuse has expanded. Notably, forensic anthropologists developed an alternate autopsy technique, pediatric skeletal examination (PSE), which is often applied in cases of suspected pediatric non-accidental injury (Love and Sanchez, 2009). PSE is performed by reflecting the musculature and periosteum from the long bones, clavicles, and scapulae. Additionally, the pleura, musculature, and periostea are removed from the internal surface of the ribs. The exposed bones are examined *in situ* for injury and/or subperiosteal new bone formation, a reaction to subperiosteal hemorrhage. Chondro-osseous junctions (COJs) are closely examined for injuries along the growth plate. Such injuries are considered highly suspicious for non-accidental injury.

Recent research has shown that utilizing the PSE increases the sensitivity of the autopsy with regard to the identification of skeletal injury. Love *et al.* (2014) compared the number of skeletal injuries identified in cases where PSE was performed (experimental group) with the number of skeletal injuries identified in cases where PSE was not performed (control group). The cause and manner of death in all cases were blunt force trauma and homicide, respectively. Skeletal injuries were identified in 34 (72%) cases of the experimental group and 30 (64%) cases of the control group. Of note, the total number of fractures identified in the experimental group was 512 compared with 198 fractures in the control group. The statistically significant difference in the number of skeletal injuries identified in the experimental group demonstrated that the PSE increased the sensitivity of an autopsy to skeletal injury.

Recognition of skeletal injury, however, is only a portion of the anthropologist's role in a medicolegal death investigation. The anthropologist must understand bone biomechanics to differentiate between accidental and non-accidental injury.

Moreno (2003:534) stated it best in her article, "Einstein on the Bench?: Exposing What Judges Do Not Know About Science and Using Child Abuse Cases to Improve How Courts Evaluate Scientific Evidence,"

> Although the medical evidence in child abuse cases may be complex, these cases almost always involve a binary decision—were the injuries caused by abuse or accident?

Differentiating between accidental and non-accidental skeletal injury is where the anthropologist's interpretation becomes acutely intertwined with foundational, interpretive, and methodological theories. Boyd and Boyd (Chapter 1, this volume; also see Boyd and Boyd, 2011) define foundational theories as broad, all-encompassing abstract explanations that are applicable to a multitude of circumstances. Interpretive theories are explanations linking foundational theories to direct observations of human behavior or natural process. Methodological theories are generalized analytical protocols, based on their successful application to multiple direct observations. In terms of child abuse interpretation, foundational theories are based on skeletal growth and development. Theories of childhood motor skill development and fracture biomechanics can be considered interpretive theory. Finally, protocols used to develop prediction models from databases and case study reports provide the foundation for methodological theory.

10.4 Foundational theory

Accurate interpretation of pediatric skeletal injury requires a firm understanding of normal bone growth and development. Healthy bone is able to perform several vital bodily functions, including protection of internal organs, body support, muscle attachment sites for locomotion, cavity for hematopoiesis, and mineral storage necessary to maintain mineral homeostasis (Rodan, 1992; Marks and Odgren, 2002; Bartl and Frisch, 2009; Rauner *et al.*, 2012; Burr and Akkus, 2013). When mineral homeostasis cannot be maintained or the bone fails to form normally, the bone and overall health are negatively affected.

Skeletal development begins during the 6th week of gestation and continues into the late teens to early adulthood. Development occurs through intramembranous and endochondral ossification (Allen and Burr, 2014). During intramembranous ossification, mesenchymal stem cells aggregate into layers, known as condensations, and differentiate into osteoblasts (Marks and Odgren, 2002). Most cranial bones, all facial bones, mandible, scapula, pelvis, and central portion of the clavicle develop by intramembranous ossification (Buckwalter *et al.*, 1995; Scheuer and Black, 2000). Endochondral ossification occurs on an anlage, a cartilage template, which is produced by chondrocytes. Weight-bearing bones form through endochondral bone formation (Marks and Odgren, 2002). Within the embryo, the first bones to form endochondrally are the long bones: femur, tibia, fibula, humerus, radius, and ulna. Elongation of the long bones, occurring through endochondral ossification, continues at the growth plates until skeletal maturity, which occurs during the late teens to early adulthood (Buckwalter *et al.*, 1995).

The mechanical properties of bone, properties that describe how the bone will behave under loading, depend on the composition of the extracellular matrix of the connective tissue, the degree of mineralization of the organic matrix, and bone's structure. Osteoblasts, chondroblasts, and fibroblasts are responsible for the synthesis of collagen, proteoglycan, and other non-collagenous proteins. Bone's response to normal loading can be altered by disturbances in collagen synthesis or ossification of the organic matrix, resulting in compromised bone strength. Osteogenesis imperfecta (OI), a widely known congenital disease, is a good example of how abnormal bone composition, resulting from the disruption of collagen production, compromises bone strength. Clinicians and geneticists recognize six distinct types of OI based on the clinical presentation and genetic features (Bullough, 2004). Fracture incidence varies significantly based on the expression of the disease (Greeley *et al.*, 2013). For example, in OI type I, the structure of type I collagen is normal, but the amount of collagen is reduced. Individuals affected with OI type I have mild manifestations of the disease, such as gray-blue sclera and moderate osteoporosis; these individuals may experience no or few fractures throughout their lifetime. In contrast, the structure of type I collagen is abnormal in OI type II. Individuals affected with OI type II have severe manifestations of the disease, such as intrauterine fractures, and often die during the perinatal period.

In addition to genetic conditions, compromised bone strength can be acquired through nutritional deficiencies, such as scurvy and rickets (Bullough, 2004). Scurvy results from ascorbic acid (vitamin C) deficiency, an essential nutrient for the intracellular synthesis of collagen. In cases of scurvy, spontaneous epiphysiolysis, separation of the epiphysis from the growth plate, has been reported (Nerubay and Pilderwasser, 1984). Rickets or osteomalacia results from a deficiency of vitamin D, an important nutrient for calcium homeostasis. Common sources of vitamin D disturbance are dietary deficiency, intestinal malabsorption, and chronic renal failure. In children, rickets may cause irregularities in the growth plates, swelling of the costochondral junctions, and curvature of the long bones and spinal column. Both osteomalacic and rachitic bones are predisposed to fracture.

10.5 Interpretive theory

Bone biomechanics and childhood motor skill development are additional areas of research that are central to the proper interpretation of skeletal injury. No fracture type is pathognomonic for physical abuse; the classification of a fracture as accidental versus non-accidental depends on fracture type and location, as well as the level of motor skill development achieved by the child. A child that is able to run, jump, and climb is more likely to sustain accidental injury than a child that is unable to roll over. Furthermore, developing bone responds differently to force (e.g., compression, tension, torsion) than mature bone. The joint consideration of the biomechanical properties of developing bone and normal motor skill development supports an accurate interpretation of skeletal injury as accidental or non-accidental.

10.5.1 Bone biomechanics

Bone's response to stress (amount of force exerted over an area) depends on the force (amount, direction, area, and loading rate) and the mechanical properties of the bone (density, tissue composition, gross geometric shape, collagen orientation, and rigidity) (Love and Symes, 2004). Biomechanical studies show that bone is stronger in compression (pushing together) than tension (pulling apart) (Frost, 1973). As a result, when force is applied to a bone, the bone will first fail at the point of greatest tension.

In children, some fracture types are considered suspicious for non-accidental injury, while others are considered more likely to be accidental in nature. Posterior rib fractures are considered highly suspicious for inflicted injury (Kleinman, 1998). The posterior region of the rib lies deep within the skeletal musculature and is less susceptible to direct impact. Biomechanical studies have shown that posterior rib fractures tend to occur at the rib tubercle and result from the posterior levering of the rib over the transverse process of the vertebra as the ribcage is compressed in an anterior/posterior direction (Tsai *et al.*, 2012). A metaphyseal fracture, also known as a classic metaphyseal lesion, bucket fracture, or corner fracture, is another fracture type considered highly suspicious for inflicted injury (Kleinman, 1998). Metaphyseal fractures are fractures through the metaphyseal regions of long bone growth plates. These fractures involve the osseous component of the growth plate and not the cartilage. Biomechanical research has shown that metaphyseal fractures of the proximal tibia and distal femur can result from varus, laterally directed, and valgus, medially directed, forces applied to the knee (Thompson *et al.*, 2015). The application of significant varus and valgus forces to the knee, elbow, wrist, and ankle is inconsistent with normal handling of an infant. These biomechanical understandings form the theoretical foundation for interpreting posterior rib fractures and metaphyseal fractures as non-accidental injury (Kleinman, 1998; Tsai *et al.*, 2012; Thompson *et al.*, 2015).

Biomechanical studies have focused on pediatric skull fractures as well. Skull fracture patterns are influenced by the level of force, impact surface area and type, and impact location on the skull (Hipp and Haues, 1998). Studies have tried to identify cranial fracture patterns specific to non-accidental injury. For example, Meservy *et al.* (1987) reviewed the radiographs of 132 children under 2 years of age with skull fractures in order to identify distinguishing features between accidental and non-accidental fracture patterns. The authors found that multiple fractures, bilaterally located fractures, and fractures that cross sutures were more common in non-accidental injury than accidental injury.

In an attempt to fully understand how pediatric cranial bone responds to blunt force trauma, researchers have examined cranial fracture patterns produced by controlled impacts. Baumer *et al.* (2010) and Powell *et al.* (2012, 2013) conducted a series of studies exposing infant porcine skulls to controlled blunt force impacts. The researchers evaluated impacts using compliant and rigid impact surfaces, at low- and high-level impact forces as well as fracture characteristics of entrapped (head on supported surface) and free falling impacts (Baumer *et al.*, 2010; Powell *et al.*, 2012; Powell *et al.*, 2013). In each study, the authors measured impact force and duration and mapped the resulting fracture pattern recording fracture length and location. These studies reported several important findings. In general, the energy required to initiate a skull fracture increased with the age of the individual, and a high energy impact with a rigid impact surface produced more fractures than an impact of equal energy on a compliant surface (Baumer *et al.*, 2010). High energy impacts to the parietal bone resulted in fractures of the parietal and occipital bones (Powell *et al.*, 2012). An impact to an entrapped head resulted in a more extensive fracture pattern than a free-fall impact. Free-fall impacts to the parietal resulted in fractures of the parietal bone that often crossed into the frontal bone, while impacts of equal force to an entrapped head resulted in multiple fractures of the parietal, occipital, and frontal bones (Powell *et al.*, 2013). Perhaps most importantly, the researchers found that a single focal impact often created fractures that did not initiate at the impact site, created multiple fractures that did not communicate, and at times these fractures were on separate bones (Baumer *et al.*, 2010; Powell *et al.*, 2012; Powell *et al.*, 2013). In contrast, biomechanical studies of controlled impacts to adult human skulls showed that fractures initiated at and propagated outward from the impact site (Kroman *et al.*, 2011) *if* the impact was from an object with a small surface area (see Berryman *et al.*, Chapter 11, this volume).

The aforementioned examples of biomechanical research formulate the foundation of the interpretive theory that is relied upon during pediatric non-accidental injury interpretation. The scientific basis for these theories circles back to the foundational theory of bone growth and development and cannot be separated from it. Young bone is more elastic than older bone. Therefore, developing bone is structurally different than mature bone and, as a result, responds differently to trauma than adult bone. For example, the COJ of long bones, the site of metaphyseal fractures, are the weakest part of a growing bone in young infants (Kleinman, 1998). During early development, long bone growth occurs rapidly at the COJ, and newly mineralized spicules of bone (primary spongiosa) are weaker than the adjacent epiphysis. This newly-formed weak bone is susceptible to failure when forces are applied to the extremities. The longitudinal growth rate decreases in older children, allowing the newly forming spicules to thicken as they elongate, increasing the strength of the structures. Concurrent with the change in skeletal development is a shift from fractures of the primary spongiosa to fractures of the physeal cartilage (Kleinman, 1998). The structure of cranial bones also changes during skeletal development. With skeletal maturity, the occipital, parietal, and frontal bones transform from a single layer of bone to two layers of compact bones sandwiching a layer of cancellous, erythropoietic diploë between them. As a result of this developmental difference, infant cranial bone responds differently to impacts than adult cranial bone as illustrated by the previously mentioned studies (Baumer *et al.*, 2010; Kroman *et al.*, 2011; Powell *et al.*, 2012; Powell *et al.*, 2013).

10.5.2 Motor skill development

Theoretical understanding of childhood motor skill development is also critical to interpretation of skeletal injury. Age-related developmental milestones are well-defined. The American Academy of Pediatrics (2016) lists motor skill milestones for each month of infancy. Infant activity and associated injury risk directly reflect these developmental milestones. Injury risk changes as children age. Argan *et al.* (2003) examined mortality and morbidity data and found that, within the first year of life, age-related differences in major causes of injury could be narrowed to 3-month age intervals. Specifically, the leading cause of injury for infants aged 0–2 months was a fall from height, 3–5 months was battering, 6–8 months was falls from furniture, and 9–11 months was non-airway foreign body.

Differentiating between accidental and non-accidental injuries cannot be made solely on a fracture type and location, because no skeletal injury is pathognomonic for abuse. Therefore, the classification of a non-accidental fracture in a child undergoing normal growth and development is dependent on the type of fracture, injury history, and motor skill development of the child. The case study leading this chapter demonstrates the need to examine the complete case with the understanding of motor skill development and fracture biomechanics. The injury history was inconsistent with the expected development of the child; 2-month-old infants typically do not roll over (American Academy of Pediatrics, 2016). Additionally, posterior rib fractures and metaphyseal fractures are inconsistent with a history of a fall.

10.6 Methodological theory

Case studies and injury databases inductively built from direct observations of non-accidental injury form the foundation for methodological theory of child abuse. Practitioners recognize certain types of fractures as highly suspicious for non-accidental trauma because the fracture types are seen nearly exclusively in non-accidental injury cases. For example, Barness *et al.* (2003) found that the positive predictive value of rib fractures for non-accidental injury in children under the age of 3 years was 97%. Upon consideration of the injury history and clinical circumstances, the predictive value increased to 100% (Barness *et al.*, 2003). No instances of rib fractures were observed in young, healthy patients with minor accidental trauma. In contrast, a study conducted by Scherl *et al.* (2000) cautions against viewing specific types of femoral shaft fracture as indicative of non-accidental injury. Scherl *et al.* (2000) retrospectively reviewed the records of 207 patients under the age of 6 years with femoral shaft fractures. Child abuse investigations were initiated for 76 of the 207 patients, and the findings for 13 of these patients were positive for abuse. The medical records were specifically examined for femoral shaft fracture type: transverse, spiral, or oblique. The researchers found no significant difference in the type of shaft fractures between the cases of accidental and non-accidental injuries and caution against viewing specific types of femoral shaft fractures as suspicious for non-accidental injury. These two studies illustrate how direct observation is an important methodology in theory development. The grounds for considering an injury suspicious for abuse are often based on the prevalence of various types of skeletal injury within the pediatric population.

Much of the pediatric trauma research is built on injury databases maintained by trauma centers. Using a database of nearly 3000 children assessed for possible abuse in a hospital setting between the years of 1997 and 2012, Fagen *et al.* (2015) calculated the frequency of skeletal injuries in children with inflicted burns. Of the 3000 children, 112 children were diagnosed with a burn and received a skeletal survey. Ultimately, 17 of the 112 children had fractures and 15 of these children were diagnosed with non-accidental trauma. Accidental versus non-accidental trauma could not be determined for the remaining two children with fractures. No fractures were observed in the children with accidental burns.

A low-level fall is the most common story provided by caretakers when non-accidental trauma has occurred (Carter and Moulton, 2016). Carter and Moulton (2016), using a trauma database compiled from two level-one regional pediatric trauma centers, attempted to identify differences between abdominal injury patterns resulting from non-accidental and accidental trauma (Carter and Moulton, 2016). The authors found that victims of non-accidental trauma were typically younger than 5 years and had higher injury severity scores. In general, the history of a low-level fall was inconsistent with the extent of the injury.

Case studies also serve an important role as methodological tools in developing the theoretical knowledge of child abuse. For example, Murphy *et al.* (2014) presented a case study of a 3-year-old child with a traumatic hip dislocation and no clear explanation for the mechanism of injury. The anatomical characteristics of the hip joint in young children, such as ligamentous laxity and incomplete fusion of the acetabulum, predispose it to accidental injury. However, hip dislocations are more commonly observed in school-age children. In addition to the hip dislocation, there were several bruises in different stages of healing. When the case was viewed in totality, a diagnosis of non-accidental trauma was made. The authors emphasized that the specific case circumstances, such as the child's age, level of motor skill development, and numerous bruises at different stages of healing, underscored the need to consider non-accidental trauma even when the skeletal injury is often recognized as accidental. This case study is an excellent illustration of how the interpretation of non-accidental injury was not only based on methodological theory of prevalence of injury by age but also contingent on the underlying foundational theory of anatomy and skeletal growth and development.

10.7 Conclusion

The anthropologist's role in recognizing non-accidental skeletal injury is firmly grounded in all forms of theory. Foundational theory encompasses our understanding of normal skeletal growth and development and the impact abnormal growth and development have on fracture propensity. Interpretive theory of bone biomechanics provides the tools to compare reported injury history with observed skeletal injury for the purpose of recognizing inconsistencies between them. Fracture interpretation is also built on the interpretive theory of childhood motor skill development and age-specific injury risk. Finally, methodological theory indicates when skeletal injuries are suspicious for non-accidental injury using injury prevalence in the pediatric population as a basis of comparison.

Circling back to the case study in the introduction of the chapter, the multilevel theoretical foundation of child abuse recognition provides the necessary tools to classify the child's injuries as non-accidental. First, posterior rib fractures and metaphyseal lesions are inconsistent with the forces associated with a fall from a changing table. Second, a 2-month-old child is not expected to roll over. Third, these fracture types are observed more frequently in non-accidental injury than accidental injury. The interpretation of case findings using the theoretical understandings presented in this chapter provides the pathway to classifying these injuries as non-accidental.

References

Allen, M.R. and Burr, D.B. (2014) Bone modeling and remodeling. In: *Basic and Applied Bone Biology* (eds. D.B. Burr and M.R. Allen). Academic Press, Amsterdam, pp. 75–90.

American Academy of Pediatrics (2016) *Developmental Milestones: 1 Month*. https://www.healthychildren.org/English/ages-stages/baby/Pages/Developmental-Milestones-1-Month.aspx (last accessed March 8, 2016).

Argan, P.F., Anderson, C., Winn, D., *et al.* (2003) Rates of pediatric injuries by 3-months intervals for children 0 to 3 years of age. *Pediatrics*, **111**(6), 683–692.

Barness, K.A., Cha, E.S., Bensard, D.D., *et al.* (2003) The positive predictive value of rib fractures as an indicator of non-accidental trauma in children. *Journal of Trauma*, **54**(6), 1107–1110.

Bartl, R. and Frisch, B. (2009) Biology of bone. In: *Osteoporosis: Diagnosis, Prevention, Therapy* (eds. R. Bartl and B. Frisch). Springer-Verlag, Berlin, pp. 7–28.

Baumer, T.G., Passalacqua, N.V., Powell, B.J., *et al.* (2010) Age-dependent fracture characteristics of rigid and compliant surface impacts on the infant skull-a porcine model. *Journal of Forensic Sciences*, **55**(4), 993–997.

Boyd, C. and Boyd, D. (2011) Theory and the scientific basis for forensic anthropology. *Journal of Forensic Sciences,* **56**(6), 1407–1415.

Buckwalter, J.A., Glimcher, M.J., Cooper, R.R., *et al.* (1995) Bone biology 2. Formation, form, modeling, remodeling, and regulation of cell-function. *Journal of Bone & Joint Surgery-American Volume,* **77A**(8), 1276–1289.

Bullough, P.G. (2004) *Orthopaedic Pathology,* 4th edn. Mosby, Edinburgh.

Burr, D.B. and Akkus O. (2013) Bone morphology and organization. In: *Basic and Applied Bone Biology* (eds. D.B. Burr and M.R. Allen). Academic Press, Amsterdam, pp. 3–25.

Carter, K.W. and Moulton, S.L. (2016) Pediatric abdominal injury patterns caused by falls. A comparison between non-accidental and accidental trauma. *Journal of Pediatric Surgery,* **51**(2), 326–328.

Fagen, K.E., Shalaby-Rana, E., and Jackson, A.M. (2015) Frequency of skeletal injuries in children with inflicted burns. *Pediatric Radiology,* **45**(3), 396–401.

Frost, H.M. (1973) *Orthopaedic Biomechanics.* Charles C. Thomas, Springfield.

Greeley, C.S., Donaruma-Kwoh, M., Vettimatten, M., *et al.* (2013) Fractures at diagnosis in infants and children with osteogenesis imperfecta. *Journal of Pediatric Orthopaedics,* **33**(1), 32–36.

Hipp, J.A. and Haues, W.C. (1998) Biomechanics of fractures. In: *Skeletal Trauma: Fractures, Dislocations, Ligamentous Injuries* (eds. B.D. Browner, A.M. Levine, J.B. Jupiter, and P.G. Trafton). Saunders Company, Philadelphia, PA, pp. 97–129.

Kleinman, P.K. (1998) *Diagnostic Imaging of Child Abuse,* 2nd edn. (ed. P.K. Kleinman). Mosby, St. Louis, MO.

Kroman, A., Kress, T., and Porta, D. (2011) Fracture propagation in the human cranium: a re-testing of popular theories. *Clinical Anatomy,* **24**(3), 309–318.

Lewis, M.E. (2007) *The Bioarchaeology of Children: Perspectives from Biological and Forensic Anthropology,* Cambridge University Press, Cambridge.

Love, J.C. and Sanchez, L.A. (2009) Recognition of skeletal fractures in infants: an autopsy technique. *Journal of Forensic Sciences,* **54**(6), 1443–1446.

Love, J.C. and Symes, S.A. (2004) Understanding rib fracture patterns: incomplete and buckle fractures. *Journal of Forensic Sciences,* **49**(6), 1153–1158.

Love, J.C., Wiersema, J.M., Derrick, S.D., *et al.* (2014) The value of the pediatric skeletal examination in the autopsy of children. *Academic Forensic Pathology Journal,* **4**(1), 100–108.

Marks, S.C. and Odgren, P.R. (2002) Structure and development of the skeleton. In: *Principles of Bone Biology* (eds. J.P. Bilezikian, L.G. Raisz, and G.A. Rodan). Academic Press, San Diego, pp. 3–15.

Meservy, C.J., Towbin, R., McLauring, R.L., *et al.* (1987) Radiographic characteristics of skull fractures resulting from child abuse. *American Journal of Roentgenology,* **149**(1), 173–175.

Moreno, J.A. (2003) Einstein on the bench?: Exposing what judges do not know about science and using child abuses cases to improve how courts evaluate scientific evidence. *Ohio State Law Review* **64**(531), 532–585.

Murphy, S., Naranje, S.M., Kelly, D.M., *et al.* (2014) Non-accidental traumatic dislocation of the hip in a 3-year-old child: a report of a rare pediatric injury. *American Journal of Orthopedics,* **43**(8), 374–376.

Nerubay, J. and Pilderwasser, D. (1984) Spontaneous bilateral distal femoral physiolysis due to scurvy. *Acta Orthopaedica Scandinavica,* **55**(1), 18–20.

Powell, B.J., Passalacqua, N.V., Baumer, T.G., *et al.* (2012) Fracture patterns on the infant porcine skull. *Journal of Forensic Sciences,* **57**(2), 312–317.

Powell, B.J., Passalacqua, N.V., Fenton, T.W., *et al.* (2013) Fracture characteristics of entrapped head impacts versus controlled head drops in infant porcine specimens. *Journal of Forensic Sciences,* **58**(3), 678–683.

Rauner, M., Stein, N., and Hofbauer, L.C. (2012) Basics of bone biology. In: *Principles of Osteoimmunology: Molecular Mechanisms and Clinical Applications* (ed. P. Pietschmann). Springer-Verlag, New York, pp. 1–26.

Rodan, G.A. (1992) Introduction to bone biology. *Bone*, **13**(S1), S3–S6.

Scherl, S., Miller, L., Lively, N., *et al.* (2000) Accidental and nonaccidental femur fractures in children. *Clinical Orthopaedics and Related Research*, **376**, 96–105.

Scheuer, L. and Black, S. (2000) Bone development. In: *Developmental Juvenile Osteology* (eds. L. Scheuer and S. Black). Academic Press, Amsterdam, pp. 18–31.

Thompson, A., Bertocci, G., Kaczor, K., *et al.* (2015) Biomechanical investigation of the classic metaphyseal lesion using an immature porcine model. *American Journal of Roentgenology*, **204**(5), W503–W509.

Tsai, A., Coats, B., and Kleinman, P.K. (2012) Stress profile of infant rib in the setting of child abuse: a finite element parametric study. *Journal of Biomechanics*, **45**(11), 1861–1868.

Walker, P.L., Cook, D.C., and Lambert, P.M. (1997) Skeletal evidence for child abuse: a physical anthropological perspective. *Journal of Forensic Sciences*, **42**(2), 196–207.

CHAPTER 11

Bone trauma analysis in a forensic setting: Theoretical basis and a practical approach for evaluation

Hugh E. Berryman[1], John F. Berryman[2] and Tiffany B. Saul[1]

[1] *Forensic Institute for Research and Education, Middle Tennessee State University, Murfreesboro, TN, USA*

[2] *Mechanical Engineering Consultant, Nashville, TN, USA*

11.1 Introduction

Concern for the validity of scientific evidence presented in court first became formalized in 1923 with *Frye v. United States*, where general acceptance was held as the standard for admissibility. However, it was the 1993 *Daubert v. Merrell Dow Pharmaceuticals, Inc.* case that forced forensic scientists to seriously examine their court-offered opinions for scientific validity. Forensic anthropologists became concerned about their own expert testimony and whether they, if called upon, could demonstrate the scientific basis for the particulars to which they would testify.

A courtroom opinion is based on science when it is derived from evidence with a solid theoretical underpinning. A theory is considered valid only when it can be supported by numerous observations and experiments. However, it must also be understood that theories do not require proof to be accepted as fact or to be applied for their utility by the scientific community. For example, both *evolution* and *gravity* are generally accepted as theoretical facts and are used to explain and understand natural phenomena, yet neither can unequivocally be proven.

Scientific theories—whether it is gravity, evolution, or bone trauma—are continually challenged and refined by scientists who eliminate inaccurate elements so that the parts remaining solidly encapsulate whatever truths actually exist. Hypotheses are formulated relative to bone trauma theories and tested to identify conditions where the theory does not hold and where no valid judicial opinion can be formulated. In essence, exceptions to a theory are identified through this process and eliminated, strengthening the theory. Any judicial opinion derived from a theory that has remained intact after repeated scientific challenge *is* based on science.

Forensic Anthropology: Theoretical Framework and Scientific Basis, First Edition.
Edited by C. Clifford Boyd Jr and Donna C. Boyd.

Boyd and Boyd (2011) borrowed a hierarchical model from Schiffer (1988) involving archaeological theory (high-level, middle-range, and low-level theory) to encompass the many diverse areas within forensic anthropology. Boyd and Boyd (2011) stated that high-level theory is more broad-ranging and abstract; middle-range theory involves relating forensic observations with the varying forces responsible for them; and low-level or methodological theory is comprised of recovery, analytic, and inferential theories. Boyd and Boyd (Chapter 1, this volume) further state that all these types of theory "...are linked together and provide necessary feedback for each other in the process of theory building." It is considered that, because of this linkage, the hierarchical model may be revised to refer to three *forms* of theory—foundational, interpretive, and methodological—to more accurately depict their interaction and interdependence (Boyd and Boyd, Chapter 1, this volume). Regardless of form, theory is created through three lines of logical reasoning: abductive, deductive, and inductive (Boyd and Boyd, Chapter 1, this volume).

In this chapter, we discuss three related topics. First, the theoretical basis for bone trauma analysis is scrutinized through the three theoretical levels outlined in the first chapter of this book, coupled with the various lines of logical reasoning used in science. Next, the fundamental assumption used in bone trauma analysis is presented, and the three commonly held principles in fracture production are explored. These three principles coupled with a knowledge of intrinsic properties and extrinsic forces provide the theoretical concepts needed for the interpretation of bone trauma, as well as the fundamental building blocks for bone fracture theory and courtroom opinion. Finally, a practical approach—consisting of a trauma assessment triad and thought experiments—is promoted as a means of facilitating bone trauma evaluation and hypothesis building.

11.2 Theory

Material science and engineering is a field involving research—both theoretical and experimental—that focuses on the properties of materials and their application or use. A subspecialty of material science and engineering that deals with material failure (fractures) is biomechanics of orthopedic implants. This specialty focuses heavily on the load-bearing capacity of various materials. Aspects of physics, chemistry, and engineering are used in this field, often to explore the magnitude of load various materials can withstand before failure. Historically, there have been many studies involving load-bearing capacity with bone as the material in question, some dating back 30 years or more (White *et al.*, 1973; Hartman, 1974; Carter and Hayes, 1976; Pearcy *et al.*, 1983). Biomechanics research of orthopedic implants has examined multiple variables involving bone grafts, reparative strategies, and materials used in implant devices (Klawitter and Hulbert, 1971; Smith and Cody, 1993; Staiger *et al.*, 2006; Ballo *et al.*, 2007; Smith *et al.*, 2014).

Studies such as those outlined earlier are primarily concerned with the functionality of materials or best outcomes from surgical interventions and have a theoretical basis in physics. Those involving load-bearing capacity of test materials are designed to determine at what point the material will fail, under what conditions the material will fail, or perhaps where the failure will occur. The emphasis is on when and where, not *how*, failure occurs. In these fields, once a crack appears in a material, the interest in the fracture itself ends with no concern regarding how the fracture behaves. Generally, the forensic anthropologist's interest begins where the material scientist's interest ends. Research on bone fracture from an engineering perspective is limited, with little concern for fracture propagation or the pattern of the fracture. Forensic application of bone fracture focuses on how the fracture behaves and what influences fracture behavior.

Fracture formation in bone, especially complex fracture patterns, may seem random; however, this is not the case. There are no random fractures in bone; each fracture doggedly obeys the laws of physics. When a fracture changes direction as it propagates across the cranial vault, or when it bifurcates to form a butterfly fracture, or when it ratchets leaving secondary fractures across tubular bone or completes the fracture leaving a breakaway spur, it does so for a reason. There is nothing random in the way a fracture forms.

The foundational assumption in bone trauma analysis is the nonrandomness of fracture configuration or more specifically fracture behavior; it is this nonrandomness that allows fracture analysis and bone trauma interpretation. Intuitively, fracture patterns are repeatable when subjected to similar influences. To avoid confusion, it must be stressed that fracture behavior is highly repeatable; however, the actual fracture will be slightly different from one specimen to the next. Although the general shape of a tibia is the same between humans, its micromorphology, elasticity, density, and so on may vary considerably, resulting in variation in the subtlest aspects of fracture behavior. The greater the knowledge and experience of the practitioner, the greater their success in associating the fracture pattern presented with the force that produced it. However, analysis cannot rely on intuition, but rather knowledge based on sound theory coupled with the experience necessary to validate the theory. The theoretical basis for bone trauma analysis in a forensic setting can best be explored through an examination of foundational, interpretive, and methodological theory.

11.2.1 Foundational theory

The terms *hard science* and *soft science* are informal expressions that popularly categorize disciplines relative to their *perceived* scientific rigor and objectivity. Hard science disciplines customarily include fields such as chemistry, physics, and biology, while social science disciplines are often considered soft science. Within the hard sciences, there is a gradient of disciplines based upon standards, with physics and chemistry providing more clearly delineated standards than biology or biological anthropology. Compared with standards in biological anthropology, standards related to concrete and steel are clearly distinct in the degree of objectivity with which they are measured. The inherent nature of biology is much more susceptible to extraneous influences than concrete and steel. Objective, measurable standards can be developed for concrete and steel. In the industry, instruments in one job site can evaluate concrete and steel to determine whether appropriate building specifications are met. A laboratory a continent away can derive the same findings void of subjectivity. This is not always the case with biology. For example, hospital pathologists have, for decades, determined the presence of cancer by examining stained cells microscopically and subjectively making a determination. However, current-day technology has removed much of yesterday's subjectivity from biology. DNA applications provide a much more objective approach in this field.

Objectivity alone cannot be used to rank the contribution of a specialty. In fact, it is not the objectivity within a field that determines its theoretical virtues; it is the theory upon which a specialty is based that defines its scientific rigor and establishes the validity of its contributions. Anthropology, with its four subfields, is listed among the social sciences and is generally considered a soft science, while forensic anthropology, specifically osteologically-based applications, is rooted in biology. More specifically, bone trauma interpretation has its roots and research in disciplines such as physics and the field of biomechanics—clearly viewed as hard science. Those who popularly categorize disciplines would never question the solid theoretical basis of physics and biomechanics. Bone trauma interpretation possesses the solid theoretical underpinning that would surely satisfy any Daubert hearing. But why is this so? What gives physics and biomechanics the gravitas?

The answer may rest in the high-level theory associated with physics and biomechanics. According to Schiffer (1988) and reiterated by Boyd and Boyd (2011:1408), "Theories that serve as broad, all-encompassing abstract explanations for a multitude of specific circumstances are designated as High-Level." In physics and biomechanics, these high-level foundational theories are attributed to historic figures such as Leonardo da Vinci, who studied the biomechanics of flight; Galileo Galilei, who examined bone architecture and strength; and Sir Isaac Newton with his laws of inertia, acceleration, and reaction (Kieser *et al.*, 2013). The theoretical basis for physics and biomechanics stretches far back in history and serves as broad, comprehensive explanations for many of the phenomena frequently encountered in these and related fields. The weight of history places a profound level of scientific acceptance to these two fields, and, by association, it provides an overarching theoretical basis for bone trauma analysis in a forensic anthropology setting.

11.2.2 Interpretive theory

As Boyd and Boyd (Chapter 1, this volume) have noted, interpretive theory is "... clearly more applied, focusing on the development of observation-based explanations and improved inferences about events of significance." Forensic fracture research originated in medical examiner morgues where fracture patterns began to be recognized and associated with specific causes. A circular defect with an internal bevel became associated with gunshot entrance wounds, which could be borne out by simple experiments. Breakaway spurs in tubular bone were observed in autopsy, and experiments found that they always occur on the compression side of the bone. Fracture pattern observations at autopsy provided raw data and led to hypotheses and experiments to determine how and why. Hypothesis testing involving the laboratory production of bone fractures produced more data and led to findings that could be applied when examining actual forensic cases (Berryman and Gunther, 2000; Gunther *et al.*, 2000; Symes *et al.*, 2002; Love and Symes, 2004; Passalacqua and Fenton, 2012; Powell *et al.*, 2013; Berryman and Saul, 2015).

Three forms of logical reasoning (abduction, deduction, and induction) are used in the interpretation of bone trauma and in the building of hypotheses. Abductive may represent the initial logic applied when examining bone trauma. It is the simple *suggestion* that some particular force may be at work. For example, massive trauma to the skull suggests that the energy was of a magnitude that could not be absorbed by the bone, causing the catastrophic failure. This *suggests* a massive amount of force with a low rate of application (e.g., a fall from a great distance, impact from a vehicle, multiple-blow blunt trauma), or a high rate of application (e.g., high velocity gunshot injury) *may* be at work. It would also eliminate such causes as small-caliber gunshot trauma or single-blow blunt trauma.

Deductive reasoning can be used to prove the existence of something. If reconstruction of the skull described earlier resulted in the following observations—the cranium exhibits (i) no evidence of plastic deformation, (ii) a large circular defect that is internally beveled with an irregularly notched margin, (iii) multiple small penetrating defects with internal beveling are found near the large circular defect, and (iv) multiple small points of lead wipe—then it can be *deduced* with some level of confidence that the force producing the trauma was a shotgun. Such observations may be used to build hypotheses that may lead to identifying the force responsible for specific patterns of injury.

Inductive reasoning is the opposite of deductive reasoning. It allows researchers to identify elements associated with a force (e.g., magnitude, direction, rate of application, mass of the object, and size of impact surface) and hypothesize the resulting fracture or fracture pattern. For example, a researcher may inductively reason the effects of the size of an impact surface on blunt trauma fracture patterns and then test that hypothesis by holding constant magnitude, direction, rate of application, and mass while varying the size of the impact surface.

11.2.3 Methodological theory

Methodological theory provides the basis for establishing appropriate methodological approaches and protocols. The Scientific Working Group Anthropology (SWGANTH) was an organization that existed from 2008 to 2014 with the goal of developing "...consensus best-practice guidelines and [establishing] minimum standards for the Forensic Anthropology discipline..." (SWGANTH, 2013) and disseminating these guidelines to the forensic community. One area covered by SWGANTH was bone trauma. These guidelines outlined "...procedures for describing, documenting and interpreting skeletal trauma" (SWGANTH, 2011).

In 2014, the Scientific Area Committee's (SAC) Anthropology Subcommittee within the Organization of Scientific Area Committees (OSAC) was formed. OSAC is currently referencing the best practice guidelines developed by the SWGANTH to develop standards for the various subspecialties within forensic anthropology, including bone trauma. Boyd and Boyd (Chapter 1) note, "Appropriate methodology guides the observation and collection of data and influences the interpretation (explanation) of *any* past event." Methodology developed by the SWGANTH for trauma, and refined by the OSAC, is founded in practical experience and research design from countless laboratory experiments. This methodology directs the types of observations (data) to be made, how the observations are made, and how these observations are to be interpreted. Methodology, as seen in the SWGANTH trauma document and soon to be codified as standards by OSAC, is foundational for any theories developed in bone trauma analysis.

11.3 Fundamental principles in bone fracture interpretation

According to the Merriam-Webster (2015) Online Dictionary, a principle is "a law or fact of nature that explains how something works or why something happens." Fundamental laws or facts of nature form the foundation upon which hypotheses are constructed and theories are ultimately based. In order to understand the fundamentals of fracture production, the modes of loading must first be understood. Wescott (2013:84) stated, "Loads can be applied in tension (stretching), compression (compaction), bending (angulation), torsion (twisting), shear (sliding), or a combination of these basic components." Although these means of loading exist in the broader, more general sense, a closer view of the fracture tip reveals only two significant types of load—tension and shear. In regard to bone fracture production, an understanding of tension and shear is foundational in trauma interpretation. As principles they can be stated as follows:

- *All bone fractures initiate under tension.*
- *Shear forces direct fracture propagation in bone.*

Collectively, these two principles make it possible to reason about the formation of a fracture and the basic influences that caused it. A cantilevered bone specimen, loaded as shown in Figure 11.1, serves as an illustration of this. Here the left side of the specimen is firmly fixed, while the right side is free to move. Upon application of a load as shown in the figure, the specimen tends to bend, placing the

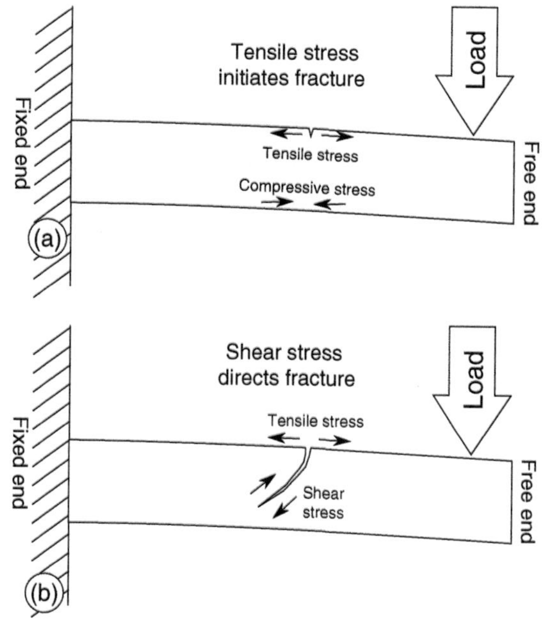

Figure 11.1 Cantilevered material with (a) initial fracture occurring under tension at the site of least resistance and (b) shear forces directing the fracture toward the fixed end of the material.

upper surface under tension, while the lower surface is in compression. Bone can withstand compressive forces to a greater amount than tensile forces. As the load is increased, at some point the tension in the upper surface of the specimen will exceed the strength of the material. At that point, the fracture will initiate and begin to propagate downward through the bone as shown in Figure 11.1a. The exact location where the fracture initiates may be a point of weakness in the surface of the bone and/or a point where the stress is more highly concentrated (e.g., due to local imperfections in the surface of the bone). The important thing to note is that the fracture will initiate in tension on the upper surface of the bone (as depicted in Figure 11.1) and will not form on the lower surface, which is in compression—this is the essence of the principle of tension.

Referring to Figure 11.1b, as the fracture begins to propagate, the applied load causes a shearing effect in the material. The load on the right side causes the material on the right side of the fracture to be pressed downward. At the same time, the fixed end of the bone rigidly holds the specimen in place, causing an equivalent and opposite force to push upward on the material on the left side of the fracture. As stated in the shear principle earlier, these shear forces influence the direction of the fracture as it propagates through bone. In particular, a load that applies a *clockwise* shearing effect (as depicted in Figure 11.1) will lead to clockwise angulation in the fracture. The fracture propagates at an angle toward the fixed end. Additionally, the greater the shear stress, the greater the corresponding fracture angulation.

In order to clarify both axioms and show how they are related, consider Figure 11.2, which depicts a close-up of Figure 11.1 just after the fracture has begun to propagate through the bone. As shown in Figure 11.2a, shear stress and tensile stress are both present at the leading end of the fracture. As shown in Figure 11.2b, it is the combination of these two stresses that pulls the material apart. On the right side of the fracture tip, the tensile stress pulls the material toward the right, while the shear stress pulls material downward. Combined, this causes the material to be pulled at an angle down and to the right. Likewise, on the left side of the fracture tip, the tensile stress pulls the material toward the left, while the shear stress pulls the material upward. Combined, this causes the material to be pulled at an angle up and to the left. The overall effect, as indicated by the dark arrows in Figure 11.2b, is that the material is pulled apart by these resulting stresses. Thus, a closer look into the actual tip of the fracture reveals that the material is still being pulled apart under tension. Specifically, the fracture will propagate in the direction where the tensile *stress* exceeds the tensile *strength* of the material. This example also demonstrates exactly how shear forces influence the fracture angulation. Figure 11.2b illustrates that increasing the shear stress

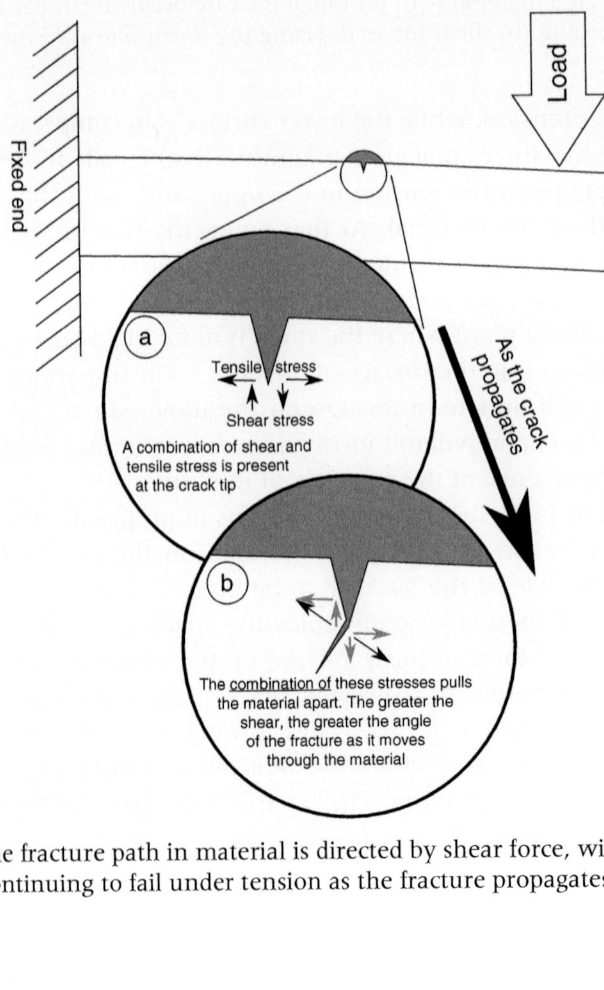

Figure 11.2 The fracture path in material is directed by shear force, with the active end of the fracture continuing to fail under tension as the fracture propagates.

(while keeping tensile stress constant) causes the combined stress to pull the material at a sharper angle, resulting in an even more angulated fracture pattern.

A generally accepted concept states that *gunshot entrance wounds are internally beveled.* Forensic science practitioners who deal with trauma interpretation hold this as a fact, with the principles of tension and shear presented earlier providing a solid underpinning. Tension and shear forces define the primary fracture to cantilevered tubular bone (Figure 11.3a), and the same dynamics can be seen with a gunshot entrance wound to the cranial vault (Figure 11.3b). When the bullet strikes the bone, it represents a dynamic load (a load that keeps advancing), like that exerted to the free end of a cantilevered bone (Figure 11.3a). As the bullet begins to compress the area of impact, the unaffected bone around it acts like cantilevered or fixed bone in the tubular bone example (Figure 11.3a). Tensile forces should develop first around the area of impact to produce a circular defect. As the bullet continually depresses the bone, shear forces expand the fracture continually as it propagates in an ever-increasing, concentric fashion producing the characteristic internal bevel (Figure 11.3b). The major contributions of tensile and shear forces are undeniable, and the overall patterns seen in a fracture to tubular bone are also reflected in gunshot entrance wounds.

Another concept rooted in tension and shear involves the termination of a fracture. Fractures form as a means of absorbing energy. Each individual fracture in a complex of fractures terminates when the tensile strength of the material exceeds

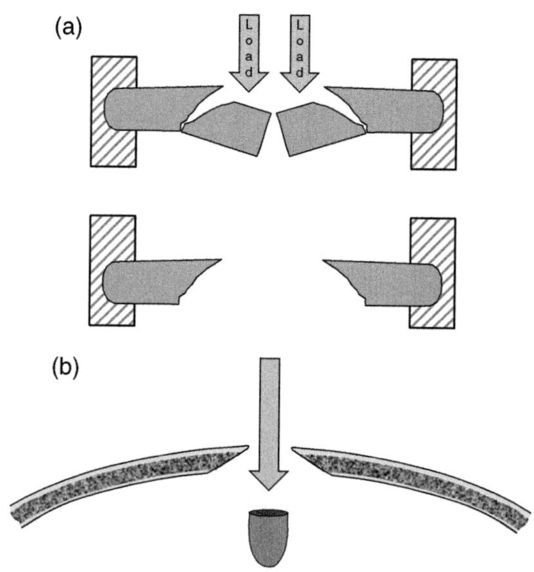

Figure 11.3 Tension and shear forces acting upon bone. (a) Cantilevered tubular bone fracturing under tension with shear forces directing the fracture. (b) Gunshot entrance wound to the cranial vault (cross-sectional view) with the dynamic load of a bullet depressing the bone upon impact, the surrounding vault acting as a cantilever, and shear forces directing the fracture, just as in tubular bone, to produce the classic internal bevel.

the tensile stress. This leads to the concept that *bone fractures terminate into preexisting bone fractures*. Blacksmiths and farriers have known this concept for years; a crack in metal or a split in a horse's hoof can be terminated by drilling a hole at its tip. This hole allows the energy to be absorbed and will terminate the crack unless the energy exceeds the capability of the hole to absorb it. This same concept holds true for fractures in bones, but instead of a hole being drilled, a preexisting fracture will terminate the advance of a fracture by dissipating and absorbing its energy. If the amount of energy cannot be absorbed in the preexisting fracture, the preexisting fracture may elongate to absorb the energy, or a new fracture may open in the preexisting fracture. The point of interest here is the fact that the fracture in question *terminated* into a preexisting fracture. Any fracture initiating in the preexisting fracture as a result of the energy dump from the terminating fracture is a new fracture, not a continuation of the old. Fractures terminating into preexisting fractures result in the familiar T-shaped fracture configuration that allows the sequencing of multiple gunshot wounds or multiple blunt trauma. Rooted in tension and shear, the generally accepted concept of fractures terminating into preexisting fractures—as with the concept that gunshot entrance wounds are internally beveled—provides another valuable tool when examining fracture behavior.

In fact, there are numerous "generally accepted concepts" used to interpret bone trauma. For example, the breakaway spur associated with a fracture to tubular bone is always located on the compression side of the bone and on the fixed end. Thumbnail fractures are the concentric fractures often seen on tubular bone after thermal damage. The direction the heat progressed on the bone is from the convex side of the concentric fracture to the concave side. A ring fracture to the base of the skull is caused by blunt trauma that depresses the cranium onto the cervical vertebrae or elevates the cranium away from the cervical vertebrae. Whether the ring fracture is internally beveled or externally beveled may indicate the direction the cranium was displaced to produce the fracture.

Admittedly, the complex of influences responsible for the specific shape of an internally beveled gunshot entry defect or for a complex of fractures produced in a multiple blunt trauma case is exceedingly complicated. Exactly how the principles of tension and shear affect fracture behavior varies in response to influences inside and outside of the bone. These influences are defined by the following:

- *Fracture behavior is dictated by the interplay of intrinsic and extrinsic factors.*

Extrinsic factors involve forces outside the bone, such as the magnitude of the load, the area and rate of application, the mass of the object impacting the bone, the duration of the load, and the direction of the load. Intrinsic factors are those inside the bone that contribute to the way a bone behaves when subjected to a load. Bone, as a material, is far more complicated than many of the homogeneous materials tested for load-bearing capacity in biomechanics studies. Intrinsic factors include a bone's viscoelastic and anisotropic properties. Viscoelasticity is the capability of bone to possess both viscous (a quality between a solid and a liquid) and elastic qualities (the ability to return to its original shape after a load is removed). Anisotropicity is the condition where the physical properties of bone are not constant, but vary depending upon the direction of the force. For example, the shaft of a femur can accommodate much greater load when it is applied axially as opposed to laterally.

Another intrinsic factor of bone is morphology, both macro morphology and micromorphology. Long bones are not simple cylinders; rather, their macromorphology or shape varies according to the specific bone. For example, a tibia shaft possesses a much more complicated shape than a femur shaft. However, a specific bone from one individual, such as a humerus, is very similar in its macromorphology to that of another individual, but may vary more in its micromorphology (e.g., haversian system, cortical thickness and shape, trabeculae configuration, etc.). It is these micro- and macromorphology variations—variations that are often difficult to measure—that can result in different outcomes in the *finest details* of bone fracture pattern. However, the finest details in a fracture pattern usually hold less value in fracture interpretation than the more conspicuous fractures.

Lastly, biological factors (e.g., age, sex, pathology, drugs, alcohol, medications, etc.) will influence the viscoelasticity of bone in ways that can make it more elastic or more brittle, affecting its susceptibility to fracture. Although bone is exceedingly complicated in its composition and morphology, and it is susceptible to many intrinsic influences, it does exhibit behavior that can be demonstrated using simple material models. Models that use diverse materials can be tested so that the intrinsic quantities are known and can be varied, and the failure characteristics can be studied by altering the extrinsic factors. Predicting a specific fracture pattern, void of any consideration of the extrinsic and intrinsic factors involved, is not feasible.

In a general sense, fracture patterns are predictable at a macroscopic level, but not at the smallest level of detail. The overall behavior *is* predictable because it adheres to simple principles. This predictable behavior lends itself well to understanding circumstances under which a fracture might occur in a given bone. As previously demonstrated, when one end of a tubular bone is cantilevered and a load is continuously applied to the free end, an angular fracture will form that propagates toward the cantilevered end (Figure 11.4a). However, in this same example, it is impossible to predict how many secondary fractures (Figure 11.4c) there will be or even if a secondary fracture will occur at all. Secondary fractures appear to form as the primary fracture moves across the bone and encounters resistance to its advance due to subtitles in bone morphology, composition, microstructure, or any number of factors (Figure 11.4a). When this happens, the primary fracture will terminate; however, the dynamic load will continue to force the free end of the bone down. Tensile forces now build on the newly exposed surface of the primary fracture (i.e., the surface of the new fracture) until stress risers build at its weakest point (Figure 11.4b). When this occurs, a new fracture

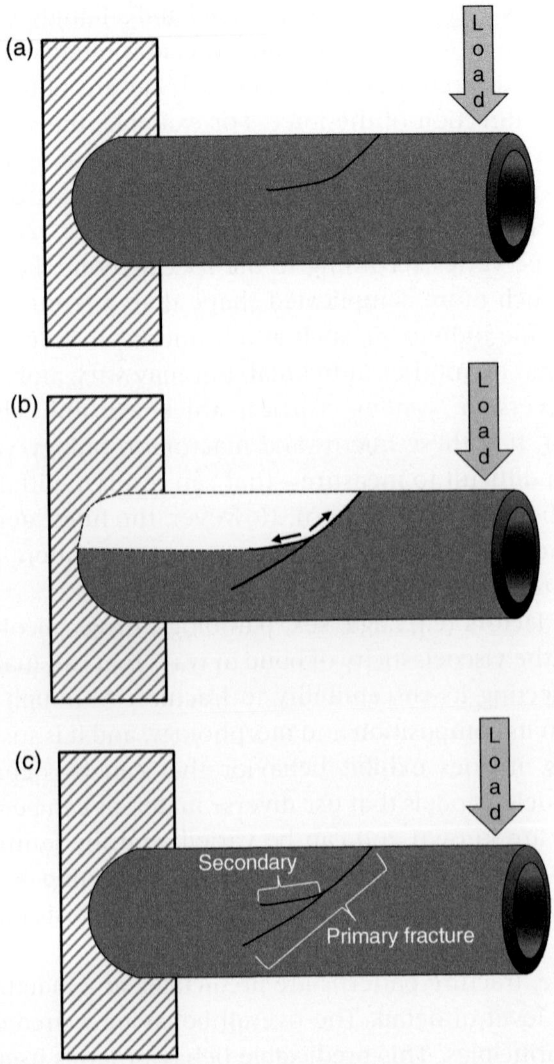

Figure 11.4 Illustration of the development of secondary fractures. (a) The formation and termination of a primary fracture. (b) Dynamic loading on the free end of the bone forces it downward, building tensile forces on the exposed surface of the primary fracture until stress risers build at the weakest point and a new fracture opens. (c) The new fracture is a continuation of the primary fracture and the short portion of the primary fracture that terminated remains as the secondary fracture.

will open under tension, and shear forces will direct it toward the cantilevered end. This new fracture becomes a continuation of the primary fracture, and the short portion of the primary fracture that terminated (i.e., remnant of the initial primary fracture) will remain as the secondary fracture (Figure 11.4c).

The absence, existence, or number of secondary fractures is dictated by the intrinsic (e.g., elastic component, density, morphology, micromorphology, etc.) and extrinsic (e.g., area and rate of application, direction, etc.) factors present during the fracture formation. When examining bone fractures in the absence of a strictly controlled laboratory experiment, there is no way of accounting for all of the internal and external factors involved in their production. However, with an examination of the fracture pattern and a basic comprehension of the intrinsic factors at play, an anthropologist can make a reasonable estimation of the extrinsic factors required to cause the traumatic event. This determination, when founded on sound and accepted scientific principles, can represent a powerful analytical tool. Although the fracture is not predictable at small scales, the overall behavior is predictable and lends itself well to understanding circumstances leading to the fracture.

Anne Kroman (2007, p. vii) was correct when she stated that:

> ...bone trauma is best viewed as a continuum (rather than discrete independent categories), with the variables of force, acceleration/deceleration, and surface area of impacting interface governing the appearance of the resulting fractures.

Sharp trauma, blunt trauma, and gunshot trauma are discrete categories assigned according to their apparent form of delivery; however, the fractures produced in each of the categories are again dictated by the interplay of intrinsic and extrinsic factors. Kroman's comment may be exemplified by comparing blunt trauma characteristics to a cranial vault from a ball-peen hammer versus a .50 caliber bullet. A ball-peen hammer has two striking surfaces. The first is a circular flat surface consistent with most hammers, but the second is a spherical-shaped surface, close in size to a .50 caliber bullet. If the ball-peen striking surface of the hammer impacts the cranial vault at a slow rate of application (~30 feet/second), it will produce a fracture pattern typical of blunt force trauma. However, if a steel ball .50 inch in diameter impacts the cranium at a rate of application consistent with a sniper rifle (~2800 feet/second), the fracture pattern is totally different even though the impact area is the same. On the Kroman bone trauma continuum, the only variable in this example is the rate of application, but, with the lower and rapid rates of application, the impact site is typical of blunt trauma and gunshot trauma, respectively. At what point along this rate of application continuum does blunt trauma begin to look like gunshot trauma?

This also applies to sharp trauma injury. The area of impact is an exceedingly thin surface, much thinner than the striking surface of a 2×4 board, and both may be applied at a slow rate (~30 feet/second), but the end results are very different. To borrow a statement from blood pattern analysis, "...stabbing events are considered a beating with a sharp object" (James *et al.*, 2005:123). This statement aligns somewhat with Kroman's view of a bone trauma continuum. To be more specific, with all other intrinsic and extrinsic factors held constant, and the knife-edge striking surface is slowly increased to that of a 2×4, at what point does sharp trauma begin to look like blunt trauma? Clearly, the variation of any one of the intrinsic properties or extrinsic forces can have a profound impact on fracture behavior.

11.4 A practical approach to bone trauma evaluation and hypothesis building

The authors propose a two-step approach that facilitates fracture analysis and hypothesis building by using a *fracture assessment triad* in conjunction with *thought experiments*. A *fracture assessment triad* is composed of (i) fracture behavior (i.e., principles of tension and shear form the basis for evaluation as guided by various generally accepted concepts regarding bone trauma), (ii) intrinsic properties, and (iii) extrinsic circumstances, which represent the totality of information needed to evaluate bone trauma. *Given any two items in the triad, the remaining item can be determined* (Figure 11.5) *through deductive reasoning*. It must be noted that, outside of a laboratory setting, it is impossible to "know" every intrinsic and extrinsic variable that influences fracture production. Nonetheless, if the dominant extrinsic causes and the intrinsic properties can be estimated, the resultant fracture behavior can be postulated. In like manner, when fracture behavior and the extrinsic cause are known, the intrinsic properties of the bone that influence fracture behavior can be surmised. However, in a medical examiner's morgue and ultimately a judicial setting, the most pertinent component of the triad is the cause of the trauma (i.e., extrinsic forces). Determining the cause of bone trauma requires that fracture behavior be evaluated and intrinsic properties be surmised. The anthropologist must first evaluate the fracture by using principles of tension and shear along with the shape of fracture lines as they traverse a bone, angle of each fracture relative to the bone surface, angle of the fracture surface relative to the bone surface, secondary fracture orientation, and so on along with generally accepted concepts (e.g., bevel direction in gunshot wounds, preexisting fractures, breakaway spurs, etc.). Locating where each fracture initiated is exceedingly useful and should be routinely undertaken in fracture analysis. Next, every attempt should be made to understand the intrinsic properties of the bone containing the fracture. For example, a very old adult will likely have bones that are much more brittle than those of a very young adult. Deductive reasoning of these two areas (fracture behavior and intrinsic characteristics) will illuminate the extrinsic properties responsible for the fracture pattern. From these extrinsic properties, the source of the trauma (e.g., hammer, gunshot wound, ball bat, stab wound, etc.) may be deduced or eliminated.

Given any one item in the triad, elements of the remaining two items can be determined (Figure 11.5) *through inductive reasoning*. The fracture assessment triad, through inductive reasoning, facilitates the development of hypotheses that can be tested under controlled settings. For example, fracture shape may be of interest. Since the remaining two areas are responsible for the fracture shape, inductive reasoning can be used to identify specific elements from the intrinsic properties and the extrinsic forces to hold constant or to vary in an attempt to experimentally reproduce the fracture shape.

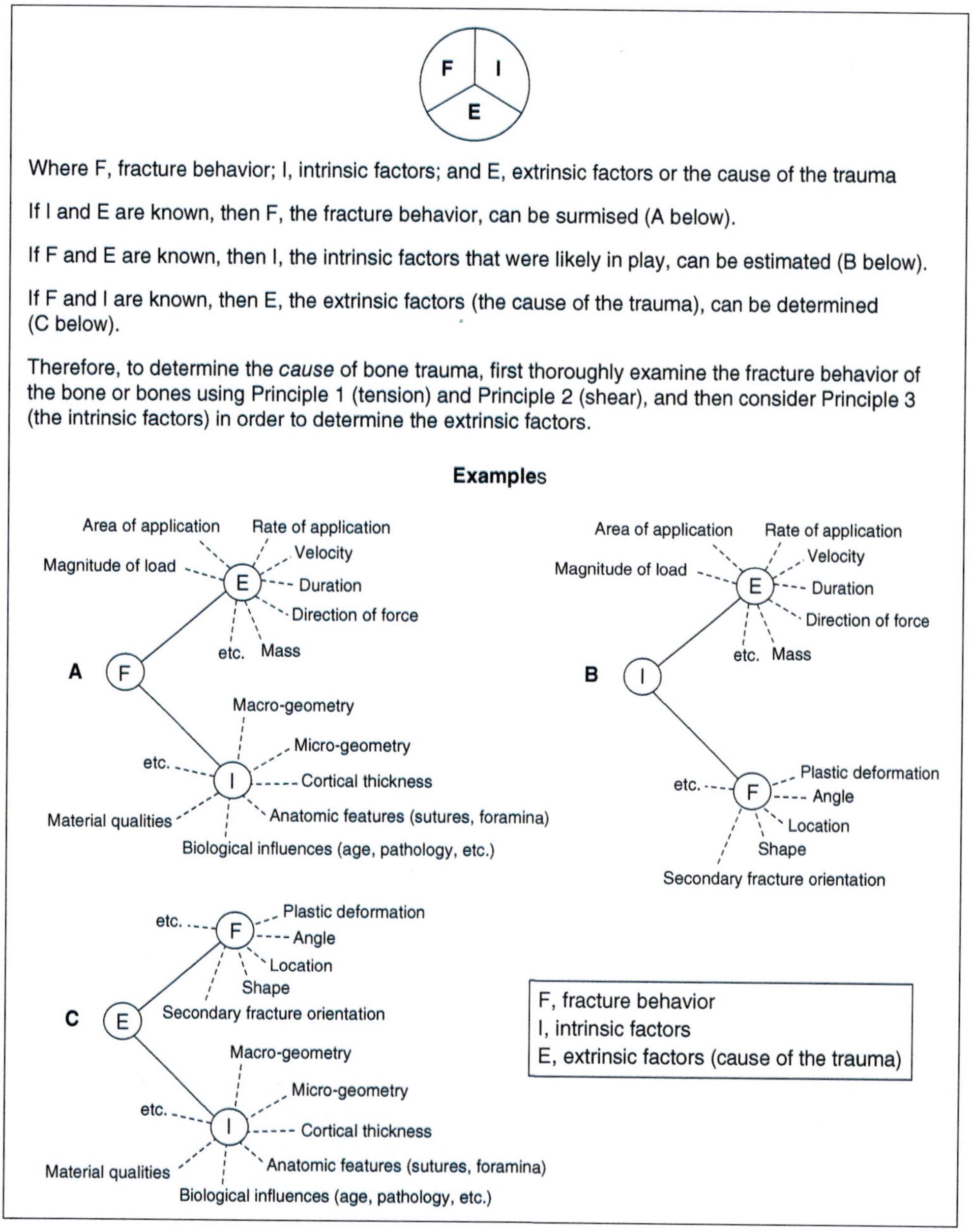

Figure 11.5 The fracture assessment triad provides a simplified approach that facilitates trauma analysis.

The fracture assessment triad provides the necessary information to identify the cause of perimortem trauma as well as postmortem damage and taphonomic influences. This information can then be subjected to *thought experiments*, which can be accomplished without the cost of equipment and laboratory space and in much less time. Admittedly, an exercise termed "thought experiments" seems trivial or frivolous; however, they have long been a powerful analytical tool used by philosophers and scientists from Galileo to Albert Einstein (Brown, 1993). In fact, Einstein's theory of special relativity derived from his thought experiments as a youth. According to the Brown and Yiftach (2016):

> Thought experiments are devices of the imagination used to investigate the nature of things. They are used for diverse reasons in a variety of areas, including economics, history, mathematics, philosophy, and the sciences, especially physics. Most often thought experiments are communicated in narrative form, frequently with diagrams.

The paramount findings needed by medical examiners and the courts involve extrinsic factors, specifically the identification or physical explanations regarding the weapon. Thought experiments used in conjunction with the fracture analysis triad would pair the observed findings (i.e., fracture appearance) with the likely intrinsic influences (i.e., bone morphology, elasticity, plasticity, brittleness, anatomic features affecting fracture behavior, etc.) and subject them to the influence of potential extrinsic factors (e.g., area of impact, direction of force, rate of impact, mass of object impacting bone, etc.). This deductive exercise will not only facilitate interpretation but also produce hypotheses where inductive reasoning can provide answers regarding extrinsic factors that influence fracture patterns. This represents interpretive theory as described by Boyd and Boyd (2011; Chapter 1, this volume), which is observation-based and clearly more applied. Thought experiments serve as a tool to mentally examine how the fracture(s) in question could have originated, as well as effects of various intrinsic and extrinsic influences on fracture behavior. Thought experiments frequently use extreme, even farcical experiments to more clearly delineate the salient elements responsible for the fracture. As a cautionary note, it must be emphasized that mental laboratory conclusions are not sufficient for the courts, but these thought experiments can lead to accepted physical explanations or research designs and testing that can be used in a judicial setting.

The utility of the proposed two-step approach can be demonstrated through the following examples taken from blunt force cranial trauma research. Gurdjian *et al.* (1947, 1950a, b) proposed a theory that, with blunt force cranial trauma, the fracture can initiate at a distance from the impact site. However, Smith *et al.* (1991) stated that cranial fractures initiate at and radiate from the impact site. Kroman *et al.* (2011) tested this theory using five cadaver heads and high-speed photography and found that fractures radiated from the impact site in all five cases, thus refuting Gurdjian *et al.* (1947, 1950a, b). However, Fenton *et al.* (2015) used high-speed photography to examine fractures to fresh crania when struck by an object and demonstrated that fractures can originate distantly to the impact site. To further complicate matters, both researchers produced video evidence clearly supporting their conclusions. In essence, it can be clearly seen that these two seemingly inconsistent conclusions are both apparently true. How can well-structured research conducted by highly capable researchers (Kroman *et al.*,

2011; Fenton *et al.*, 2015) produce opposite findings? The specific force that produced the disparate results can be viewed using the fracture assessment triad and thought experiments.

For this example, inductive reasoning may be used to examine each of the fracture patterns independently. The pattern with fractures radiating away from the impact site may be examined first. Something in either the intrinsic or extrinsic components of the triad must be responsible and that "something" must be different between the two research protocols. In the intrinsic component, bone brittleness is a concern; however, for the purpose of the thought experiment, it can be assumed that the heads used are basically similar with some degree of elasticity. In the extrinsic component, many factors can vary. Since the original experiments involved blunt trauma, both used slow loading, which can be held as a constant in the thought experiment. Of the extrinsic factors that could have made a difference, abductive reasoning suggests the size of the impact area as a factor. For the thought experiment, extremes can be used; two hammers are visualized—one with a striking surface 1 foot in diameter and the other with a striking surface of 1/8th inch in diameter and each with the same mass. The visual image of each striking the skull at the same slow rate produces two distinctly different visual results. The smaller striking surface penetrates the skull immediately, with the possibility of fractures radiating from the site of penetration, whereas the larger striking surface does not penetrate the skull, but rather deforms it. No logical means exist that enables fractures to initiate remotely from the penetrating impact site produced by a small striking surface.

This leads to a second thought experiment that focuses on the remote fracture in Fenton's experiment. In this thought experiment, the remote fracture initiation point can be set to open in the squamosal suture, and the fracture can be set to advance to the impact site on the superior aspect of the parietal bone. The bone will be assumed to possess a more elastic than brittle character. The fracture characteristics and the various intrinsic factors will serve as constants and each of the extrinsic factors can be varied individually to allow the mind's eye to observe the effects on the fracture. Abductive reasoning points to the slow rate of loading that allows the bone to deform before fracturing.

For this second thought experiment, a malleable cylinder (e.g., a marshmallow provides a farcical, but useful, mental image) will serve as a suitable model (Figure 11.6). The purpose of this experiment is to examine how surface tension behaves when the cylinder is deformed. First, the mind's eye may allow ink dots to be placed around the equator of the cylinder, and then the cylinder may be held between thumb and index finger (Figure 11.6a) and compressed (Figure 11.6b). With axial loading, the circumference expands, resulting in tensile forces increasing on the external surface perpendicular to the long axis of the cylinder (Figure 11.6c), and the dots placed around the imaginary equator will begin to separate. This simple thought experiment becomes much more complex when applied to a cranial vault, but the same basic dynamics exist. When a cranium (Figure 11.7a)

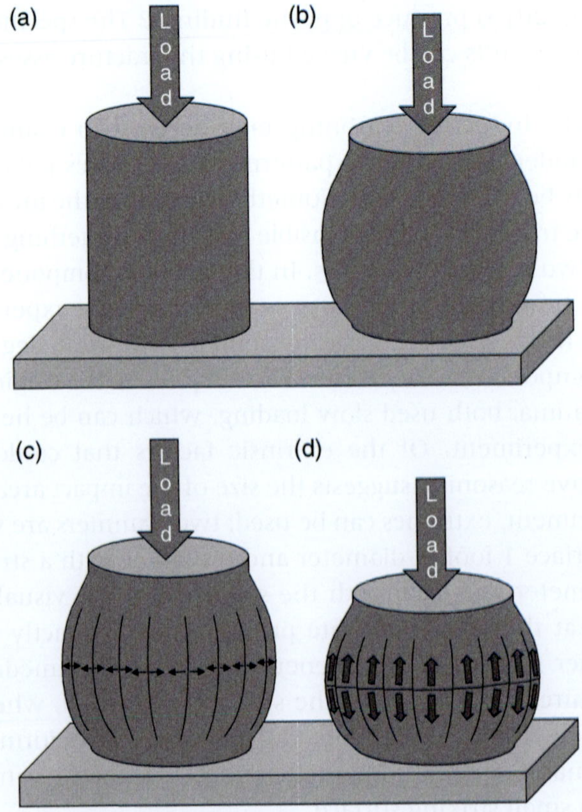

Figure 11.6 An example of a simple thought experiment in which a malleable cylinder with a static load (a) is compressed with a dynamic load (b). The circumference of the cylinder expands, causing increased tensile forces on the external surface perpendicular to the axial load, producing radiating fractures (c). As the dynamic load continues, tensile forces continue to increase on the external surface parallel to the axial load, producing concentric fractures (d).

with a relatively high elastic component is impacted by a blunt object with a broad striking surface (e.g., a 2-by-4 board) and at a slow rate of application, the vault will slowly bend outward with tension being exerted on the external surface as seen in Figure 11.6c. As the compressive load continues to increase, tensile stress will continue to rise, and a fracture will initiate at the weakest site (the squamosal suture in this example) and may advance along areas defined by bone morphology, bone composition, bone thickness, and so on, toward the impact site (Figure 11.7a). As the load continues, tensile forces will increase on the external surface parallel to the long axis of the cylinder (Figure 11.6d). As the plates of bone defined by these fractures bend outward, fractures appear across the plates, perpendicular to the radial fractures. Figure 11.6 clearly illustrates how radiating (Figure 11.6c) and concentric fractures (Figure 11.6d) can occur with blunt trauma to a cranial vault.

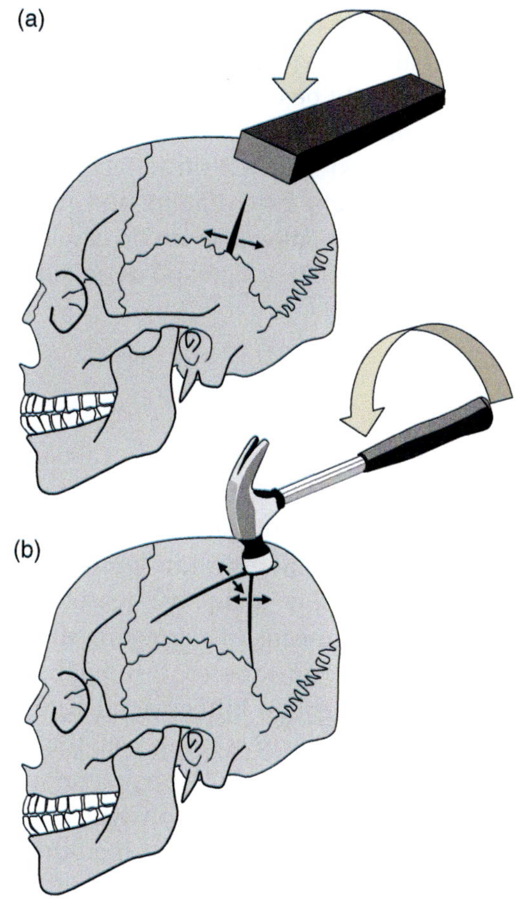

Figure 11.7 Blunt trauma to cranium by (a) a blunt object with a broad striking surface results in the vault being deformed and the fracture initiating at a point distant to the impact site, while trauma inflicted with (b) a blunt object with a narrow striking surface fractures the vault at the impact site and results in fractures radiating away from the site of impact.

The thought experiment has allowed the realization that bone elasticity and the ability for the bone to deform during the impact can explain how a fracture can radiate from the impact site and also form at a site remote to the impact site. When a cranium (Figure 11.7b) with a relatively low elastic component is impacted by a blunt object (high mass, like a hammer) with a constricted impact surface and at a slow rate of application, the blunt object will tend to fracture the vault at the impact site and fractures will tend to radiate away from the impact site (Figure 11.7b). On the other hand, when a cranium (Figure 11.7a) with a relatively high elastic component is impacted by a blunt object (moderate mass, like a 2 × 4 board) with a broad impact surface and a slow rate of application, the blunt object will tend to deform the skull, increasing surface tension perpendicular to the axis of impact and causing fractures to initiate remotely.

The fracture assessment triad serves as a means of facilitating research design and the thought experiment allows hypotheses to be constructed through inductive reasoning, where the goal might be to produce specific fracture characteristics (e.g., fractures occurring remote to the impact site) by varying intrinsic qualities of bone (e.g., elasticity, brittleness) with extrinsic factors (e.g., surface area of impact, rate of application). Thought experiments and the fracture assessment triad are tools for the forensic anthropologist to use in case assessment, as a guide in hypothesis formulation and research design and as an aid in the classroom.

11.5 Conclusion

The foundational theoretical assumption required to validate bone trauma analysis as a functional specialty within forensic anthropology is the nonrandomness of fracture configuration. The laws of physics dictate fracture behavior, which allows a measure of predictability and permits interpretation. Within interpretive theory, forensic anthropologists apply abductive reasoning during the initial examination of a trauma case as a means of suggesting the force that may have produced the trauma (blunt, sharp, gunshot, etc.). Inductive reasoning is used to identify intrinsic and extrinsic factors that influence fracture patterns and to construct and test hypotheses. Deductive reasoning can then be used to further narrow the possibilities and ultimately identify the precise source of the trauma.

A fracture assessment triad used in conjunction with thought experiments is proposed as a valuable tool for fracture analysis, hypothesis formulation, and research design. If any two of the three areas of the triad are known, deductive reasoning can be used to determine the third. The fracture assessment triad, along with inductive reasoning, can be used to develop hypotheses and construct research designs to test them. Thought experiments are proposed as an expedient, cost-free means of testing these hypotheses using either deductive or inductive reasoning. Thought experiments, though often absurd, can lead to a deeper understanding of proposed questions and, in so doing, can lead to more appropriate research design and testing.

References

Ballo, A.M., Lippo, V.L., Vallittu, P.K., and Närhi, T.O. (2007) Load bearing capacity of bone anchored fiber-reinforced composite device. *Journal of Materials Science: Materials in Medicine*, **18**, 2025–2031.

Berryman, H.E. and Gunther, W.M. (2000) Keyhole defect production in tubular bone. *Journal of Forensic Sciences*, **45**(2), 483–487.

Berryman, H.E. and Saul, T.B. (2015) Skeletal evidence of violent sexual assault in remains with excessive evidence of scavenging. In: *Skeletal Trauma Analysis—Case Studies in Context* (ed. N. Passalacqua and C. Rainwater), John Wiley & Sons, Ltd, Chichester, pp. 118–129.

Boyd, C.C. and Boyd, D.C. (2011) Theory and the scientific basis for forensic anthropology. *Journal of Forensic Sciences*, **56**(6), 1407–1415.

Brown, J.R. (1993) *Laboratory of the Mind: Thought Experiments in the Natural Sciences*. Routledge, Florence, KY.

Brown, J.R. and Yiftach, F. (2016) Thought experiments. In: *The Stanford Encyclopedia of Philosophy* (ed. E. Zalta). Stanford Encyclopedia of Philosophy, Stanford, CA. http://plato.stanford.edu/archives/spr2016/entries/thought-experiment/ (last accessed October 5, 2016).

Carter, D.R. and Hayes, W.C. (1976) Bone compressive strength: the influence of density and strain rate. *Science*, **194**(4270), 1174–1176.

Daubert v. Merrell Dow Pharmaceuticals, Inc. (1993) 509 US 579. United States Supreme Court.

Fenton, T.W., Isa, M.I., Vaughan, P.E., and Haut, R.C. (2015) Experimental and computational validations of the initiation and propagation of cranial fractures in the adult skull. *Proceedings of the 67th American Academy of Forensic Sciences*, **XXI**, 180–181.

Frye v. United States. (1923) 293F, 1013, 1014. District of Columbia Court of Appeals.

Gunther, W.M., Symes, S.A., and Berryman, H.E. (2000) Characteristics of child abuse by anteroposterior manual compression versus cardiopulmonary resuscitation. *The American Journal of Forensic Medicine and Pathology*, **21**(1), 5–10.

Gurdjian, E.S., Lissner, H.R., and Webster, J.E. (1947) The mechanism of production of linear skull fracture: Further studies on deformation of the skull by the stresscoat technique. *Surgery, Gynecology & Obstetrics*, **85**, 95–210.

Gurdjian, E.S., Lissner, H.R., and Webster, J.E. (1950a) The mechanism of skull fracture. *Journal of Neurosurgery*, **2**, 106–114.

Gurdjian, E.S., Lissner, H.R., and Webster, J.E. (1950b) The mechanism of skull fracture. *Radiology*, **54**, 313–339.

Hartman, W.F. (1974) Deformation and failure of spinal materials. *Experimental Mechanics*, **14**(3), 98–103.

James, S.H., Kish, P.E., and Sutton, T.P. (2005) *Principles of Bloodstain Pattern Analysis: Theory and Practice*, 3rd edn. CRC Press, Boca Raton, FL.

Kieser, J., Taylor, M., and Carr, D. (2013) *Forensic Biomechanics*, John Wiley & Sons, Ltd, Chichester.

Klawitter, J.J. and Hulbert, S.F. (1971) Application of porous ceramics for the attachment of load bearing internal orthopedic applications. *Journal of Biomedical Materials Research*, **5**(6), 161–229.

Kroman, A.M. (2007) *Fracture Biomechanics of the Human Skeleton*. Dissertation. The University of Tennessee, Knoxville.

Kroman, A., Kress, T., and Porta, D. (2011) Fracture propagation in the human cranium: a re-testing of popular theories. *Clinical Anatomy*, **24**, 309–318.

Love, J.C. and Symes, S.A. (2004) Understanding rib fracture patterns: incomplete and buckle fractures. *Journal of Forensic Sciences*, **49**(6), 1153–1158.

Merriam-Webster. (2015) Merriam-Webster Online Dictionary: Principle. http://www.merriam-webster.com/dictionary/principle (last accessed October 5, 2016).

Passalacqua, N.V. and Fenton, T.W. (2012) Developments in skeletal trauma: blunt force trauma. In: *A Companion to Forensic Anthropology* (ed. D. Dirkmaat). Blackwell Publishing, Ltd, Chichester, pp. 400–411.

Pearcy, M.J., Evans, J.H., and O'Brien, J.P. (1983) The load bearing capacity of vertebral cancellous bone in interbody fusion of the lumbar spine. *Engineering in Medicine*, **12**(4), 183–184.

Powell, B.J., Passalacqua, N.V., Fenton, T.W., and Haut, R.C. (2013) Fracture characteristics of entrapped head impacts vs. controlled head drops in infant porcine specimens. *Journal of Forensic Sciences*, **58**(3), 678–683.

Schiffer, M.B. (1988) The structure of archaeological theory. *American Antiquity*, **53**(3), 461–485.
Smith, M.D. and Cody, D.D. (1993) Load-bearing capacity of corticocancellous bone grafts in the spine. *Journal of Bone and Joint Surgery (American Volume)*, **75**(8), 1206–1213.
Smith, O.C., Berryman, H.E., Symes, S.A., and Moore, S.J. (1991) Bone fracture I: The physics of fractures. *Presented at the American Academy of Forensic Sciences 43rd Annual Scientific Meeting*, Anaheim, CA, February 18–21, 1991.
Smith, S.D., Wijdicks, C.A., Jansson, K.S., *et al.* (2014) Stability of mid-shaft clavicle fractures after plate fixation versus intramedullary repair and after hardware removal. *Knee Surgery, Sports Traumatology, Arthroscopy*, **22**, 448–455.
Staiger, M.P., Pietak, A.M., Huadmai, J., and Dias, G. (2006) Magnesium and its alloys as orthopedic biomaterials: a review. *Biomaterials*, **27**(9), 1728–1734.
SWGANTH (2011) Trauma analysis. https://www.nist.gov/oles/scientific-working-groups (last accessed October 5, 2016).
SWGANTH (2013) Home. https://www.nist.gov/oles/scientific-working-groups (last accessed October 5, 2016).
Symes, S.A., Patton, S.B., Campbell, T.A., *et al.* (2002) Child abuse: it's all in the recognition. *Proceedings of the 54th American Academy of Forensic Sciences*, **VIII**, 251–252.
Wescott, D.J. (2013) Biomechanics of bone trauma. In: *Encyclopedia of Forensic Sciences*, 2nd edn. (ed. J. Siegel and P. Saukko). Elsevier, New York, pp. 83–88.
White, A.A., Jupiter, J., Southwick, W., and Panjabi, M. (1973) An experimental study of the immediate load bearing capacity of three surgical constructions for anterior spine fusions. *Clinical Orthopaedics and Related Research*, **91**, 21–28.

CHAPTER 12

Thinking outside the box: Theory and innovation in sharp trauma analysis

John A. Williams[1] and Ronald W. Davis[2]

[1] *Department of Anthropology and Sociology, Western Carolina University, Cullowhee, NC, USA*

[2] *Department of Geosciences and Natural Resources, Western Carolina University, Cullowhee, NC, USA*

12.1 Introduction

At first glance, theory and innovation don't sound like they should be compatible at all. Theory is generally thought of in the abstract. A theory is a possibility not yet proven or even tested. Biological evolution is often spoken of as theoretical even though it is accepted as a factual process in natural science. When something is spoken of as innovative, it is generally described as novel, new, or even a departure from the norm. Innovation is within the realm of the practical, an application. Yet where does innovation come from? It originates as a new idea or theory, an untried idea, something not yet attempted or being attempted in a manner not originally conceived of. This chapter will explore a very old but venerable theory in forensic science and apply it to the interpretation of sharp trauma on bone. This will be done in a manner that is "thinking outside the box."

12.2 Transfer of evidence

In the brief history of forensic science, numerous personalities stand out in their importance to the field. During the late nineteenth and early twentieth centuries, these first forensic theorists took the then-existing scientific knowledge base and applied it to the investigation of criminal actions. Matthew Orfila and his work with toxins and Alphonse Bertillon and criminal human identification are widely known early examples in every recounting of the origins of the discipline (Saferstein, 2007). Edward Locard also emerged as one of the pioneers of modern forensic science. Locard had his start in the new field of forensic

Forensic Anthropology: Theoretical Framework and Scientific Basis, First Edition.
Edited by C. Clifford Boyd Jr and Donna C. Boyd.

science rather inauspiciously in an attic space in the Lyon, France, police department. There he focused his attention on connections, connections between the criminal and the crime scene. His breakthrough, so to speak, came with his study of dust. Working with almost invisible dust particles, he was able to demonstrate that a person brought dust to a crime scene and removed dust from the crime scene. This observation became the essence of his principle of the transfer of evidence that every contact leaves behind a trace (Crispino and Houck, 2013).

Locard's theory of the transfer of evidence, as simple and intuitive as it is to us today, is the foundation for all of the forensic sciences. Forensic science is all about making connections, or linkages, between a person and event, a person and a person, a person and an object, or an object and another object. This holds true if a questioned document, DNA, fingerprints, structural failure, biological profile of a skeleton, or interpretation of trauma and pathology is being examined. All hinge on some form of transfer of evidence.

Locard's focus was on the individual criminal. His work with dust particles illustrates his theory that the criminal brings evidence to the scene and takes away evidence as well. While Locard focused on the individual person as the unit of transfer, it is a simple extension that any item in contact with an individual can likewise transfer evidence into and out of a crime scene. This is the basis of all trace evidence analysis, from rifling marks on bullets to tool marks produced on the surface of a lock. Most of criminalistics hinges on Locard's theory.

12.3 Theory connections

Forensic science is historically young and does not have the same test of time that fields like mathematics and chemistry have experienced. This is not too surprising given that forensic science as a field is, by its nature, an applied one. This is not an excuse for the lack of scientific rigor, but it conceivably explains why some elements of the forensic sciences have recently received significant negative reviews. Concerns with the scientific rigor and integrity of the discipline, as voiced in the 2009 National Academy of Science report, are perhaps a reflection of its youth (NAS, 2009). It could be argued that forensic science, as an applied discipline, out of necessity often bypassed the theoretical dimension of hypothesis testing. In the pre-Daubert era, expert testimony might hinge as much on the expert's reputation as on any technique used by that expert. Peer review and demonstration of the theoretical basis for a forensic procedure were not strict requirements for legal acceptance.

Forensic anthropology suffers from the same bias. One author (Williams) regularly teaches a course on human osteology method and theory. This course is long on method and short on theory. We practice but often do so without a firm theoretical basis for what we do.

Boyd and Boyd (2011) argue that forensic anthropology is at a crossroads. The discipline has its roots as an applied science. This applied approach can no longer be accepted without question. Forensic anthropology has advanced beyond simple applications of the comprehension of the human skeleton's biological parameters. Today, forensic anthropology embraces a vastly wider range of endeavors and audiences, ones that the founders of our discipline perhaps could not have imagined or foreseen. If the discipline is to move out of the nineteenth century's pure application, then the theories behind its applications need to be addressed. Boyd and Boyd (see Chapter 1 of this volume), drafting from various disciplines including sociology and archaeology, describe three forms of forensic anthropological theory: foundational, interpretive, and methodological. Foundational theory refers to all-encompassing theories that form the basis for a multitude of applications. Darwinian evolution as the foundation for human biological evolution is one example. There is interpretive theory that uses observations such as those derived from case studies and experimentation. Even if we don't recognize it as theoretical, this is what forensic anthropology bases much of its application on. Methodological theory includes recovery protocols and statistical interpretation of experimentation (Schiffer, 1988).

This isn't to say that forensic anthropology (and forensic science in general) has been entirely lacking in a theoretical disposition. In its early days, the late nineteenth and early twentieth centuries, the discipline was very much theoretical. George Dorsey, like the other founders, was employing elements of interpretive theory, in applied court testimonies (Stewart, 1978). Like Locard and his dust particles, early forensic anthropologists were inventors, taking a theory and applying it to forensic questions. It wasn't long, however, before theory took a back seat to application.

12.4 The human skeleton as transfer evidence

Frank Saul coined the term "osteobiography" when referring to the human skeleton (Saul and Saul, 1989). By Saul's definition, the human skeleton is a person's life history recorded in their bones. At the time of death, the human skeleton is a snapshot of the person, encompassing physical characteristics of that person up to that point in time. This osteobiography does suffer from one drawback-memory. Much like human memory, the skeleton "remembers" recent events better than past ones. Bone remodeling is constantly rewriting the story of the skeleton, but, of course, some life events never even enter the realm of skeletal memory.

Another way of thinking about the human skeleton is as 206 individual pieces of potential transfer evidence. A person's age, sex, and ancestry are transferred from themselves to their skeleton. From this perspective, the forensic anthropologist ultimately then is a trace or transfer evidence specialist. The forensic anthropologist is trained in the interpretation of the one particular class of Locard's theory, lifetime changes, both removal and additions, to human bone and the human skeleton.

When viewing the human skeleton as transfer evidence, it can be conveniently divided into two classes or categories. The first is that which is intrinsic to the individual. This includes the biological profile of the person as well as genetic and developmental anomalies and pathological conditions. These elements are generally immutable though subject to some level of interpretation. For example, what pubic symphysis phase does an adult possess? The other class of transfer evidence is extrinsic and far more ephemeral and individual. This represents the unique life experiences of the person and includes such things as healed broken bone, orthopedic surgeries and appliances, markers of occupational stress, and perimortem and taphonomic events (i.e., dismemberment). This second class, while extrinsic, is highly individual in nature; no two persons will react in the same manner to the same life events. Extrinsic features are also more temporally fragile. If it was possible, a snapshot or osteobiography of a person taken even a year before death may present a totally different picture of that person compared with the picture at the time of death.

12.5 A primer on saws and dismemberment

As Boyd and Boyd (see Chapter 1, this volume) discuss, forensic anthropology has a theoretical basis that has gone unrecognized for the most part. Locard's theory as it applies to saw cut marks in bone is a case in point. Without directly referencing Locard, the transfer of saw class characteristics to bone is a fundamental premise of this aspect of sharp trauma analysis.

Taphonomically speaking, it is generally accepted that purposeful body dismemberment occurs for one of two reasons: to dispose the body and to preclude identification (Symes *et al.*, 2002; Ortner, 2008). Experience has shown that, when the goal is ease of body disposal, the limb bones are targeted for dissection. The bone or bones in question are bisected. It is also common to find knife cut marks and false starts associated with limb dissection (Reichs, 1996). In fewer instances, a body is dismembered to destroy or alter evidence, usually to hinder identification of the remains. For obvious reasons, decapitation and removal of the hands form the pattern for this type of dismemberment. This additionally means that the remains will not be found together in one location but rather will be scattered or not totally recovered (Symes *et al.*, 1996, 2002).

Saws are ancient tools and, while they have undergone improvements in technology, today's handsaws are not appreciably different from those of 400 years ago (Symes, 1992). All modern handsaws possess a basic design–a function of their use. There is, of course, a handle; as handsaws are of the reciprocating variety, there must be a means for the user to move the saw back and forth. A frame to hold the blade varies by design. In a carpenter's saw, the blade is the frame. With hacksaws, which are designed for ease of blade removal, the blade is mounted on an adjustable frame. The frame functions to hold the blade true as it moves back and forth in the medium. The most diagnostic or identifiable feature of a saw is its teeth, which do the actual work of the saw. Teeth range in size, number, and design. The greater the number of teeth, the easier it is to move the saw through the material, but it is also easier for the material to lodge between the teeth, thereby reducing cutting efficiency. Tooth number and size vary with the medium being cut. A 32-teeth-per-inch hacksaw would be a very poor choice to cut firewood just as a 4-teeth-per-inch bow saw would be a poor choice to cut plastic. Saws with standard teeth have teeth designed as either rip or cross cut. Ripsaws have teeth shaped like a chisel and, when cutting wood, function to cut along and between the wood fibers. Crosscut saw teeth are knife-shaped and designed to slice through fibers of wood or other media. Another feature of saw teeth is their set. This is the arrangement of the teeth on the saw blade. Set is designed to assist in removing the kerf material as the saw cuts through its medium. There is the alternating set in which the teeth are bent or offset from the midline of the blade in a specific angle or degree. Some saws have a third tooth called a raker. It is a chisel-shaped tooth that sweeps away the kerf material cut by the preceding teeth. The raker tooth also reduces blade drift or the side-to-side movement of the blade as the alternating teeth move through the medium. In the case of very high teeth per inch blades, the teeth are usually arranged in a wavy set. This is akin to the alternating format, but here a bank of teeth is progressively moved laterally and then medially and then laterally on the opposite side of the blade center. There are also saws that, while possessing teeth, are not traditionally designed. The Gigli saw, essentially a chain of teeth with two handles, is an example (Williams, 2008).

As a saw cuts through its medium, it creates various characteristic features (Bonte, 1975; Symes, 1992; Symes *et al.*, 1996). While the expression of each of these characteristics will vary depending on the medium—wood, metal, plastic, or bone—their presence is universal, or nearly so. The first and most obvious is the cut itself. The distance across the cutting edges of the teeth establishes how much material is removed by the teeth. This creates the kerf, the amount of material removed from the medium after the cut has been completed. The greater the distance across the teeth, the wider the kerf. There is a direct relationship between blade functional width, the lateral distance across adjacent teeth, and kerf thickness. A 32-teeth-per-inch hacksaw creates a much smaller kerf than a 4-teeth-per-inch bucksaw used to cut through logs. Tooth design and set create the shape of the kerf as the saw progresses through the medium. Establishing kerf thickness is heavily dependent on the presence of incomplete saw cuts or false starts, once referred to as hesitation marks. While these would be rare in the normal use of a saw in cutting wood or another medium, they are a common occurrence in cases of dismemberment (Reichs, 1996; Symes *et al.*, 1996). A false start represents an incomplete bisection of the bone, and, in terms of transfer of evidence, represents an optimal application of Locard's principle. When a false start is present, it is a simple procedure to measure the width of the kerf. False starts also provide another form of class feature, kerf profile. When viewed laterally, the base of the false start will take on one of several shapes based on the tooth type, size, number, and set. This is the tooth profile. Each class of saw is associated with its own particular though not necessarily unique kerf profile.

Love *et al.* (2015) recently discussed the functionality of microscopic saw cut mark analysis. Not surprisingly, they found kerf width and kerf profile to be reliable indicators of saw class. The problem, as they very clearly point out, is that many additional saw class identifiers (i.e., exit chipping) are not routinely present on cut bone surfaces. Even the highly diagnostic kerf width and kerf profile are not immune from being absent on a cut bone surface. It is this lack of consistency in saw cut marks in bone that make saw class diagnosis tenuous at times. Saw dismemberment can create everything from a wealth of diagnostic morphometric data in the form of multiple false starts on a humerus to a nearly impossible to interpret decapitation through the body of a cervical vertebra. No two cases of dismemberment are the same.

This brings us to the most visible of saw cut characteristics of bone: the striations created on the kerf wall. As the saw teeth reciprocally progress through the bone, they leave behind grooves in the wall. Generally speaking, the higher the teeth per inch, the finer these striations will be, and, conversely, the lower the teeth per inch, the coarser these grooves will be. That said, striation patterns do not provide the same level of specificity that saw kerf thickness or profile do in linking the saw cut to a specific class of saw. This is unfortunate given that nearly every saw-cut bone will have kerf wall striations. Despite being nearly universal in presence, striations are the least useful characteristic to link a saw to a saw cut. This isn't to say that striations are totally useless. They can establish whether a powered saw or handsaw was used. They can assist in establishing the direction of saw cut and on rare occasions may lead to the determination of teeth per inch (Symes, 1992). But despite their high visibility, striations lack the level of diagnostic specificity other aspects of the cut may have.

In reviewing the literature of sharp trauma analysis, especially saw cut mark interpretation, there is little reference to the theoretical basis for any conclusions reached concerning instrument identification. It has been generally accepted that saw class can be identified from transfer marks (Love *et al.*, 2015). Much has been published regarding analysis and interpretation but few, if any, comments exist concerning the theoretical basis for the interpretation (Bonte, 1975; Reichs, 1996; Symes *et al.*, 1996; Love *et al.*, 2015). Only recently have attempts been made to validate the error rate of saw class identification and the ability to link a specific saw to saw cut marks.

12.6 Geographic information system

A geographic information system (GIS) is a suite of software tools for creating, editing, and analyzing spatial data representing earth features. GIS tasks can range from simple display and location queries to statistical analyses and predictive modeling. Spatial data generally take two forms: (i) *vector*, consisting of georeferenced points, lines, and polygons, and (ii) *raster*, consisting of numeric pixels. Vector data are user-created or derived, whereas raster data are at least initially sensor-derived. Sensors like those in digital cameras produce pixels where numeric values indicate the level of light reflected from a surface. Differences in the composition and texture of any given surface will produce variation in light reflectance and hence pixel values. Variation and patterns of such light reflectance are the basis of most spatial image analyses (Lillesand and Kiefer, 2004). While GIS may be thought of as a very recent technology, it had its beginnings in the late 1960s. It is only with recent advances in computer technology that GIS has become more widespread in its application.

Geographic features differ in their surface composition, color, shape, and texture and thus will reflect light from their surfaces in unique ways. Evaluating this variation in light reflectance is the core of remote sensing, which has been applied for decades to study earth features at scales ranging from local to global (Lillesand and Kiefer, 2004). The use of image analyses has practical applications throughout the sciences and has seen increased use within the anthropological disciplines in recent years (Anemone *et al.*, 2011).

The GIS program was designed to interpret patterns for large geographic areas. However, pattern recognition knows no size limitations—smaller areas are just a matter of scale. From a state the size of North Carolina to a single county within the state, both can be analyzed using GIS. The only difference is in the size of the area under study. Nor are there any limitations as to what can be mapped; while GIS was designed to recognize geographic patterns, there is nothing that restricts GIS to the geographic domain.

12.7 Applications of GIS in forensic anthropology and human osteology

The application of GIS to the spatial analysis of human remains is by no means novel (Herrmann 2002; Anemone *et al.*, 2011; Herrmann *et al.*, 2014). GIS is a tool designed to map the spatial distribution of objects. Archaeological, fossil, and forensic sites are routinely mapped. Marean *et al.* (2001), for example, developed an ArcGIS (Environmental Systems Research Institute) software subroutine for mapping individual bones at archaeological sites.

A number of anthropologists have gone beyond the traditional use of GIS in mapping patterns other than the distribution of skeletal remains within a site. The earliest use of GIS in what would be termed a nontraditional approach was that of Zuccotti *et al.* (1998), who mapped molar cusps of several extant and extinct hominoids. They topographically mapped cusps as they related to diet, comparing the extant to the extinct species. Herrmann and Devlin (2008) used GIS to map fragmentary cremated human remains from a Woodland bioarchaeological site in

Kentucky. Their goal was to improve upon the estimation of the minimum number of individuals (MNIs) by observing how many fragments shared locations in the same virtual bone space. Parkinson *et al.* (2014) used GIS to map canid damage on bones. In a similar line of inquiry, using immature porcine skulls, Powell *et al.* (2012, 2013) and Deland *et al.* (2015) used GIS to plot blunt force trauma fracture patterns. In their protocol, immature pig skulls were traumatized in different locations. The resulting fractures were then mapped to demonstrate the causal link between force application site and resultant fractures. In all of these applications, while based on small spaces, the goal was spatial mapping of the distribution of events: molar cusps, bone fragments, canid tooth marks, or fracture locations. GIS mapping was a tool but in a secondary role to the overarching questions of each analysis. Rose *et al.* (2012) went deeper, both analytically and figuratively, in examining bone microstructure. The use of GIS was the focus of their study: cross-sectional images of a right first metatarsal were processed using ArcGIS to establish patterns of osteon remodeling. While Rose and colleagues' approach is mapping, it is on a different level from simply compiling patterns. They clearly showed that applications of GIS are "all a matter of scale" and that the technology has utility in nontraditional mapping situations.

12.8 GIS: innovation in cut mark striation interpretation

These studies serve as the inspiration to "think outside the box" and use GIS as a mapping tool for sharp trauma analysis of dismemberment cut marks. They have also demonstrated that GIS can be used for more than traditional mapping of bone distribution within a site.

Once tool-specific patterns have been recognized, interpretation and identification of an unknown pattern is a matter of comparison to known patterns. Currently, in most situations, the analysis of class-specific cut mark patterns relies on morphometric characteristics like kerf thickness and kerf profile. As Symes (1992) has demonstrated, this is a highly effective method. Yet there are times when morphometric analysis is hindered, if not rendered useless, by the absence of observable class-specific characteristics (Love *et al.*, 2015). As noted earlier, there is one feature of tooth-instrument transfer that is nearly universally present–striations on the cut surface or kerf wall. Despite their visibility, they have proven to have limited diagnostic power in pattern analysis using traditional morphometric methods.

To test the utility of GIS in the interpretation of saw cut striations, an experimental design was created. Two classes of saws were chosen to represent the extremes of saw blade classes that might normally be encountered in dismemberment cases, 11 and 32 teeth per inch. Simply put, the 11-teeth-per-inch saw blade creates relatively large striations and the 32-teeth-per-inch saw blade creates very fine striations. While a less dramatic difference in teeth per inch might provide a better test of the discriminating power of GIS, the purpose of this design was to determine if GIS could distinguish in a reasonable manner two very different patterns of saw cut striations.

Long bones of *Odocoileus virginianus* (white-tailed deer) were used as the experimental medium. The methodology for making these cuts is outlined in Williams and Davis (2014). It involved making complete single cuts through each bone. In making each saw cut, each bone was stabilized in an autopsy bone histology sectioning device. To account for any variations in bone cross section and sawing technique, multiple trials were performed using each saw. Each trial consisted of a single complete saw cut. As each trial created two saw cut surfaces, essentially duplicates of each other, only one surface was used for each trial. Love *et al.* (2015) demonstrated how lighting affects the visualization of striae on the cut bone surface. As it was critical for the surface topography of the cut surface to be visible, every effort was made to use fiber optic illumination to maximize shadows across the striations.

The cut surfaces were then examined using digital microscopy (Figures 12.1 and 12.2). It is very easy to see the topographic differences between the 11-teeth-per-inch saw cut with its deep (relatively speaking) ridges and furrows and the 32-teeth-per-inch surface with significantly less surface relief. Digital microscopy has the added benefit of storing the resulting image in a jpeg format. Digital imagery is one of the two bases for GIS applications. The creation of a color digital image requires at a minimum three bands (selected portions of the electromagnetic spectrum), typically red, blue, and green, although numerous sensors also include infrared and other wavelengths. Variations in surface characteristics (i.e., texture)

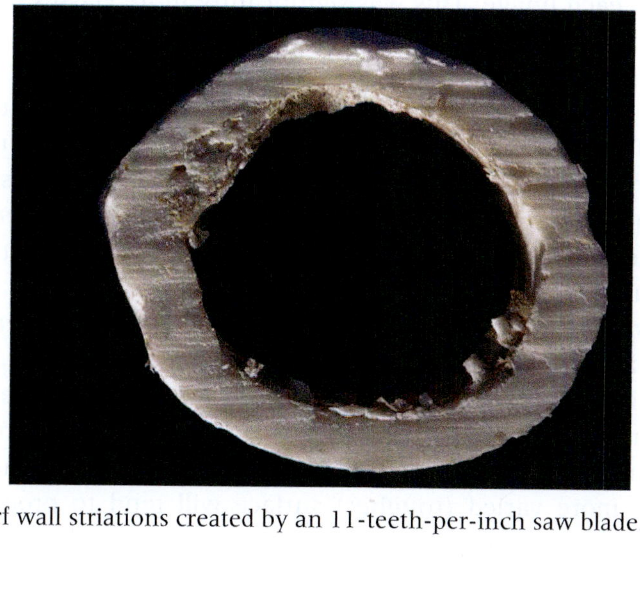

Figure 12.1 Kerf wall striations created by an 11-teeth-per-inch saw blade.

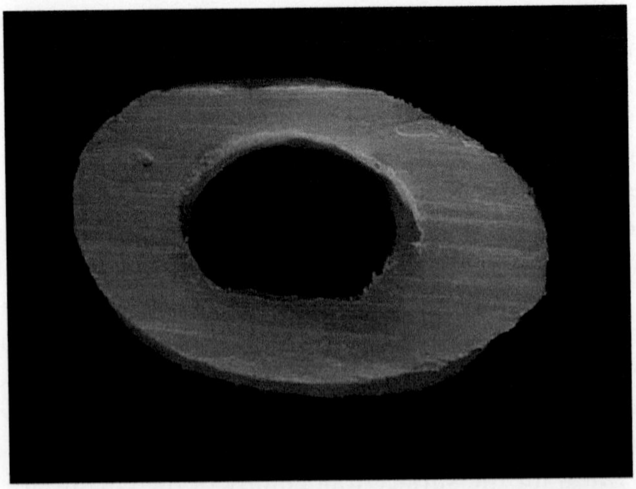

Figure 12.2 Kerf wall striations created by a 32-teeth-per-inch saw blade.

will produce different reflectance values across these bands and the spectral variation contained within an image can be very high.

To analyze the variation within each bone cut image, an *unsupervised classification* in ArcGIS 10.3.1 was applied (ESRI, Redlands, California). The unsupervised approach is used to identify groups of pixels having statistically similar reflectance patterns. The more homogeneous the surface being analyzed (i.e., smooth with low texture), the fewer statistical classes are required to represent the spectral variation in the image (Lillesand and Kiefer, 2004).

As the goal of this research was to evaluate the overall heterogeneity, the minimum class number was set to 50. This maximized the number of classes detected within each image. This was significantly more classes than required, making the number of resulting classes a true indicator of the inherent variation in reflectance and not the result of an arbitrary distinction. Figures 12.3 and 12.4 are screenshots from ArcGIS after applying the unsupervised classification. The colors applied to the cut surface topography are created by ArcGIS and have no specific interpretative meaning. Each color simply represents a different distinguished class. The number of colors and therefore classes is clearly greater for the 11-teeth-per-inch cut surface than for the 32-teeth-per-inch cut surface.

To examine spectral heterogeneity, measures of class richness were first evaluated. Richness is simply the number of statistical classes produced by the unsupervised classification and is an indicator of the overall heterogeneity in reflectance values within a given image. Images having a smoother and more homogenous surface will tend to result in fewer classes (lower richness), whereas those having a more varied (rougher) surface will tend to produce a higher number of classes.

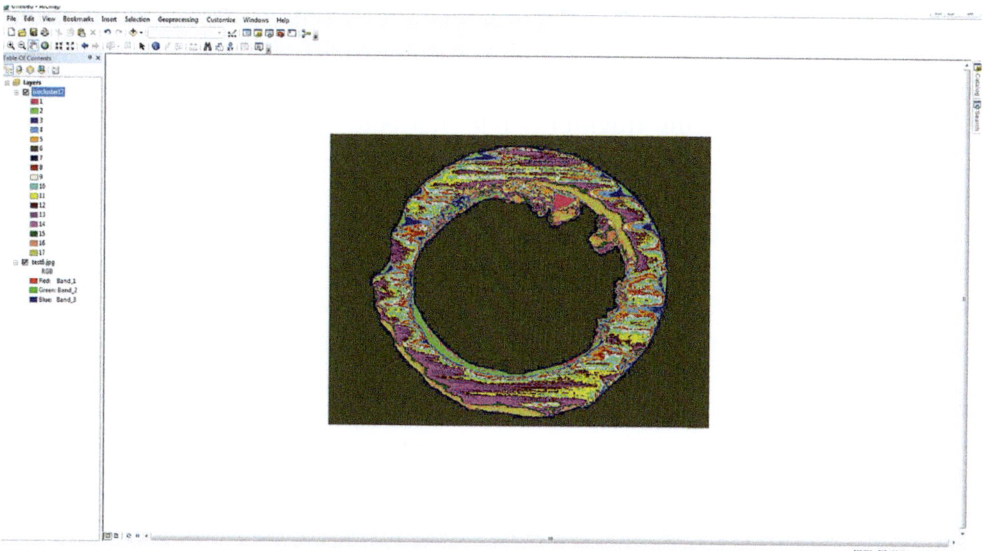

Figure 12.3 Screenshot from ArcGIS unsupervised classification of the 11-teeth-per-inch saw blade striations (jpeg image).

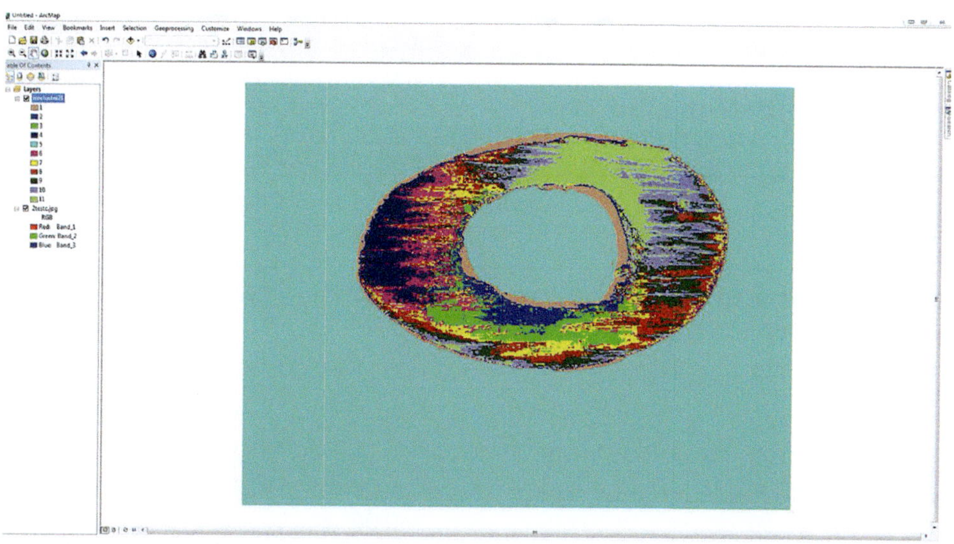

Figure 12.4 Screenshot from ArcGIS unsupervised classification of the 32-teeth-per-inch saw blade striations (jpeg image).

Because richness considers only the number of classes, indices of class diversity were also examined in order to reflect the relative abundance of each class. The widely used Shannon diversity index (SHDI) was applied (Shannon and Weaver, 1949; Nagendra, 2002), which evaluates both the number and proportion of classes to produce a unitless indicator, with 0 representing a single class situation (hence no diversity) and values increasing (no theoretical limit) as the number of classes increases (Table 12.1). Dominance and evenness are derived from diversity calculations and produce index scores of 0–1.0, reflecting how uniformly distributed the classes are in terms of area. In all cases, the number of classes obtained from bone fragments fell well below 50 attempted, indicating that the statistical variation produced by each blade was captured by the classifications.

The 11-teeth-per-inch saw blade produced an average of 26 classes (range 20–38) while the 32-teeth-per-inch saw blade produced an average of 11 classes (range 9–12) (Table 12.2). Both blades produced nearly identical values for dominance and evenness with the amount of area distributed quite evenly among

Table 12.1 GIS metrics

Metric	Formula	Output	Interpretation
Diversity	$1-\Sigma(P_i \times \ln(P_i))$	0–unlimited	A value of 0 (no diversity) is assigned when only one class is represented. Values increase as richness and/or proportional distribution of classes becomes more even
Evenness	$1-\Sigma(P_i \times \ln(P_i))/\ln(n)$	0–1.0	A score of 1.0 indicates a completely even distribution of classes based upon the proportion of area occupied by each
Dominance	1 – Evenness	0–1.0	A score of 1.0 indicates an image comprised of only a single (dominant) class

Table 12.2 GIS metrics for the 11- and 32-teeth-per-inch saw blade cut surfaces

Image	Attempted classes	Resulting classes (richness)	Dominance	Evenness	Diversity (SHDI)
11 tpi					
Test 1	50.00	29.00	0.10	0.90	3.28
Test 2	50.00	38.00	0.03	0.97	3.54
Test 3	50.00	26.00	0.05	0.95	3.21
Test 4	50.00	20.00	0.06	0.94	2.82
Test 5	50.00	20.00	0.10	0.90	2.61
			0.07	**0.93**	**3.09**
32 tpi					
Test A	50.00	9.00	0.04	0.96	2.11
Test B	50.00	12.00	0.03	0.97	2.40
Test C	50.00	11.00	0.06	0.94	2.33
Test D	50.00	12.00	0.01	0.99	2.36
			0.04	**0.96**	**2.30**

classes in both cases. As with richness, the 11-teeth-per-inch blade produced greater diversity values with an average SHDI of 3.09 compared with 2.30 for the 32-teeth-per-inch blade (Table 12.2). While sample sizes are small, consistent differences in the number and diversity of patches produced by these blades were found.

12.9 Locard and the twenty-first century: It's all a matter of scale

A little more than 100 years ago, forensic science and forensic anthropology were both in their infancies. The forensic sciences were inventing themselves. It was a time of novel thinking, a time of theory and theoretical application. Locard's theory of the transfer of evidence, while so obvious in today's world, was innovative in his day. One hundred years later, Locard's theory is just as relevant as it was then. It would not be too sweeping a generalization to state that all of forensic science hinges in some manner on what Locard first observed with dust particles in his attic laboratory in Lyon. Forensic science is in its essence the interpretation of how evidence is transferred from person to person, person to object, or object to object.

Using Saul's osteobiography, the human skeleton is one large accumulation of transfer evidence. Trauma to the skeleton is, of course, a classic application of evidence transfer. Sharp trauma, and in this case saw dismemberment, involves the transfer of saw class characteristics to bone. This is precisely what Locard envisioned–that every criminal leaves behind evidence. Saws used to dismember create unique patterns of cut marks. Traditionally, these patterns have been interpreted based on direct saw-to-bone transfer (i.e., kerf thickness and saw blade width). The traditional approach has weaknesses, especially when only one cut surface or kerf wall is present.

Locard's theory was applied by "thinking outside the box" and using GIS as a tool. Other anthropologists have also used GIS in what could be called nontraditional applications. Normally, GIS is used to map large surfaces, to find patterns on the Earth's surface. But what is the cut surface of a bone? It is nothing more than a pattern of saw tooth striations. Inspired by the innovative work of others, the saw cut surface was approached as any other surface. GIS took the cut surface of bone and reduced it to a pattern of bands. Choosing two highly discordant saws, 11 and 32 teeth per inch, GIS demonstrated that striation band patterns are easily distinguished. Rather than being relegated to the occasionally useful, kerf wall striations do produce demonstrably useful information for identifying saw class in cases of dismemberment. Using GIS and following Locard's theory, it is all just a matter of scale.

References

Anemone, R.L., Conroy, G.C., and Emerson, C.W. (2011) GIS and paleoanthropology: Incorporating new approaches from the geospatial sciences in the analysis of primate and human evolution. *Yearbook of Physical Anthropology*, **54**, 19–46.

Bonte, W. (1975) Tool marks in bone and cartilage. *Journal of Forensic Sciences*, **20** (2), 315–325.

Boyd, C. and Boyd, D.C. (2011) Theory and the scientific basis of forensic anthropology. *Journal of Forensic Sciences*, **56**, 1407–1415.

Crispino, F. and Houck, M.M. (2013) Principles of forensic science. In: *Encyclopedia of Forensic Sciences* (2nd edn.) (eds. J.A. Siegel and P.J. Saukko). Academic Press, Waltham, pp. 278–281.

Deland, T.S., Niespodziewanski, E., Fenton, T.W., *et al.* (2015) The role of interface on the impact characteristics and cranial fracture patterns using the immature porcine head model. *Journal of Forensic Sciences*, **61**, 1–7.

Herrmann, N.P. (2002) GIS applied to bioarchaeology: An example from the Rio Talgua Caves in northeast Honduras. *Journal of Cave and Karst Studies*, **64**, 17–22.

Herrmann, N.P. and Devlin, J.B. (2008) Assessment of commingled human remains using a GIS-based approach. In: *Recovery, Analysis, and Identification of Commingled Human Remains* (eds. B. Adams and J. Byrd). Humana Press, Totowa, pp. 257–269.

Herrmann, N.P., Devlin, J.B., and Stanton, J.C. (2014) Bioarchaeological spatial analysis of the Walker-Noe Crematory (15GD56). In: *Commingled and Disarticulated Human Remains: Working toward Improved Theory, Method, and Data* (eds. A.J. Osterholtz, K.M. Baustian, and D.L. Martin). Springer, New York, pp. 51–66.

Lillesand, T.M. and Kiefer, R.W. (2004) *Remote Sensing and Image Interpretation*. John Wiley & Sons, Inc., Hoboken.

Love, J.C., Derrick, S.M., Weirsema, J.M., *et al.* (2015) Microscopic saw mark analysis: An empirical approach. *Journal of Forensic Sciences*, **60**, S21–S26.

Marean, C.W., Abe, Y., Nilssen, P.J., *et al.* (2001) Estimating the minimum number of skeletal elements (MNE) in zooarchaeology: A review and a new image-analysis GIS approach. *American Antiquity*, **66**, 333–348.

Nagendra, H. (2002) Opposite trends in response for the Shannon and Simpson indices of landscape diversity. *Applied Geography*, **22**, 175–186.

National Academy of Sciences (2009) *Strengthening Forensic Science in the United States: A Path Forward*. National Academies Press, Washington, DC.

Ortner, D. (2008) Differential diagnosis of skeletal injuries. In: *Skeletal Trauma: Identification of Injuries Resulting from Human Rights Abuse and Armed Conflict* (eds. E.H. Kimmerle and J.P. Baraybar). CRC Press, Boca Raton, pp. 21–93.

Parkinson, J.A., Plummer, T.W., and Bose, F. (2014) A GIS-based approach to documenting large canid damage to bones. *Palaeogeography, Palaeoclimatology, Palaeoecology*, **409**, 57–71.

Powell, B.J., Passalacqua, N.V., Baumer, T.G., *et al.* (2012) Fracture patterns on the infant porcine skull following severe blunt impact. *Journal of Forensic Sciences*, **57**, 312–317.

Powell, B.J., Passalacqua, N.V., Baumer, T.G., *et al.* (2013) Fracture characteristics of entrapped head impacts versus controlled head drops in infant porcine specimens. *Journal of Forensic Sciences*, **58**, 678–683.

Reichs, K.J. (1996) Postmortem dismemberment: Recovery, analysis, and interpretation. In: *Forensic Osteology: Advances in the Identification of Human Remains* (2nd edn.) (ed. K.J. Reichs). Charles C. Thomas, Springfield, pp. 353–388.

Rose, D.C., Agnew, A.M., Gocha, T.P., *et al.* (2012) Technical note: The use of geographical information systems software for the spatial analysis of bone microstructure. *American Journal of Physical Anthropology*, **148**, 648–654.

Saferstein, R. (2007) *Criminalistics: An Introduction to Forensic Science* (9th edn). Pearson, Upper Saddle River.

Saul, F.P. and Saul, J.A. (1989) Osteobiography: A Maya example. In: *Reconstruction of Life from the Skeleton* (eds. M.Y. Iscan and K.A.R. Kennedy). Wiley-Liss, New York, pp. 287–302.

Schiffer, M.B. (1988) The structure of archaeological theory. *American Antiquity*, **53**, 461–485.

Shannon, C.E. and Weaver, W. (1949) *The Mathematical Theory of Communication*. University of Illinois Press, Chicago.

Stewart, T.D. (1978) George A. Dorsey's role in the Luetgert case: A significant episode in the history of forensic anthropology. *Journal of Forensic Sciences*, **23**, 786–791.

Symes, S.A. (1992) *Morphology of Saw Marks in Human Bone: Identification of Class Characteristics*. Doctoral thesis, University of Tennessee, Knoxville.

Symes, S.A., Berryman, H.E., and Smith O.C. (1996) Saw marks in bone: Introduction and examination of residual kerf contour. In: *Forensic Osteology: Advances in the Identification of Human Remains* (2nd edn.) (ed. K.J. Reichs). Charles C. Thomas, Springfield, pp. 389–409.

Symes, S.A., Williams, J.A., Murray, E.A., *et al.* (2002) Taphonomic context of sharp-force trauma in suspected cases of human mutilation and dismemberment. In: *Advances in Forensic Taphonomy* (eds. W.D. Haglund and M.H. Sorg). CRC Press, Boca Raton, pp. 404–434.

Williams, J.A. (2008) Saw cut marks in bone created by atypical saws. *Proceedings of the 60th American Academy of Forensic Sciences*, **XIV**, 323.

Williams, J.A. and Davis, R.W. (2014) The utility of GIS in the spatial analysis of saw cut marks on bone. *Proceedings of the 66th American Academy of Forensic Sciences*, **XX**, 429–430.

Zuccotti, L.F., Williamson, M.D., Limp, W.F., *et al.* (1998) Technical note: Modeling primate occlusal topography using geographic information systems technology. *American Journal of Physical Anthropology*, **107**, 137–142.

CHAPTER 13

The forensic anthropologist as broker for cross-disciplinary taphonomic research related to estimating the postmortem interval in medicolegal death investigations

Daniel J. Wescott

Forensic Anthropology Center at Texas State, Department of Anthropology, Texas State University, San Marcos, TX, USA

13.1 Introduction

Estimating the postmortem interval (PMI) is often a primary objective in criminal investigations and therefore an issue of interest shared by numerous disciplines, including anthropology, botany, entomology, geoscience, medicine, microbiology, and others. Professionals in these fields understand the complexity of decomposition and strive to uncover the underlying similarities and rules governing how carrion is recycled (i.e., how dead animals decompose and the chemicals from the bodies are recycled into the environment). In the past, scientists have attempted to understand this complexity using methods and theories from their own disciplines. However, new models and approaches are needed in the wake of recent criticisms of the scientific basis of forensic science (National Research Council, 2009) and the need for reproducible and valid methods with known error rates (Dirkmaat *et al.*, 2008; Christensen and Crowder, 2009; Christensen *et al.*, 2014). This cannot be accomplished if the various disciplines approach the topic separately.

Complex issues that are driven by multiple forces, such as carrion recycling, require integrated cross-disciplinary approaches where multiple disciplines cooperate to develop new methods and theories that transcend each discipline and solve real-world, multifaceted problems. Cross-disciplinary approaches to research

Forensic Anthropology: Theoretical Framework and Scientific Basis, First Edition.
Edited by C. Clifford Boyd Jr and Donna C. Boyd.

involving forensic taphonomy, and especially estimations of the PMI, are the only means to fully understand carrion recycling and ultimately to accurately estimate the PMI in medicolegal death investigations. Knowledge from various fields must be integrated and data, methodologies, perspectives, and concepts combined in order to develop unified methods and theories in forensic taphonomy that predict all the phenomena observed and take into account the needs of the various stakeholders. At a minimum, multidisciplinary research is required. However, to move beyond our simple understanding of carrion recycling and to accurately estimate the PMI with the precision needed in medicolegal death investigations, forensic scientists need to employ inter- and transdisciplinary approaches, and forensic anthropologists are ideally situated to broker the necessary cross-disciplinary research. Forensic anthropology is traditionally holistic, often borrowing and utilizing theory and methodologies from both the natural and social sciences in research and evidence interpretation, has a long history of conducting taphonomic research, and already frequently serves as an intermediary in medicolegal investigations and research.

The goals of this chapter are to (i) define taphonomy and the current theoretical and scientific basis for taphonomic studies, (ii) show how taphonomy relates to all the forensic science disciplines examining the PMI, (iii) summarize the knowledge of carrion recycling and how it relates to estimations of PMI, (iv) describe cross-disciplinary research, (v) highlight the need for cross-disciplinary approaches for the development of integrated theories in forensic taphonomy as they relate to estimating the PMI, and (vi) convincingly argue that forensic anthropologists are optimally prepared to broker this research that will result in new knowledge, tools, and practices necessary to fully comprehend the complex issues and questions arising in forensic taphonomy, especially the estimation of the PMI.

13.2 Taphonomy and taphonomic theory

Taphonomy is the study of the accumulated effects of the physical, chemical, and mechanical processes biological organisms undergo from the moment of death until discovery (Lyman, 1994). Initially defined as "the study of the transition (in all its details) of animal remains from the biosphere into the lithosphere" (Efremov, 1940:85), taphonomy is concerned with the phenomena involved in biostratinomy (preburial biological processes) and diagenesis (postburial geological and chemical processes) (Lyman, 1994, 2010). Taphonomic processes are often used to understand information loss or taphonomic bias (e.g., bone loss), but taphonomy has also been used to evaluate and reconstruct the postmortem record and to address questions dealing with disarticulation, dispersion, and bone modification (Lyman, 1994, 2002; Haglund and Sorg, 2002).

The goals of taphonomic analysis are to identify the diagnostic taphonomic effects that result from processes caused by agents. A taphonomic agent can be defined as the immediate cause of modification to the carcass (e.g., dog, insect, human, or water), while a taphonomic process is the dynamic action of an agent. Examples of taphonomic processes would include gnawing of bone by a dog, cutting a bone by a human, and movement of the carcass by water (Lyman, 1994). The static result of a taphonomic process is a taphonomic effect. What taphonomists must determine is the ultimate cause of a particular modification and identify the diagnostic features of taphonomic agents to develop a taphonomic history. In other words, taphonomists must determine the chronology of agents and processes (Lyman, 1987, 1994).

Theoretically and methodologically, taphonomy relies on rules "concerning cause–effect relations of various properties of an organism's tissues and how those tissues will respond to a particular taphonomic process" (Lyman, 1994:463) based on actualism (i.e., argument by analogy) or the principle of uniformitarianism (Lyman, 1994). Actualism is the "documentation of modern processes and the visible effects and patterns they produce" (Lyman, 2002:xix) and is therefore both a scientific theory and a methodological principle. Actualistic research is used in taphonomy to build models, control for important independent variables, and systemize dependent variables (Sorg and Haglund, 2002). The principle of uniformitarianism states that processes observed in the present function the same and have the same effects as those in the past, although the world may not be uniform.

While there is a need for a more integrated theory of taphonomy, taphonomists already rely on many principles, laws, and theories for the foundation of taphonomic analyses and interpretations. The decomposition process itself is accounted for by laws and theories in biology, chemistry, and physics (Schiffer, 1988). For example, temperature, humidity, solar radiation, and other factors affect the rate of chemical reactions and the activities and development of necrophagous microorganisms and insects, which are explained by theories in these fields. Furthermore, many interpretive and methodological theories are used in taphonomy. Some examples include recovery, analytical, and statistical induction theories (Boyd and Boyd, 2011). Methodological theory (Schiffer, 1988; Boyd and Boyd, 2011, Chapter 1, this volume) provides the underlying protocol for the proper collection, analysis, and interpretation of taphonomic data. Recovery theory provides the principles for the collection of evidence and the documentation of unrecoverable taphonomic data that must be conducted in the field. These data are then used to determine the depositional context and the association of objects (man-made or natural) with human remains. Analytical theory is used to assess the physical and contextual information obtained in the field and laboratory, and statistical induction theory may be used to determine the probability or likelihood of taphonomic histories.

13.3 Forensic taphonomy

As defined by Haglund and Sorg (1997a:3), forensic taphonomy is:

> the use of taphonomic models, approaches, and analyses in forensic contexts to estimate the time since death, reconstruct the circumstances before and after deposition, and discriminate the products of human behavior from those created by the earth's biological, physical, chemical, and geological subsystems.

As noted by Boyd and Boyd (2011:1408; Chapter 1, this volume), forensic taphonomy primarily uses interpretive theory that links "static observations to the dynamic natural and cultural processes in the past that created them." That is, forensic taphonomy is concerned with the "processes of decomposition and decay, animal and plant disturbance, and a host of environmental influences" to understand and interpret forensically important events (Boyd and Boyd, 2011:1408). Forensic taphonomic studies are generally experimental or case-based. Experimental research relies primarily on hypothetico-deductive reasoning and actualism, while case-based studies are normally a combination of inductive and deductive reasoning (Bristow *et al.*, 2016; Boyd and Boyd, Chapter 1, this volume). As with the archaeological and paleontological record, in medicolegal cases, taphonomic processes can alter or destroy evidence (Dirkmaat *et al.*, 2008), but in other cases it can be evidence in and of itself that aids in locating clandestine bodies, determining the manner of death, estimating the PMI, and reconstructing postmortem events (Haglund and Sorg, 1997b; Kalacska and Bell, 2006; Kalacska *et al.*, 2009; Lyman, 2002, 2010; Isaacks, 2015).

There are some differences between more traditional taphonomy (often referred to as paleotaphonomy) and forensic taphonomy. The differences are primarily related to time depth, the almost exclusive focus on a single species (humans), and often the analysis of a single individual rather than populations in forensic taphonomy. Relative to more traditional paleotaphonomy, forensic taphonomy is especially concerned with the early stages of the taphonomic record that can affect the interpretation of biological evidence during a medicolegal investigation (Haglund and Sorg, 1997a, 2002; Pokines, 2013). The precision of PMI estimations in forensic cases is "frequently in terms of days, weeks, or months, whereas the margin of error in [paleo]taphonomy may encompass hundreds of years" (Haglund and Sorg, 1997a:4). As a result, decomposition of soft tissue and periodic changes such as seasonal precipitation patterns or necrophagous insect succession are more critical to forensic taphonomists than the paleotaphonomists (Haglund and Sorg, 1997a; Pokines, 2013). Due to the relatively shorter PMI, forensic taphonomy is also less reliant on the principle of uniformitarianism since the processes that form the taphonomic history in medicolegal cases can be witnessed during the lifetime of the investigator (Beary and Lyman, 2012). In fact, Komar and Buikstra (2008) argue that the use of uniformitarianism in forensic taphonomy may not be valid because taphonomic processes observed in the present do not always have an analog to the past.

Traditional taphonomic research has also tended to focus on vertebrate skeletal assemblages made up of multiple species and individuals. Forensic taphonomy, on the other hand, is primarily concerned with a single species (*Homo sapiens*) and often a single individual. However, forensic taphonomy may involve multiple individuals in mass graves. While forensic taphonomists may examine the remains of multiple species, the goal is generally to determine if the remains are human or nonhuman (i.e., of forensic significance).

Forensic taphonomic analyses are more greatly affected by behavioral processes, especially human behavior or humans as a taphonomic agent, than traditional taphonomic investigations. Most forensic scenes are formed at least in part by human processes. While actualism and uniformitarianism govern mechanical, chemical, and physical processes, they do not necessarily govern behavioral processes (Lyman, 1994). For example, while the consumption of soft tissues by maggots and scavenging by vultures may leave diagnostic characteristics (i.e., static taphonomic effects), the succession of scavengers to the body may vary due to seasonal migration and activity patterns. As Haglund and Sorg (1997a:14) point out: "The behavior of human killers, for example, may introduce extreme variation of transport, dismemberment, and other disturbances of remains." However, it is often the taphonomic effects that allow us to differentiate between human behavior and those caused by other species or natural processes (Micozzi, 1991; Forbes, 2008; Boyd and Boyd, 2011).

While forensic taphonomy is often cited as a branch of anthropology (Haglund and Sorg, 1997a; Sorg and Haglund, 2002; Dirkmaat and Passalacqua, 2012; Pokines, 2013), taphonomy is used by all forensic science disciplines involved with the recovery and examination of human remains, the estimation of the PMI, and outdoor scene interpretation (Forbes, 2008; Sorg *et al.*, 2012). Taphonomy has been traditionally used by paleontologists and archaeologists, but, because of the shortened PMI examined in most medicolegal death investigations, forensic taphonomy has an important role to play in creating new approaches and actualistic models associated with the early stages of decomposition. To understand the shortened taphonomic history requires knowledge from many fields of science.

13.4 Taphonomy and the estimation of time since death

While taphonomic time is relative and only correlated with chronological time, taphonomic methods are used by forensic scientists to reconstruct the time since death or the PMI of unwitnessed deaths. Accurate and precise estimation of the PMI with known error rates can provide critical information regarding not only when the individual died but also when evaluating the alibis of suspects. The estimation of PMI relies on reconstruction of the taphonomic history. Taphonomic theory aids in determining the timing of alteration to the remains (e.g., stages of decomposition, effects of environmental exposure, succession of scavengers, and postburial interval) necessary for estimating the PMI. The insects, microbes, plants, and fungi associated with deceased individuals and the soils surrounding them provide a "biological clock" that can be used to estimate the time since death (Sorg *et al.*, 2012).

The scientific techniques used by a forensic practitioner to estimate the PMI are often dependent on the length of time since death (Forbes, 2008; Wells and LaMotte, 1995; Sharma *et al.*, 2015). For example, in the first hours after death, processes caused by chemical reactions, thermal transfer, and gravity cause rigor, algor, and livor mortis, respectively. In the first weeks of the PMI, the succession and development rates of necrophagous insects and microbes are often used to determine the taphonomic history. After skeletonization, however, methods examining bone weathering, deposition, and bone chemistry may be more appropriate.

13.5 The necrobiome

The estimation of PMI requires an understanding of carrion recycling (Haglund and Sorg, 1997b, 2002; Carter *et al.*, 2007). As Lyman (1994) points out, after death, the constituent parts of an organism are recycled, and therefore taphonomic research observes and documents this recycling. Dead organisms are a rich source of nutrients that are consumed and released into the ecosystem (Carter *et al.*, 2007; Metcalf *et al.*, 2016). If we think back to our high school biology courses, we remember the importance of understanding ecosystems and how energy, water, and organisms all interact. During carrion recycling, scavenger species (microbial, invertebrate, and vertebrate) compete, and sometimes cooperate, to obtain nutrients and energy from this transitory but valuable resource (Haglund and Sorg, 2002; Pechal *et al.*, 2014b; Metcalf *et al.*, 2016). These various species form the necrobiome. The chemical nutrients and water released by these necrophagous species, especially microbes, are then used by plants and other organisms, which are then consumed by other living species.

The sequence of events occurring during the decay of a body are generally universal (Micozzi, 1991; Galloway, 1997; Goff, 2000; Love and Marks, 2003; Megyesi *et al.*, 2005), but understanding decomposition rates requires knowledge of how the various species compete for this resource and respond to environmental variables such as temperature, moisture, and seasonal variation. Figure 13.1, for example, shows two individuals seven days (left) and 20 days (right) after death that were placed on the ground surface in Central Texas. For the individual on the left, vultures were able to take advantage of the resource before microbial and insect communities could be established. In contrast, the body on the right was protected from avian and mammalian scavengers and decomposition is primarily driven by insect and microbial consumption. This example illustrates how important it is to be able to reconstruct the taphonomic history of the remains before estimating the PMI. What is necessary for forensic

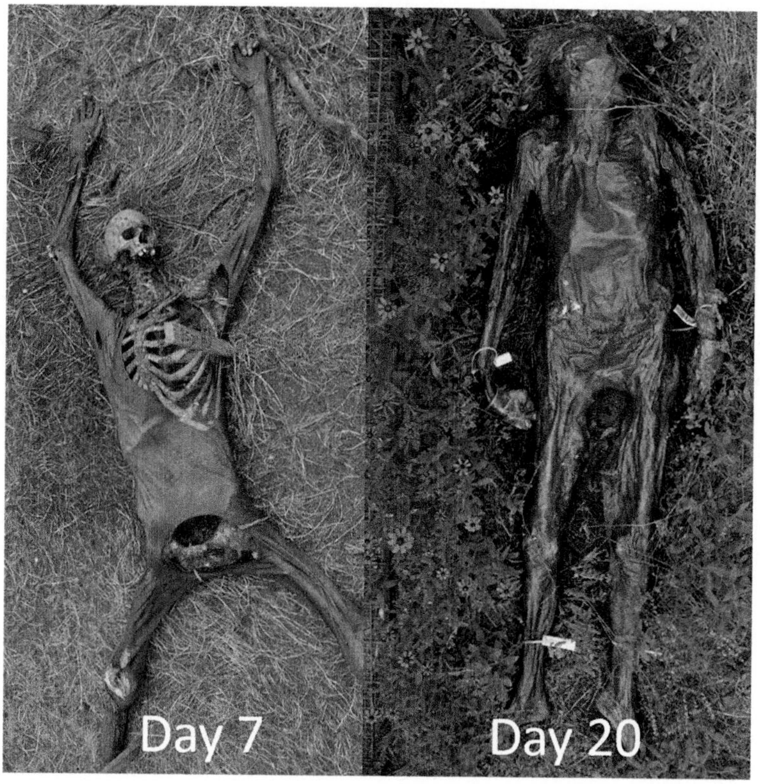

Figure 13.1 Variation in decomposition between two individuals placed on the ground surface in Central Texas. The body on the left is seen at 7-day PMI and is mainly skeletonized with desiccated skin. This body was uncaged and therefore available to large scavengers. The body on the right is seen 20-day PMI and is still in wet decomposition with a significant amount of soft tissue remaining. This body was caged and protected from large scavengers. The difference between the two bodies illustrates the importance of reconstructing the taphonomic history of human remains in medicolegal death investigations to accurately estimate the PMI.

scientists to accurately estimate the time since death is an understanding of the competition between the various trophic levels and how they interact with the environment. Forensic scientists must understand not only the taphonomic processes involved in decomposition but also how they influence one another (Lyman, 1994).

13.6 Cross-disciplinary research

13.6.1 Need for cross-disciplinary research in PMI estimation

In 1980, Dr. William Bass established the first human decomposition facility at the University of Tennessee to facilitate the understanding of human decomposition in a semi-controlled, scientific manner while maintaining a natural outdoor setting (Shirley *et al.*, 2011). Prior to this, most research on decomposition was case-based or focused on plant-derived and fecal matter decomposition, with very little focus on carrion recycling, especially involving human remains. Pioneering work at Tennessee's Anthropology Research Facility (ARF) concentrated primarily on physical changes in the hard and soft tissues of the body during decomposition and on the abiotic variables (e.g., temperature and humidity) that affect the rate of decomposition (Rodriguez and Bass, 1983, 1985; Rodriguez, 1984; Mann *et al.*, 1990; Bass, 1997; and others). This early work provided the initial hypothetico-deductive research foundation for methods of establishing time since death and also demonstrated what variability was due to local environmental conditions.

Dr. Bass encouraged multidisciplinary research at ARF. As a result, a variety of forensic scientists focused primarily on the role of scavengers, both invertebrate and vertebrate, in carrion recycling (Rodriguez and Bass, 1983; Rodriguez, 1984; Haskell *et al.*, 1997; Shahid *et al.*, 2003; Schoenly *et al.*, 2005; Hart and Whitaker, 2006; and others) at ARF. More recently, much of the research has focused on investigating the use of volatile organic compounds and bacteria to estimate the time since death (Vass, 1991, 2001, 2011; Vass *et al.*, 1992, 2002, 2004; Damann *et al.*, 2012, 2015). Using a multidisciplinary approach, scientists have learned a great deal from each other about the numerous phenomena that occur during decomposition and how to describe and explain them. Forensic scientists have also learned the sequence of events that occur during decomposition and how some of the natural biotic and abiotic factors affect the rate of decomposition. However, estimating the PMI is still one of the most elusive aspects of medicolegal death investigations beyond the very early postmortem period (Forbes, 2008).

Unlocking the mystery of the ecology of carrion recycling is key to understanding and interpreting the process and rate of the PMI in various geographical and ecological regions and to establishing methods that accurately and precisely estimate the PMI in any ecological region. Complex real-world problems such as carrion decomposition can rarely be understood through the lens of a single academic discipline. While forensic science has made considerable progress in uncovering the underlying similarities and rules governing how carrion is recycled using unidisciplinary and multidisciplinary tactics, new methods and approaches are needed, and this cannot be accomplished if the various disciplines approach the topic separately. To fully understand human decomposition, forensic scientists need unified theories of forensic taphonomy that describe, explain, and predict the phenomena observed in all disciplines.

13.6.2 Cross-disciplinary approaches

There are three primary cross-disciplinary approaches—multidisciplinary, interdisciplinary, and transdisciplinary (Table 13.1). Multidisciplinary efforts involve researchers from two or more disciplines working in parallel on a single scientific problem, but within each discipline, creating their own goals and research questions. Often these questions relate to how the particular discipline can contribute

Table 13.1 Cross-disciplinary approaches to research

Characteristics	**Approach/model**		
Graphical representation	*Multidisciplinary* 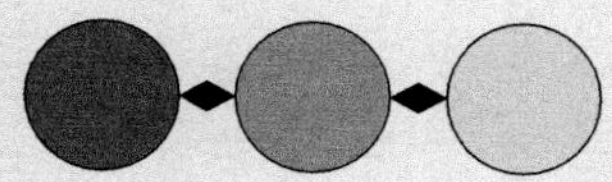	*Interdisciplinary* 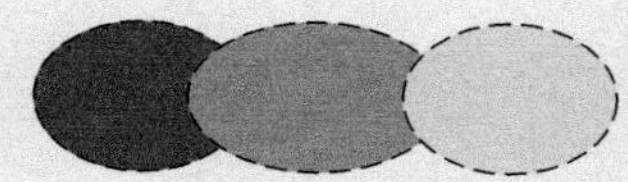	*Transdisciplinary* 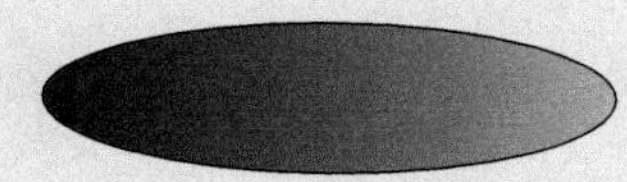
Integration	Separate	Integration	Integration, congruent
Perspective	≥2 disciplines working separately, contribution remains anchored in each discipline	≥2 disciplines working jointly, some integration of ideas, concepts, and methods	≥2 disciplines + stakeholders working jointly, synthesize discipline-specific theories, concepts, and methods
Leadership	Varied depending on PI discipline	Varied	Rotating
Team goals	Projects, sharing discipline results	Common problem, learning, new ideas	Problem-oriented, new approaches, shared framework

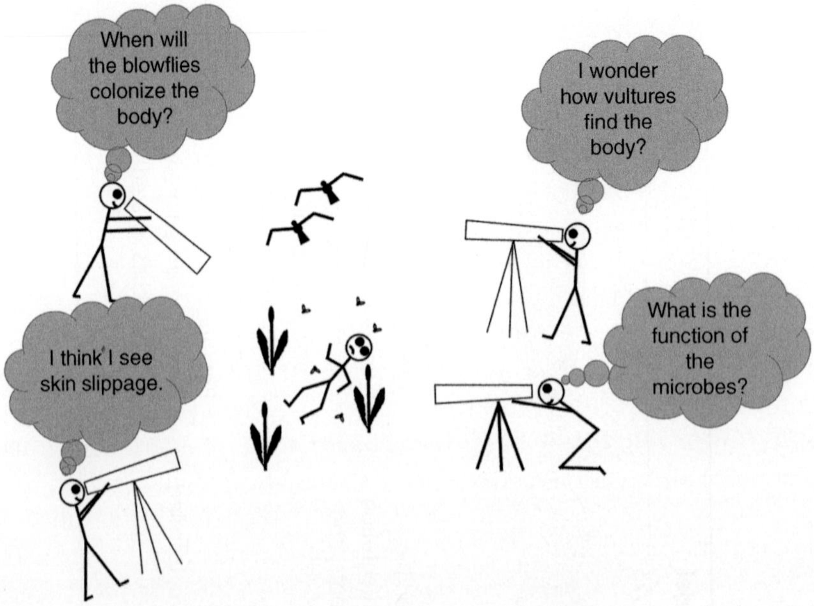
When will the blowflies colonize the body?
I wonder how vultures find the body?
What is the function of the microbes?
I think I see skin slippage.

Figure 13.2 Cartoon illustration of the multidisciplinary approach. Researchers work together, but on separate projects related to the estimation of the PMI and rarely collaborate or examine the interaction between taphonomic processes.

to a single problem such as the estimation of the PMI, but researchers may not communicate among each other or look at how factors covered in other fields affect their observations and interpretations. That is, forensic scientists often do not look at the bigger picture. This is illustrated by the cartoon in Figure 13.2.

Under a multidisciplinary approach, forensic anthropologists, for example, have commonly addressed questions related to gross morphological changes in the soft and hard tissues of a decomposing body (Micozzi, 1986; Galloway, 1997; Megyesi *et al.*, 2005), while forensic entomologists are mainly concerned with questions related to the succession, colonization, and developmental stages (Tomberlin *et al.*, 2011) of arthropods, and microbiologists focus on the diversity and quantity of microorganisms on the decomposing remains (Metcalf *et al.*, 2014, 2016). Promising multidisciplinary research examining gross morphology (Galloway *et al.*, 1989; Megyesi *et al.*, 2005, and others), soil chemistry (Carter *et al.*, 2007; Tibbett and Carter, 2008, 2009; Ritz *et al.*, 2009; and others), microbial populations (Hyde *et al.*, 2013; Pechal *et al.*, 2013, 2014a; and others), volatile organic compounds (Love, 2001; Vass *et al.*, 2002, 2004; Hoffman *et al.*, 2009; and others), and insect activity (Benbow *et al.*, 2011; Pechal *et al.*, 2014b; and others) has greatly helped in our endeavor to understand decomposition processes.

Ideas, terminology, and sometimes methods are often borrowed and shared across disciplines using a multidisciplinary approach. For example, forensic anthropologists have adopted the use of accumulated degree days (ADDs) instead of calendar days from biology and agriculture to help account for regional and even microenvironmental differences in climate (Megyesi *et al.*, 2005). However, while ADD may provide information about the thermal energy necessary for insect development rates, it does not always correlate with the thermal energy necessary for gross decomposition rates (Bates and Wescott, 2016). While multidisciplinary research is a minimal requirement for understanding the processes occurring during the PMI, this approach does not always allow us to fully understand complex problems because the various disciplines are not coordinated and there is a low level of integration.

Interdisciplinary research is the integration or synthesis of the analytical strengths of two or more often disparate scientific disciplines or bodies of knowledge to solve a problem and produce a product that is more powerful than its constituent parts (Thompson Klein, 1990; Aboelela *et al.*, 2007; Rhoten and Pfirman, 2007) (Table 13.1). During interdisciplinary research, studies are undertaken by scholars from two or more disciplines interested in a problem, but, unlike multidisciplinary research, interdisciplinary efforts involve regular discussion and collaboration among researchers from various disciplines to set goals and to jointly carry out research. Often the goal of interdisciplinary research is to form new integrated ideas about a common problem.

Transdisciplinary research is:

> the process whereby researchers from different disciplines work together to develop and use a shared conceptual framework that integrates discipline-specific concepts, theories, and methods to address a common problem (Urquhart *et al.*, 2013:20).

A transdisciplinary approach also involves input from other stakeholders (Table 13.1). In the case of forensic science, the other stakeholders would include crime scene investigators, law enforcement agents, and other professionals that apply the methods in the field and lawyers and judges that debate them in the courts. A transdisciplinary approach is best suited for the development of theoretically sound protocol and methods that can be conducted in the field and the laboratory by appropriate clinicians and technicians. The inclusion of stakeholders is a critical component to transdisciplinary research. Methods and protocol developed through research are only going to be effective if they are employed by these stakeholders. For example, protocols that require freezing samples to −80 °C within an hour after collection are unlikely to be used by field investigators no matter the accuracy of the method. As anthropologists, we have seen this phenomenon in the estimation of age at death. The popular use of aging methods associated with pubic symphysis morphology (that have moderate accuracy and low precision; Katz and Suchey, 1986; Hartnett, 2010) rather than dental cementum annulation (that has high accuracy and precision; Wittwer-Backofen *et al.*, 2004), for example, is largely because pubic symphysis morphology can be evaluated by any experienced biological anthropologist, but dental cementum requires specialized skills and equipment. Furthermore, while there is a strong need for basic research on carrion recycling, when methods are developed for estimating the PMI, they must go beyond describing postmortem changes and have applicability and reliability (Henssge and Madea, 2007). In other words, the methods must be relatively easy to apply and have low inter-observer error.

13.7 Overcoming barriers to cross-disciplinary research

While cross-disciplinary research is necessary to tackle real-world problems effectively, there are numerous barriers to its methodological and theoretical development, including the institutional structures of academia, the funding criteria, and the bureaucracy of death investigation. Bringing together different disciplines for interdisciplinary or transdisciplinary research is often a stated goal of academia, funding agencies, and forensic science organizations, but it is much more labor-intensive than unidisciplinary or even multidisciplinary approaches and requires an environment that allows for collaborative team science (Dhand *et al.*, 2016).

One of the major constraints to cross-disciplinary research is that the academic knowledge base is generally and traditionally distributed among numerous disciplines. There are often considerable differences among disciplines in theory, praxis, language, and epistemological assumptions that can serve as barriers to cross-disciplinary work (Jakobsen *et al.*, 2004). Universities often state support for cross-disciplinary research, but ingrained logistical obstacles (e.g., disciplines located in different buildings and colleges) and resource constraints (e.g., funding assignments) as well as different tenure, promotion, and merit assessment policies do not readily facilitate truly collaborative, cross-disciplinary research. As a result, researchers, especially junior researchers, often perceive cross-disciplinary research as too risky for their careers. However, universities and other organizations are increasingly giving cross-disciplinary research institutional priority and providing the support necessary to strengthen cross-disciplinary teams.

The structure of professional journals can also be a barrier to disseminating cross-disciplinary research. True cross-disciplinary journals are often difficult to find and are often not seen as prestigious as unidisciplinary journals (Jakobsen *et al.*, 2004). Even in the premier journal for forensic science, the *Journal of Forensic Sciences*, the articles are divided into disciplines. The structure of journals (often disciplinary specific) frequently constrains and directs the research questions and the methodologies used to address them. However, there is increasing acceptance of publications with multiple authors from different fields of science using integrated methods and theories.

Funding agencies also encourage cross-disciplinary research but are not always structured to turn cooperation into true collaboration (Jeffrey, 2003). Many funding agencies have programmatic emphases, which make cross-disciplinary proposals less likely to be successful, especially when evaluation is discipline-specific. Even among agencies that encourage integrated research, most of the research funding tends to support a number of independently performed projects by multiple disciplines, but coordinated by a single discipline.

The time allowed for the development of research "products" required for funding can also be a barrier to cross-disciplinary research. Building cross-disciplinary teams and conducting collaborative research often requires considerably more time than unidisciplinary or multidisciplinary research. In many cases, the full-time funding of some participants may not be feasible due to the relatively long duration of cross-disciplinary research. In addition, researchers may be both temporally and spatially separated. To overcome this barrier, formal face-to-face meetings and workshops may be necessary, but funding agencies tend to discourage large travel budgets. However, funding agencies are starting to realize the benefits of cross-disciplinary research and to provide ways of funding interdisciplinary research through interagency collaborations and partnerships and between government and private sector organizations.

The bureaucracy of death investigation can also hamper true collaborative research and the development of cross-disciplinary methods and theories. Too often, forensic investigators think of PMI estimation being divided into different specialties depending on the length of the PMI. If the PMI is minutes, hours, days, or even weeks, it is usually thought to be within the domain of the forensic pathologist, biochemist, and cell biologist. If the interval is days or weeks, the estimation may fall within entomology or microbiology. Likewise, anthropologists are usually consulted when the remains are buried or skeletonized. These discipline boundaries can affect the coordination of efforts and the integration of knowledge. In addition, the bureaucracy of death investigation can establish "power hierarchy between disciplines" (Jakobsen *et al.*, 2004:10) often associated with which discipline has the essential skills for the goals of the research. However, because of the common goals of forensic scientists and the multidisciplinary nature of organizations such as the American Academy of Forensic Sciences, forensic scientists also frequently understand the strengths and limitations of their own discipline as well as others, which paves the way for breaking down barriers to cross-disciplinary research.

While there are many barriers to cross-disciplinary research (including academic departmentalization, funding objectives, institutional bureaucracy, and others), the rewards are likely to outweigh the trouble. Furthermore, academic, governmental, and private sector organizations are increasingly seeing the benefit of truly collaborative, cross-disciplinary research and are therefore making commitments to infrastructure, career policies, and funding opportunities to facilitate integrated research. What is needed now are scientists with the commitment and skills necessary to overcome the barriers and the desire to broker cross-disciplinary research.

13.8 Forensic anthropologists as brokers for unified theories in forensic taphonomy

Forensic anthropologists are ideally situated to act as brokers for cross-disciplinary research and training in forensic taphonomy, especially in investigations involving the necrobiome and methods for estimating the PMI. Forensic anthropologists are positioned to facilitate, organize, encourage, and sometimes lead integrated inter- and transdisciplinary research. However, forensic anthropologists must keep in mind that cross-disciplinary research requires a team effort where all stakeholders collaborate and cooperate to meet the goals of the team. This also requires a rotation of leadership (Table 13.1). Following are four reasons forensic anthropologists ideally can and should serve as brokers of cross-disciplinary research in forensic taphonomy.

13.8.1 Forensic anthropologists are already major players

Anthropologists have been asked to estimate the PMI in medicolegal death investigations for about as long as anthropologists have aided in forensic cases (Bass, 1997). Forensic taphonomy and the estimation of time since death are discussed, although not in detail, in pivotal works by Krogman (1962) and Stewart (1979). Forensic anthropologists also have a long history of being invited by law enforcement to help with the recovery of remains at crime scenes and increasingly with collection of evidence, especially taphonomic evidence (Dirkmaat *et al.*, 2008; Sorg *et al.*, 2012).

In addition, the first human decomposition facility was developed by Dr. Bass to facilitate research into the processes of decomposition and the estimation of the PMI. Today there are at least six more facilities in the United States and Australia that are all operated by anthropologists and most within anthropology departments. These decomposition research facilities already have the personnel and infrastructure necessary to enable cross-disciplinary research and are currently facilitating multidisciplinary (and sometimes interdisciplinary) research in forensic taphonomy.

Forensic anthropologists are also active in multiple levels of criminal investigations, and often serve the role of intermediates and supervisors, especially in mass disasters (Mundorff, 2012). Forensic anthropologists understand and communicate effectively with other disciplines and are therefore already well-situated to act as brokers.

13.8.2 Anthropologists have a long history of conducting taphonomic research

Taphonomy has been used to evaluate and reconstruct fossil and archaeological bone assemblages since the development of the discipline (see Lyman (1994) and Dirkmaat *et al.* (2008) for an overview of the history). Furthermore, the early seminal work in forensic taphonomy was conducted by anthropologists such as William Bass (Rodriguez and Bass, 1983, 1985; Bass, 1984; Mann *et al.*, 1990; Vass *et al.*, 1992), William Haglund (Haglund, 1991, 1993; Haglund *et al.*, 1988a, b), and Marcella Sorg (Sorg, 1986; Sorg *et al.*, 1998). This long history has given forensic anthropologists the skills and necessary outlook to broker taphonomic research.

13.8.3 Anthropology is traditionally a holistic field

Carrion recycling and the estimation of PMI can only be understood with knowledge of the entire necrobiome and the interconnections between the biotic species and the abiotic factors influencing them. In other words, the problem of estimating time since death requires a holistic approach. Anthropologists are trained to look at the big picture and to approach scientific questions using numerous approaches. Anthropologists have a history of conducting multidisciplinary research and utilizing theory and methodology from other disciplines. As Boyd and Boyd (2011) and the authors of numerous chapters in this book point out, forensic anthropologists utilize theory in their everyday practice. Some of this theory is borrowed from other disciplines and some is unique to forensic anthropology.

Also, because of the holistic approach of anthropology, forensic anthropologists can often operate intellectually in multiple disciplinary areas and can help maintain a collaborative atmosphere. Many forensic anthropologists serve as committee members in other subdisciplines (e.g., cultural anthropology and archaeology) and disciplines (e.g., anatomy, biology, chemistry, geology, history, and criminal justice) that have unique terminology and often utilize methods and theories that differ from our own. This experience positions forensic anthropologists to break down some of the barriers to cross-disciplinary research.

13.8.4 Forensic anthropology has its roots in academic research

Forensic anthropologists have experience conducting experimental and retrospective actualistic research as well as using hypothetico-deductive models. In addition, many forensic anthropologists are in academic departments with researchers that use a multitude of epistemological and research methodologies. Anthropologists are therefore accustomed to conducting multi-subdisciplinary as well as multidisciplinary research and have the ability to facilitate and organize researchers with different perspectives. Finally, as an applied field, forensic anthropology has a strong history of conducting and disseminating high quality research in forensic science.

13.9 Conclusions

One of the goals of the forensic sciences should be to develop accurate and precise methods for estimating the PMI that have quantitative measures, known error rates, and confidence intervals and that have been proven to be applicable and reliable in the field. This requires cross-disciplinary field, laboratory, and retrospective studies and ultimately the development of unified terminology, methodologies, and theories related to carrion recycling that take into consideration the needs of all stakeholders. As the integrated knowledge of the necrobiome increases, estimations of PMI will naturally become more accurate and precise. Because of the epistemology of anthropology, anthropologists are the ideal brokers for the development of a unified cross-disciplinary approach to human decomposition. Haglund and Sorg (1997a:3) argue that "forensic anthropology has an important role to play, both in testing traditional taphonomic hypotheses and approaches, and also in providing actualistic models from which to create new taphonomic approaches." Forensic anthropologists also have a role to play in brokering the cross-disciplinary research of the future. What better way to stimulate our future and honor the pioneering efforts of Drs. Bass, Haglund, Sorg, and others in our discipline than by facilitating cross-disciplinary theories that allow us to accurately and precisely describe, explain, and estimate the PMI.

Acknowledgments

I thank Drs. Donna Boyd and Clifford Boyd for organizing the symposium on theory in forensic anthropology and for editing this book. I also thank Dr. Deborah Cunningham for the useful comments and edits on this chapter.

References

Aboelela, S.W., Larson, E., Bakken, S., *et al.* (2007) Defining interdisciplinary research: conclusions from a critical review of the literature. *Health Services Research*, **43**, 329–346.

Bass, W.M. (1984) Time interval since death: a difficult decision. In: *Human Identification: Case Studies in Forensic Anthropology* (eds. T.A. Rathbun and J.E. Buikstra). Charles C. Thomas, Springfield, IL, pp. 136–147.

Bass, W.M. (1997) Outdoor decomposition rates in Tennessee. In: *Forensic Taphonomy: The Postmortem Fate of Human Remains* (eds. W.D. Haglund and M.H. Sorg). CRC Press, Boca Raton, FL, pp. 181–186.

Bates, L.N. and Wescott, D.J. (2016) Not all degree days are equal in the rate of decomposition: the effect of season of death on the relationship between gross postmortem decomposition and accumulated degree days. *Proceedings of the 68th American Academy of Forensic Sciences*, **XXII**, 178.

Beary, M.O. and Lyman, R.L. (2012) The use of taphonomy in forensic anthropology: past trends and future prospects. In: *A Companion to Forensic Anthropology* (ed. D.C. Dirkmaat). Wiley-Blackwell, Chichester, UK, pp. 499–528.

Benbow, M.E., Lewis, A.J., Tomberlin, J.K., *et al.* (2011) Seasonal necrophagous insect community assembly during vertebrate carrion decomposition. *Journal of Medical Entomology*, **50**, 440–450.

Boyd, C.C. and Boyd, D.C. (2011) Theory and the scientific basis for forensic anthropology. *Journal of Forensic Sciences*, **56**, 1407–1415.

Bristow, J., Simms, Z., and Randolph-Quinney, P. (2016) Taphonomy. In: *Forensic Anthropology: 2000 to 2010* (eds. S. Black and E. Ferguson). CRC Press, Boca Raton, FL, pp. 279–317.

Carter, D.O., Yellowlees, D., and Tibbett, M. (2007) Cadaver decomposition in terrestrial ecosystems. *Naturwissenschaften*, **94**, 12–24.

Christensen, A.M. and Crowder, C.M. (2009) Evidentiary standards for forensic anthropology. *Journal of Forensic Sciences*, **54**, 1211–1216.

Christensen, A.M., Passalacqua, N.V., Schmunk, G.A., *et al.* (2014) The value and availability of forensic anthropological consultation in medicolegal death investigations. *Forensic Science, Medicine, and Pathology*, **11**, 438–441.

Damann, F.E., Tanittaisong, A., and Carter, D.O. (2012) Potential carcass enrichment at the University of Tennessee Anthropology Research Facility: a baseline survey of edaphic features. *Forensic Science International*, **222**, 4–10.

Damann, F.E., Williams, D.E., and Layton, A.C. (2015) Potential use of bacterial community succession in decaying human bone for estimating the postmortem interval. *Journal of Forensic Sciences*, **60**, 844–850.

Dhand, A., Luke, D.A., Carothers, B.J., *et al.* (2016) Academic cross-pollination: the role of disciplinary affiliation in research collaboration. *PLoS ONE*, **11**, e0145916.

Dirkmaat, D.C. and Passalacqua, N.V. (2012) Introduction to Part VI. In: *A Companion to Forensic Anthropology* (ed. D.C. Dirkmaat). Wiley-Blackwell, Chichester, UK, pp. 471–476.

Dirkmaat, D.C., Cabo, L.L., Ousley, S.D., *et al.* (2008) New perspectives in forensic anthropology. *Yearbook of Physical Anthropology*, **51**, 33–52.

Efremov, I.A. (1940) Taphonomy: a new branch of paleontology. *Pan-American Geologist*, **74**, 81–93.

Forbes, S.L. (2008) Potential determinants of postmortem and postburial interval of buried remains. In: *Soil Analysis in Forensic Taphonomy: Chemical and Biological Effects of Buried Human Remains* (eds. M. Tibbett and D.O. Carter). CRC Press, Boca Raton, FL, pp. 225–246.

Galloway, A. (1997) The process of decomposition: a model from the Arizona Sonoran desert. In: *Forensic Taphonomy: The Postmortem Fate of Human Remains* (eds. W.D. Haglund and M.H. Sorg). CRC Press, Boca Raton, FL pp. 139–150.

Galloway, A., Birkby, W.H., Jones, A.M., *et al.* (1989) Decay rates of human remains in an arid environment. *Journal of Forensic Sciences*, **34**, 587–606.

Goff, M.L. (2000) *A Fly for the Prosecution: How Insect Evidence Helps Solve Crimes*. Harvard University Press, Cambridge, MA.

Haglund, W.D. (1991) *Application of Taphonomic Models to Forensic Investigations*. Ph.D. dissertation, University of Washington, Seattle, WA.

Haglund, W.D. (1993) Disappearance of soft tissue and the disarticulation of human remains from aqueous environments. *Journal of Forensic Sciences*, **38**, 806–815.

Haglund, W.D. and Sorg, M.H. (1997a) Method and theory of forensic taphonomic research. In: *Forensic Taphonomy: The Postmortem Fate of Human Remains* (eds. W.D. Haglund and M.H. Sorg). CRC Press, Boca Raton, FL, pp. 13–26.

Haglund, W.D. and Sorg, M.H. (1997b) *Forensic Taphonomy: The Postmortem Fate of Human Remains*. CRC Press, Boca Raton, FL.

Haglund, W.D. and Sorg, M.H. (2002) *Advances in Forensic Taphonomy: Method, Theory, and Archaeological Perspectives*. CRC Press: Boca Raton, FL.

Haglund, W.D., Reay, D., and Swindler, D.R. (1988a) Tooth artifacts and survival of bones in animal-scavenged human remains. *Journal of Forensic Sciences*, **33**, 985–997.

Haglund, W.D., Reay, D., and Swindler, D.R. (1988b) Canid scavenging/disarticulation sequence of human remains in the Pacific northwest. *Journal of Forensic Sciences*, **34**, 587–606.

Hart, A.J. and Whitaker, A.P. (2006) Forensic entomology: insect activity and its role in the decomposition of human cadavers. *Antenna: Bulletin of the Royal Entomological Society of London*, **30**, 159–164.

Hartnett, K.M. (2010) Analysis of age-at-death estimation using data from a new, modern autopsy sample—part I: pubic bone. *Journal of Forensic Sciences*, **55**, 1145–1151.

Haskell, N.H., Hall, R.D., Cervenka, V.J., *et al.* (1997) On the body: insect life stage presence, their postmortem artifacts. In: *Forensic Taphonomy: The Postmortem Fate of Human Remains* (eds. W.D. Haglund and M.H. Sorg). CRC Press, Boca Raton, FL, pp. 415–448.

Henssge, C. and Madea, B. (2007) Estimation of the time since death. *Forensic Science International*, **165**, 182–184.

Hoffman, E.M., Curran, A.M., Dulgerian, N., *et al.* (2009) Characterization of the volatile organic compounds present in the headspace of decomposing human remains. *Forensic Science International*, **186**, 6–13.

Hyde, E.R., Haarmann, D.P., Lynne, A.M., *et al.* (2013) The living dead: bacterial community structure of a cadaver at the onset and end of the bloat stage of decomposition. *PLoS ONE*, **8**, e77733.

Isaacks, M.E.R. (2015) *The Use of Near-Infrared Remote Sensing in the Detection of Clandestine Human Remains*. M.A. thesis, Texas State University, San Marcos.

Jakobsen, C.H., Hels, T., and McLaughlin, W.J. (2004) Barriers and facilitators to integration among scientists in transdisciplinary landscape analyses: a cross-country comparison. *Forest Policy and Economics*, **6**, 15–31.

Jeffrey, P. (2003) Smoothing the waters: observations on the process of cross-disciplinary research collaboration. *Social Studies of Science*, **33**, 539.

Kalacska, M.E. and Bell, L.S. (2006) Remote sensing as a tool for the detection of clandestine mass graves. *Canadian Society of Forensic Science Journal*, **39**, 1–13.

Kalacska, M.E., Bell, L.S., Arturo Sanchez-Azofeifa, G., and Caelli, T. (2009) The application of remote sensing for detecting mass graves: an experimental animal case study from Costa Rica. *Journal of Forensic Sciences*, **54**, 159–166.

Katz, D. and Suchey, J.M. (1986) Age determination of the male os pubis. *American Journal of Physical Anthropology*, **69**, 427–435.

Komar, D.A. and Buikstra, J.E. (2008) *Forensic Anthropology: Contemporary Theory and Practice*. Oxford University Press, Oxford, UK.

Krogman, W.M. (1962) *The Human Skeleton in Forensic Medicine*. Charles C. Thomas, Springfield, IL.

Love, J.C. (2001) *Evaluation of Decay Odor as a Time Since Death Indicator*. Ph.D. dissertation, University of Tennessee, Knoxville.

Love, J.C. and Marks, M.K. (2003) Taphonomy and time: estimating the postmortem interval. In: *Hard Evidence: Case Studies in Forensic Anthropology* (ed. D.W. Steadman). Pearson, Upper Saddle River, NJ, pp. 160–175.

Lyman, R.L. (1987) Zooarchaeology and taphonomy: a general consideration. *Journal of Ethnobiology*, **7**, 93–117.

Lyman, R.L. (1994) *Vertebrate taphonomy*. Cambridge University Press, Cambridge.

Lyman, R.L. (2002) Forword from paleontology. In: *Advances in Forensic Taphonomy: Method, Theory, and Archaeological Perspectives* (eds. W.D. Haglund and M.H. Sorg). CRC Press, Boca Raton, FL, pp. xix–xxi.

Lyman, R.L. (2010) What taphonomy is, what it isn't, and why taphonomists should care about the difference. *Journal of Taphonomy*, **8**, 1–16.

Mann, R.W., Bass, W.M., and Meadows, L. (1990) Time since death and decomposition of the human body: variables and observation in case and experimental field studies. *Journal of Forensic Sciences*, **35**, 103–111.

Megyesi, M.S., Nawrocki, S.P., and Haskell, N.H. (2005) Using accumulated degree-days to estimate the postmortem interval from decomposed human remains. *Journal of Forensic Sciences*, **50**, 618–626.

Metcalf, J.L., Carter, D.O., and Knight, R. (2014) Characterization of Bacterial and Microbial Eukaryotic Communities (Including Fungal) Associated with Corpse Decomposition using Next Generation Sequencing. National Institute of Justice, Report No. 2011-DN-BX-K533, Washington, DC.

Metcalf, J.L., Xu, Z.Z., Weiss, S., *et al.* (2016) Microbial community assembly and metabolic function during mammalian corpse decomposition. *Science*, **351** (6269), 158–162.

Micozzi, M. (1986) Experimental study of postmortem change under field conditions: effects of freezing, thawing, and mechanical injury. *Journal of Forensic Sciences*, **31**, 953–961.

Micozzi, M. (1991) *Postmortem Change in Human and Animal Remains: A Systematic Approach*. Charles C. Thomas, Springfield, IL.

Mundorff, A.Z. (2012) Integrating forensic anthropology into disaster victim identification. *Forensic Science, Medicine, and Pathology*, **8**, 131–139.

National Research Council. (2009) *Strengthening Forensic Science in the United States*. National Academies Press, Washington, DC.

Pechal, J.L., Crippen, T.L., Tarone, A.M., *et al.* (2013) Microbioal community functional change during vertebrate carrion decomposition. *PLoS ONE*, **8**, e79035.

Pechal, J.L., Benbow, M.E., Crippen, T.L., *et al.* (2014a) Delayed insect access alters carrion decomposition and necrophagous insect community assembly. *Ecosphere*, **5** (4), 45.

Pechal, J.L., Crippen, T.L., Benbow, M.E., *et al.* (2014b) The potential use of bacterial community succession in forensics as described by high throughput metagenomic sequencing. *International Journal of Legal Medicine*, **128**, 193–205.

Pokines, J.T. (2013) Introduction: collection of macroscopic osseous taphonomic data and the recognition of taphonomic suites of characteristics. In: *Manual of Forensic Taphonomy* (eds. J.T. Pokines and S.A. Symes). CRC Press, Boca Raton, FL, pp. 1–18.

Rhoten, D. and Pfirman, S. (2007) Women in interdisciplinary science: exploring preferences and consequences. *Research Policy*, **36**, 56–75.

Ritz, K., Dawson, L., and Miller, D. (eds.) (2009) *Criminal and Environmental Soil Forensics*. Springer, New York.

Rodriguez, W.C. (1984) *Insect Activity and Its Relationship to Decay Rates of Human Cadavers in East Tennessee*. M.A. thesis, University of Tennessee, Knoxville.

Rodriguez, W.C. and Bass, W.M. (1983) Insect activity and its relationship to decay rates of human cadavers in East Tennessee. *Journal of Forensic Sciences*, **28**, 423–432.

Rodriguez, W.C. and Bass, W.M. (1985) Decomposition of buried bodies and methods that may aid in their location. *Journal of Forensic Sciences*, **30**, 836–852.

Schiffer, M.B. (1988) The structure of archaeological theory. *American Antiquity*, **53**, 461–485.

Schoenly, K.G., Shahid, S.A., Haskell, N.H., *et al.* (2005) Does carcass enrichment alter community structure of predaceous and parasitic arthropods? A second test of the arthropod saturation hypothesis at the anthropology research facility in Knoxville, Tennessee. *Journal of Forensic Sciences*, **50**, 1–9.

Shahid, S.A., Schoenly, K.G., Haskell, N.H., *et al.* (2003) Carcass enrichment does not alter decay rates or arthropod community structure: a test of the arthropod saturation hypothesis at the Anthropology Research Facility, Tennessee. *Journal of Medical Entomology*, **40**, 559–569.

Sharma, R., Garg, R.K., and Gaur, J.R. (2015) Various methods for the estimation of the postmortem interval from Calliphoridae: a review. *Egyptian Journal of Forensic Sciences*, **5**, 1–12.

Shirley, N.R., Wilson, R.J., and Meadows Jantz, L. (2011) Cadaver use at the University of Tennessee's Anthropological Research Facility. *Clinical Anatomy*, **24**, 372–380.

Sorg, M.H. (1986) *Scavenger Modifications of Human Skeletal Remains in Forensic Anthropology*. American Academy of Forensic Sciences, New Orleans, LA.

Sorg, M.H. and Haglund, W.D. (2002) Advancing forensic taphonomy: purpose, theory, and process. In: *Advances in Forensic Taphonomy: Method, Theory, and Archaeological Perspectives* (eds. W.D. Haglund and M.H. Sorg). CRC Press, Boca Raton, FL, pp. 3–29.

Sorg, M.H., David, E., and Rebmann, A.J. (1998) Cadaver dogs, taphonomy, and the postmortem interval in the northeast. In: *Forensic Osteology: Advances in the Identification of Human Skeletal Remains*, 2nd edition (ed. K.J. Reichs). Charles C. Thomas, Springfield, IL, pp. 120–144.

Sorg, M.H., Haglund, W.D., and Wren, J.A. (2012) Current research in forensic taphonomy. In: *A Companion to Forensic Anthropology* (ed. D.C. Dirkmaat). Wiley-Blackwell, New York, pp. 477–498.

Stewart, T.D. (1979) *Essentials of Forensic Anthropology: Especially as Developed in the United States*. Charles C. Thomas, Springfield, IL.

Thompson Klein, J. (1990). *Interdisciplinary: History, Theory, and Practice*. Wayne State University Press, Detroit, MI.

Tibbett, M. and Carter, D.O. (eds.) (2008) *Soil Analysis in Forensic Taphonomy: Chemical and Biological Effects of Buried Human Remains*. CRC Press, Boca Raton, FL.

Tibbett, M. and Carter, D.O. (2009) Research in forensic taphonomy: a soil-based perspective. In: *Criminal and Environmental Soil Forensics* (ed. K. Ritz). Springer, New York, NY, pp. 317–331.

Tomberlin, J.K., Mohr, R., Benbow, M.E., *et al.* (2011) A roadmap for bridging basic and applied research in forensic entomology. *Annual Review of Entomology*, **56**, 401–421.

Urquhart, R., Grunfeld, E., Jackson, L., *et al.* (2013) Cross-disciplinary research in cancer: an opportunity to narrow the knowledge-practice gap. *Current Oncology*, **20**, e512–e521.

Vass, A.A. (1991) *Time Since Death Determinations of Human Cadavers Utilizing Soil Solution*. Ph.D. dissertation, University of Tennessee, Knoxville.

Vass, A.A. (2001) Beyond the grave—understanding human decomposition. *Microbiology Today*, **28**, 190–192.

Vass, A.A. (2011) The elusive universal post-mortem interval formula. *Forensic Science International*, **204**, 34–40.

Vass, A.A., Bass, W.M., Wolt, J., *et al.* (1992) Time since death determinations of human cadavers using soil solution. *Journal of Forensic Sciences*, **37**, 1236–1253.

Vass, A.A., Barshick, S.A., Sega, G., *et al.* (2002) Decomposition chemistry of human remains: a new methodology for determining the postmortem interval. *Journal of Forensic Sciences*, **47**, 542–553.

Vass, A.A., Smith, R.R., Thompson, C.V., *et al.* (2004) Decomposition odor analysis database. *Journal of Forensic Sciences*, **49**, 760–769.

Wells, J.D. and LaMotte, L.R. (1995) Estimating maggot age from weight using inverse prediction. *Journal of Forensic Sciences*, **40**, 585–590.

Wittwer-Backofen, U., Gampe, J., and Vaupel, J.W. (2004) Tooth cementum annulation for age estimation: results from a large known-age validation study. *American Journal of Physical Anthropology*, **123**, 119–129.

PART 4

Interdisciplinary influences, legal ramifications, and future directions

CHAPTER 14

Archaeological inference and its application to forensic anthropology

C. Clifford Boyd Jr[1] and William W. Baden[2]

[1] *Department of Anthropological Sciences, Radford University Forensic Science Institute, Radford University, Radford, VA, USA*

[2] *Institutional Research, Indiana University–Purdue University, Fort Wayne, IN, USA*

14.1 Introduction

In examining archaeological inference and its influence (potential and realized) on forensic anthropology, it is important to initially address theoretical perspectives in archaeology, since they guide inferences about and interpretations of the archaeological record. Since the 1960s and 1970s, American archaeology in particular has been heavily influenced by theoretical approaches that attempt to form a stronger link between archaeology and science, ideally resulting in more scientific inferences about the past (Binford, 1972, 1983, 1989; Schiffer, 1976; South, 1977). Variously referred to as "processual archaeology" or "behavioral archaeology" by its proponents, this theoretical orientation championed "theory building" through middle-range research, linking theoretical concepts to actual, observable material objects, and through experimentation, reconstructing the past behavior that created them (Groen *et al.*, 2015a).

Middle-range research is most often based on scientific experimentation. Lithic use-wear analysis (Keeley, 1980; Vaughan, 1985), for example, provided direct microscopic evidence for stone tool use. Specialized chemical analyses, such as stable isotope analysis and X-ray fluorescence, informed archaeologists about past human diets and the sources of raw materials used in artifact production. Taphonomic research through actualistic and experimental studies of animal scavenging and decay produced observations of significance for determination of the postmortem interval (PMI) and the effects of natural forces on remains after death (Lyman, 1994; Haglund and Sorg, 2002; Pokines and Symes, 2014).

This fruitful middle-range or interpretive (see Boyd and Boyd, Chapter 1, this volume) theory building helped in the understanding of past technologies and

Forensic Anthropology: Theoretical Framework and Scientific Basis, First Edition.
Edited by C. Clifford Boyd Jr and Donna C. Boyd.

behavioral processes, but did not lead to the establishment of an overarching, unifying high-level or foundational archaeological theory that all archaeologists could agree upon. Attempts by Robert Dunnell and colleagues (Dunnell, 1978, 1980, 1989; Lyman and O'Brien, 1998) to build such a theory by reaching beyond processualism and applying Darwinian evolutionary concepts to human behavior were met with disdain by many archaeologists (Pauketat, 2010). By the 1980s and 1990s, the processual models of sociocultural systems with interlocking subsystems maintaining, or striving to maintain, equilibrium began to be seen by many archaeologists as nonexplanatory, static, and stereotypic.

Thus there began a rise in the archaeological literature of theoretical models that were referred to as "postprocessual" (Preucel, 1991). Some of these theoretical concepts, borrowed from the humanities and social sciences, emphasized the role of "meaning," human emotion, and interpretation as primary causal forces and critiqued the assumed "objectivity" and search for the "ultimate truth" of scientific investigations (Pauketat, 2010; Groen *et al.*, 2015a).

However, some of these postprocessualist archaeological theories are amenable to scientific research and possess great potential utility in enhancing our understanding of a forensic event. Specifically, these theoretical concepts address the basic interpretive forensic archaeology goal of reconstructing the sequence of events forming a forensically-significant scene, based on the available physical evidence. These theories therefore have relevance to enhancing our understanding of both perimortem and postmortem events. Two such theoretical approaches include agency theory and nonlinear systems theory (Beekman and Baden, 2005a; Dobres and Robb, 2005; Joyce and Lopiparo, 2005; Preucel and Mrozowski, 2010).

14.2 Agency and nonlinear systems theories

Agency theory grew out of the writings of several social scientists beginning in the 1970s (Bourdieu, 1977, 1992; Giddens, 1979, 1984; Foucault, 1984) and began to be applied to archaeological questions in the 1980s as part of postprocessualism. Agency theory is an interpretive theory that, for archaeologists, includes the concepts of "materiality and social reproduction" (Dobres and Robb, 2005:162), meaning the study of material objects (artifacts, features) and their production in a social behavioral context. Thus, *agency* refers to actions by individuals or groups of individuals at different scales. Agents are constrained or guided by *structure* or the overall limitations to action imposed by the society or environment in which the agents exist. Some theorists see a distinct dichotomy between agency and structure, with structure often controlling action, leading agents to reproduce structure due to this conformity. Agency is therefore guided by structure (social norms, laws, beliefs, values). Chains of repeated actions define the process of technological production of "materiality" (Dobres, 2010) and also lead to *structuration* or the social reproduction of the existing structure (Beekman, 2005). The multigenerational stability in artifact style, for example, is called a *tradition* by archaeologists and reflects acceptance of established patterns by collective agents over time (Pauketat, 2010; Preucel and Mrozowski, 2010). Others see agency and structure as intertwined (Joyce and Lopiparo, 2005), with agents, in some contextual settings, enabling the transformation of structure through actions that run contrary to the established social system (e.g., innovations in technology or political revolutions). Pauketat's (2010) "historical processualism" or "practice theory" contains elements of agency theory in its focus on human actions (practice), history, and traditions.

Several common characteristics denote agency theory. Agency is context-specific—actions are influenced by initial conditions (social, environmental), the chain of succeeding events (history, time), and (important for humans) the acceptance of actions by others. The concept of *scale* is important in agency theory, as noted earlier. The actions of individuals can shape the overall structure, but the actions of collective agents will have more effect as groups of actors acting in concert with shared goals or perceptions. While some may stress the potential impact of certain individuals or "great men" (Pauketat, 1994, 2010), agency theories predominantly take an evolutionary view toward actions and their potential for change. Charismatic individuals may be able to sway political events in their direction *only* if the contextual setting is amenable to this process and *only* if that individual and their beliefs are selected for and followed by a larger collective of many individuals (note the rise of Nazism in Germany in the 1930s and the "Arab Spring" of 2011 as examples). So, when discussing major social or behavioral changes, the scale of agency is much higher than that of the individual actor, although individuals certainly contribute to this process. Collective agents produce emergent properties far beyond the scale of the individual.

A final relevant aspect of agency theory refers to intentionality. Some actions may be reflexive physical reactions stemming from the autonomic nervous system (turning your head to locate the source of a sound, quickly removing your hand from a hot object), while others may be intentional (voting for one political candidate over another). Agents can also be nonhuman (insects, carnivorous animals) or inanimate objects (a crucifix, the American flag) that can inspire, constrict, or channel behavior in certain ways.

Agent-based models are a hallmark of nonlinear systems theory. The history of nonlinear systems theory is complex, with related developments in both the physical and social sciences (Beekman and Baden, 2005b). Elements of this approach were termed chaos theory in the 1960s and catastrophe theory in the 1970s. Complex systems theory was also a related area of theoretical development, championed by Ilya Prigogine in several publications beginning in the 1960s (Prigogine *et al.*, 1972; Nicolis and Prigogine, 1977, 1989). As noted by Beekman and Baden (2005a:4), Prigogine's writings:

> ...recognized that pivotal physical laws such as the second law of thermodynamics... only worked in a closed system, and failed to accurately describe behavior in an open

> system in which energy could be introduced from the outside. The introduction of energy produced perturbations to the system and caused it to self-organize into complex patterns far from equilibrium.

These various theoretical orientations, looking at different dynamic systemic contexts where the interaction of variables produces results that are greater than the sum of their parts (so-called *emergent* properties), were subsumed by Beekman and Baden (2005a, b) under the title *nonlinear systems theory.*

As with agency theory, nonlinear systems theory focuses on the actions of agents (individual and collective) (Congram, 2014), the initial conditions (context) of an event or behavioral trajectory, its historical sequence (chain) (see Schiffer and Skibo, 1997), and multiple potential outcomes of the interaction of variables (social, environmental) over the course of time and space (emergent properties). Unlike the general systems theory models of processual archaeology that focus on equilibrium maintenance, nonlinear systems are systems in *disequilibrium*—dissipative structures (Baden, 2005). Such systems dissipate (expend) energy and reach points in their historical trajectory where adjustments (either reduction in size or sociopolitical complexity or expansion of the resource base) have to be made due to this lack of equilibrium. Such models more accurately address and depict the dynamic, unstable reality of social organizations and their change as seen in prehistory and history. The destabilizing effects and systemic readjustments of native societies resulting from European colonial incursions in the sixteenth and seventeenth centuries come to mind as examples of nonlinear systems experiencing unforeseen (emergent) consequences from this contact (Silliman, 2001).

Nonlinear systems theory, as with agency theory, has an evolutionary component, in that behaviors or products resulting from the interaction of variables in a social setting must be selected *for* by multiple agents to become *innovations.* Behavioral and biological evolutions are therefore both important to consider in the chain of events leading to emergence (change).

Finally, nonlinear systems theory focuses on *retrodictive* explanation (Beekman and Baden, 2005b) and not prediction. One cannot predict the result of the interaction of variables; one can only explain the observed consequences. As Baden (2005:101) states "...an observed state or phase transition is one of many possible outcomes." It is therefore a historical scientific endeavor, relying on abductive logic, or inference to the best explanation, which links it to archaeology and other historical sciences. Nonlinear system theorists advocate the use of computer simulations to accurately model the historical processes of interaction among variables of interest (Beekman and Baden, 2005a).

So how do these behavioral theoretical models relate to relevant issues in forensic anthropology? First and foremost, forensic anthropology is a historical science. Whether reconstructing the biological profile of a skeleton or reconstructing a crime scene, investigators are moving backward in time from the *present* available information to say something about the *past*. Regarding issues relating to forensic archaeology and taphonomy, researchers are actively addressing the roles of multiple agents and their effects on the forensic scene and its constituent elements (Haglund and Sorg, 1997, 2002; Boyd and Boyd, 2011; Pokines and Symes, 2014). These agents can be human (decedents, perpetrators, crime scene investigators) (Congram, 2014), nonhuman (scavenging animals, insects), or inanimate (temperature, humidity). Their interactions can certainly produce emergent (unforeseen) results. Establishing the context and reconstructing the behavioral chain of events (the interaction of agents) are vital to a full understanding of the forensic past. This is the necessary first step in any forensic investigation.

Finally, as with agency and nonlinear systems, forensic anthropology and archaeology operate at different scales. Even though forensic anthropologists usually engage in the identification of a single individual, the statistical analysis and determination of aspects of the biological profile are based on the analysis of several individuals from multiple skeletal populations—a larger, more inclusive referent sample. Anthropologists who conduct human identification for mass disasters or events of genocide, involving multiple individuals and complex traumatic events, also obviously work at a larger scale. The same is true for forensic archaeologists—documenting a context involving a single victim as opposed to mass graves from human rights violations (Schmitt, 2002; Groen *et al.*, 2015b). So awareness of the different requirements and challenges of different scales is an important consideration.

Given this relationship, it is proposed that nonlinear systems theory can provide a useful framework for the interpretation and modeling of complex, emergent forensic questions. This is particularly evident in the determination of the PMI. Using data from table 1 of Megyesi *et al.* (2005), an example of nonlinear modeling of the dissipative process of decomposition and the determination of PMI is provided in the following text. Problems with the data and methods originally presented in Megyesi *et al.* (2005) have recently been noted and discussed (Moffatt *et al.*, 2016) and are not repeated here. However, because of the widely cited importance of their study, it is felt that nonlinear modeling of a selected set of their data can be a useful illustration of the potential applications of archaeological theory to forensic anthropology. It also provides a more realistic picture of the complex decomposition process in humans than seen with traditional (e.g., linear regression) models.

14.3 Nonlinear modeling of the decomposition process

The constructs of agency, emergence, chaos, and so on conceptualize underlying nonlinear processes in tangible terms applicable to archaeological scales. As will be shown, nonlinearity is not about the form of a regression or correlation measure; it's about representing the dynamics of historical events along a time line. In this analysis, the focus is on determining the time span of a decay process—the PMI. It is argued that decay is the product of a nonlinear system operating within forensic scales and conceptualized by forensic observations. Analytically, to explicate the nonlinearities, a mathematical model of decay based on these observations will be constructed.

Modeling is the formal process of encoding "reality" into a useful construct that captures the most salient aspects of the observed phenomena, converting each into "parameters," without needing to be all-inclusive. What is parameterized largely follows research paradigms—what's important and relevant? As noted earlier, archaeologists have developed a wide range of perspectives over the past several decades. Associated with each is an even larger array of tools to expedite observation, analysis, and exposition. Forensic science is no different. Both disciplines deal with innumerable observations linked together by unknown coherencies. It's the business of these sciences to delineate those coherencies in meaningful ways—to see the order within the chaos. Admittedly, this focus is on the applicability of some of the more complicated approaches inspired by nonlinear systems theory—more complicated in the sense that although most observers recognize the multidimensionality of their research subjects, they often prefer to focus on linear relationships with presumed statistical applicability. In fact, considerable energy is often expended avoiding nonlinearity. Linear analysis models offer a multitude of options that have been tested and accepted after decades of use. Clearly they offer an analytical "path of least resistance." So enticing is this linear path that researchers often transform data to conform to a more linear world. If the underlying nonlinearity is minimal, such approaches are appropriate. But the transformation cost can be a loss of resolution and explicative power. The following is a brief description of the differences between the two systems as they relate to optimal information processing.

When considering time series data, linear approaches necessarily produce *proportionality relationships*—a singular rate of change per parameter dimension. Nonlinear systems are characterized by their variable rates of change across time. For example, compound interest is mathematically an exponential function producing a "nonlinear" curve, but it is a linear system—the rate of change is always proportional to the principal, meaning, its first derivative (i.e., its rate of change) is a linear function. System classifications largely focus on the form of the first derivative (Yoshida, 2010) when time series are involved. It would be acceptable to think of interest compounding to infinity—a banking nightmare but, still, large returns are conceivable. However, a decaying body is bound by a condition of complete soft tissue decay (total body score (TBS) = 35 for a decay score, see the following). This limit implies a decelerating process where the rate of change slows to zero over time. Clearly, body decomposition and PMI estimation are derived from nonlinear systems.

Traditional linear perspectives on these subjects trigger the fairly standard application of statistical models on parameterized variables. Variables of interest are selected based on careful significance testing and demonstrated proxy values for representing the observed. The process can also incorporate less statistical testing (especially when the data fail to meet statistical criteria; see Moffatt *et al.*, 2016) and more descriptive, nonparametric, approaches. The nonlinear world can be divided into small, localized, linear regions—varying ranges of parameter subspace where linear rules can be applied. Essentially, then, the "sum" of these small linear spaces "equate to" the overall nonlinear world. It is argued that embracing the complexity of decaying subjects in this manner is an achievable and rewarding approach that can reveal details about the decay process, the relationship of decay rates to time, and guidance for future, gap-filling research.

The question of calculating PMI based on the observations from the present has been approached in a number of ways (e.g., Rodriguez and Bass, 1983; Bass, 1984; Willey and Heilman, 1987; Galloway *et al.*, 1989; Mann *et al.*, 1990; Micozzi, 1991; Schoenly *et al.*, 1991; Shean *et al.*, 1993; Bass, 1997; Sledzik, 1998). The givens generally include an observed decomposition condition, a specific locale, environmental contexts, and various other relevant observations related to the state of decay. These variables can be expressed as a decomposition index (e.g., TBS), a geographic location, weather or room environment variables, and identifiable taphonomic/insect alterations. Temperature readings spanning the period of the PMI have been recognized as a close proxy for the combined environmental–chemical–biological processes that contribute to body decomposition, especially after insect successions have ceased. By tracking the accumulation of temperature energy in some way, the rate of decomposition can be approximated and, hopefully, from that an estimate of the PMI can be obtained.

Several alternative accumulated temperature measures could be used to model decay rates. In a previous study, the authors have shown that the process of decomposition in nonhuman animals, expressed as a function of time, is a nonlinear one that can be correlated with the environmental cumulative maximum temperature (CMT) sequence of the body's environment (Boyd *et al.*, 2015). Using decomposition scores periodically made (0, 5, 10, 20, 35, and 50 days) on 29 decomposing stillborn pigs and the sum of daily maximum temperature readings up to each day's observations, interpolated scores were calculated over the 50-day PMI. A cumulative coefficient of decay (CCD) was calculated as the (**decomposition score)/CMT** for each day, observed or interpolated between two observation dates. The index expresses the changing rate of decay per accumulated maximum temperature over the PMI period. For example, the CCD on the 10th day where the CMT was 896 CMT degrees and the observed decomposition score was 17 would be

$$\text{CCD}(t=10)=\frac{17}{896}=0.018973 \qquad (14.1)$$

The analysis produced a lookup table for daily expected decomposition scores in reverse order from day 50 to day 0. Given an observed decomposition score and a CMT sequence, a similar table could be constructed for any locale and period of time. The day the observed TBS score most closely equaled the expected value would provide a PMI estimate. Although perhaps not directly applicable to human contexts (see Dautartas *et al.*, 2016), the changing rates of decay clearly describe a nonlinear, nonproportional process, with the highest decay rates occurring the first 5 days of the PMI (Figure 14.1).

Ideally, a time series of daily observed scores on a sufficient sample of human bodies under variable environmental conditions would provide an optimal set of data points. In the absence of such a dataset, this work will extrapolate a decay model based on end-point observations from independent cases with known or highly likely PMI periods. Each case and its final TBS measure become a substitute for sequential TBS observations on singular subjects over time. This is recognized as a major weakness in model construction, especially given the original data gaps in the TBS scale. But, if there is an underlying relationship between temperature parameters and the decay process, parameterized as a TBS measure, the use of these data should approximate it. Therefore, what follows should be viewed as

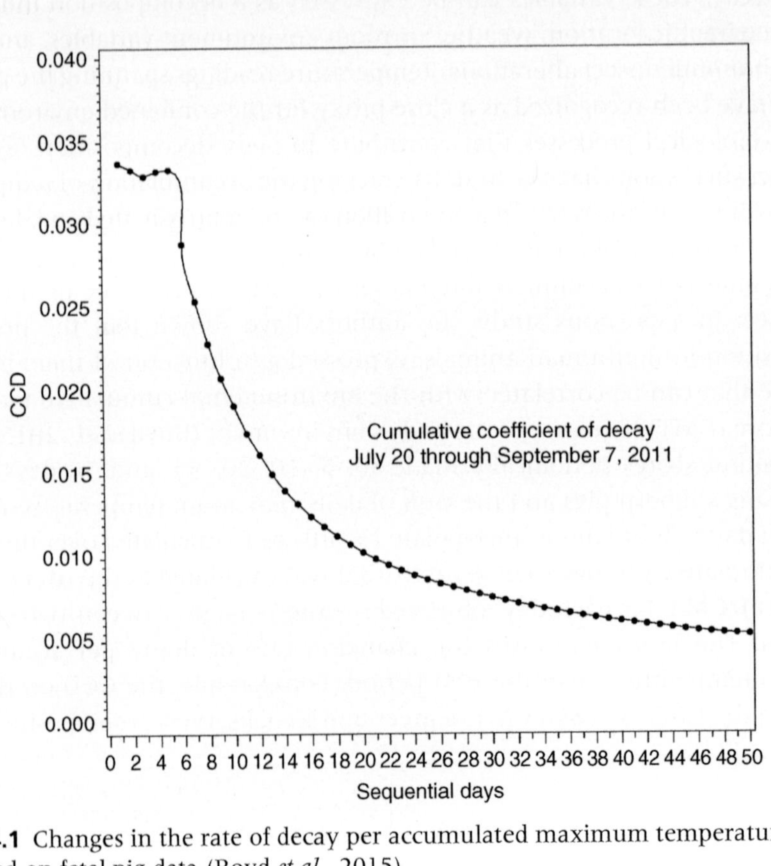

Figure 14.1 Changes in the rate of decay per accumulated maximum temperatures over time based on fetal pig data (Boyd *et al.*, 2015).

a preliminary argument for the viability of this approach to PMI modeling and a call for more systematic observations relating temperature to TBS rates and their associated PMIs under a nonlinear paradigm.

The data analyzed are derived from studies looking at the accumulated degree days (ADD) over the PMI period (Megyesi, 2001; Megyesi *et al.*, 2005) and will be referred to as the original data. ADD is defined as the sum of daily average temperature minus a base temperature across the PMI period:

$$\mathrm{ADD} = \sum_{t=1}^{\mathrm{PMI}} \frac{T_{\max_t} + T_{\min_t}}{2} - T_{\mathrm{base}} \quad \left(\text{when } \frac{T_{\max_t} + T_{\min_t}}{2} > T_{\mathrm{base}} \right) \tag{14.2a}$$

$$\mathrm{ADD} = 0 \quad \left(\text{when } \frac{T_{\max_t} + T_{\min_t}}{2} \leq T_{\mathrm{base}} \right) \tag{14.2b}$$

The base temperature is selected using criteria related to the rate of decomposition versus various temperatures. In Megyesi (2001), that temperature was 10 °C based on the minimum blowfly activity temperature. In Megyesi *et al.* (2005), it was 0 °C, reflecting the slowed decomposition below water's freezing point.

The data provided in table 1 of Megyesi *et al.* (2005) will be used as the model-building sample. The original data consist of 68 case studies in which US county location, observed TBS score, PMI period (known or strongly suspected) expressed as a date range, clothing status, indoor versus outdoor contexts, and calculated ADD value for this PMI period and location were recorded. The authors selected, for their models, a subset from this table in which weather data were available for time periods and the bodies were found in outdoor contexts during warm PMI periods (i.e., the max/min temperatures never fell below the base temperature). Further, following observations by Vass *et al.* (1992) that indicate soft tissue decomposition ceases above ADD values of 1285, only cases where the summed degree days were below this limit were used. This reduces the subjects to 30 cases, 16 clothed and 14 not (Table 14.1). The PMIs of the excluded 12 outdoor cases spanned cooler time periods and will be used to test the robustness of the models. Although previous studies have found no significant difference in the decomposition rates between clothed and unclothed specimens (Card *et al.*, 2015), the potential of two underlying decay processes differentiating clothed versus not clothed contexts led the authors to construct an analysis model for each, separately.

Using these details, daily maximum and minimum temperature readings (°C) were acquired from National Oceanic and Atmospheric Administration's (NOAA's) National Centers for Environmental Information web database (http://www.ncdc.noaa.gov/data-access/land-based-station-data) for each locale and time period. In those situations where a county had more than one weather station with a complete series of readings, the average across all stations, for each day, was calculated. From these data, for each case, variation on the ADD calculation could be derived. Using 0 °C as the base temperature, heat energy is parameterized by calculating a daily cooling degree day (CDD) index, much as the energy industry uses to estimate air conditioning demand versus a base temperature of 65 °F. Such a degree day parameter allows for nonzero measures on days when the minimum temperature, alone, is below the base temperature. It also compares temperatures with a base value empirically defined based on decay processes. Since temperature versus cooling needs is not being indexed, the parameter could more appropriately be thought of as decay degree days. The daily calculation follows this logic (http://www.vesma.com/ddd/ddcalcs.htm):

$$\text{CDD} = \frac{T_{\text{max}} + T_{\text{min}}}{2} - T_{base} \quad \text{where } T_{\text{min}} > T_{\text{base}} \tag{14.3a}$$

$$\text{CDD} = \frac{T_{\text{max}} - T_{\text{base}}}{2} - \frac{T_{\text{base}} - T_{\text{min}}}{4} \quad \text{where } T_{\text{min}} \leq T_{\text{base}} \tag{14.3b}$$

$$\text{CDD} = \frac{T_{\text{max}} - T_{\text{base}}}{4} \quad \text{where } \frac{T_{\text{max}} + T_{\text{min}}}{2} < T_{\text{base}} \tag{14.3c}$$

$$\text{CDD} = 0 \quad \text{where } T_{\text{max}} < T_{\text{base}} \tag{14.3d}$$

Because $T_{\text{base}} = 0\,°\text{C}$, these equations reduce to simpler forms:

$$\text{CDD} = \frac{T_{\text{max}} + T_{\text{min}}}{2} \quad \text{where } T_{\text{min}} > T_{\text{base}} \tag{14.4a}$$

$$\text{CDD} = \frac{T_{\text{max}}}{2} + \frac{T_{\text{min}}}{4} \quad \text{where } T_{\text{min}} \leq T_{\text{base}} \tag{14.4b}$$

$$\text{CDD} = \frac{T_{\text{max}}}{4} \quad \text{where } \frac{T_{\text{max}} + T_{\text{min}}}{2} < T_{\text{base}} \tag{14.4c}$$

$$\text{CDD} = 0 \quad \text{where } T_{\text{max}} < T_{\text{base}} \tag{14.4d}$$

Note that Equation 14.4a is the equivalent of the original ADD when the base temperature is 0 °C. Equation 14.3a represents the commonly used cooling degree calculation when max and min temperatures are both above the base. As noted, one advantage of this more complicated version of a cooling day measure is its ability to deal with occasional temperatures below the base. Heat energy drives the decay process in all situations, not just those where both the max and min temperatures are above some baseline. The refinement of this point using controlled observations will be discussed later.

The subset data along with our summed CDD calculations are presented in Table 14.1. Though not significantly different, the summed CDD values across each PMI period did not always agree precisely with the original ADD sums. Also, the PMI values are one day less than the original table 1 estimates. It is felt that

Table 14.1 Model input data from Megyesi *et al.* (2005)

Case no.	County, state	Date died	Date found	PMI[a]	TBS	Clothed?	ADD	Cumulative cooling degree days[b]
5	Bartholomew, IN	08/15/1998	09/17/1998	33	27	Yes	763.8	764.5
39	Lucas, OH	08/14/1995	09/07/1995	24	27	Yes	605.7	605.55
43	Will, IL	09/22/1994	09/29/1994	7	11	Yes	123.9	125.8
52	Fayette, PA	06/06/1995	06/13/1995	7	19	Yes	149.4	150.1
56	Will, IL	07/05/1997	08/10/1997	36	24	Yes	884.9	803.3
57	Franklin, MO	06/23/1996	08/01/1996	39	26	Yes	629.1	979.3
58	Knox, TN	09/17/1990	09/20/1990	3	6	Yes	80.2	75
72	Pasco, FL	06/09/1999	06/13/1999	4	15	Yes	133.1	130.5
80	Seminole, FL	09/15/1996	09/17/1996	2	11	Yes	87.9	81.95
82	Jefferson, WA	10/03/2000	10/13/2000	10	18	Yes	120.5	121.5
87	Cumberland, PA	08/02/1980	08/06/1980	4	17	Yes	131.4	131.1
89	Morris, NJ	07/28/1995	08/02/1995	5	20	Yes	173.1	152.3
94	Dallas, TX	06/03/1995	06/07/1995	4	12	Yes	104.8	139.2
97	La Porte, IN	04/15/1995	04/16/1995	1	3	Yes	27.1	21.1
102	Hendricks, IN	06/30/2000	07/11/2000	11	22	Yes	270.6	268
4	Owen, IN	09/01/1995	09/13/1995	12	22	No	276.3	252.55
11	Hendricks, IN	07/14/1999	08/30/1999	47	29	No	1108.7	1116.05
37	Kankakee, IL	07/13/1995	07/15/1995	2	15	No	91.7	92.75
44	Richland, SC	10/27/1996	11/03/1996	7	13	No	142.3	141.95
63	Abbeville, SC	08/25/1995	08/28/1995	3	9	No	94.8	101.4
65	Blaine, MT	08/14/1998	08/24/1998	10	23	No	239.8	205.3
78	Daviess, IN	08/31/2000	09/11/2000	11	17	No	264.1	291.8
79	Columbia, NY	09/16/2000	09/30/2000	14	22	No	213.5	187.62
85	Portage, OH	08/21/1994	08/25/1994	4	10	No	100.9	99.2
92	Largo, FL	11/01/1995	11/18/1995	17	24	No	325.8	338.05
93	Essex, NJ	10/21/1995	10/25/1995	4	3	No	74.9	73.6
95	Largo, FL	10/26/1994	10/29/1994	3	15	No	85.4	90.5
101	North Port, FL	03/01/1996	03/07/1996	6	14	No	135.8	134.95

Source: Reproduced with permission of ASTM International.
[a] PMI is one day less than originally reported.
[b] Variable added for this study.

this is a more accurate PMI number. For example, for Case 87, death was presumed to have occurred on August 2, 1980, with discovery on August 6, 1980; the authors interpret this as a PMI of 4 and not the originally reported 5.

The selected cases were divided into two groups: clothed and not clothed. The observed TBS scores were plotted against their associated CDD sums across each PMI period. Using the nonparametric LOESS regression technique, underlying trend lines can be constructed that empirically, rather than statistically, demonstrate the decay rates as a function of increasing CDD. LOESS regression creates a series of localized, linear regression lines that represent the trend of data points within sequential "regions" or "neighborhoods" of the scatterplot space (Cleveland, 1979; Cleveland *et al.*, 1988; Jacoby, 2000). The number of regression segments will vary according to the number of points and the smoothing parameter, which defines the proportion of the points within a neighborhood that is used for each local regression. Sample size ultimately affects the smoothing parameter by limiting the possible sample regions. This study's sample is relatively small, especially when clothing contexts divide it into two groups. The smoothing parameters, [0.0–1.0], can be arbitrarily selected based solely on inspection. In this analysis, given the small samples, the coefficients that produced the smallest residual differences between predicted and observed TBS values while displaying a smoothed line—a pseudo R^2 stand-in—were adopted. The smoothing parameter for the clothed cases is 0.6 and for the not clothed, 0.9. The linked linear segments represent the decomposed nonlinear system that underlies the decay process.

The analysis and graphs were executed using the LOESS and GPLOT procedures from SAS/GRAPH® (SAS Institute, Inc., 2015a) and SAS/STAT® (SAS Institute, Inc., 2015b) software versions 9.4 and 14.1, respectively. The resulting models are shown in Figures 14.2 and 14.3 along with their 90% confidence intervals (CIs). Figure 14.4 provides a comparative look at the predicted TBS sequences between the two samples. The predicted results of the LOESS regression on the model cases are presented in Table 14.2. Based on these trends, Table 14.3 is a simplified lookup table of CDD measures with expected TBS scores for each clothing context. As an example of its use, if the observed TBS for an outdoor, clothed case was 15, the expected CDD sum would be around 123 and more likely within a 90% range of 108–186. By aggregating the NOAA meteorological data on max/min temperatures for the period preceding discovery, the days associated with these CDD values would be the estimated range for time of death.

14.4 Discussion

Looking at Figures 14.2 and 14.3, there are substantial gaps in the CDD sequences between 300 and 600 and over 1000. Given that the original data are treated like a sequential set of observations, it is important that a full range of TBS possibilities are represented. There are significant gaps in the observed TBS scores above 20

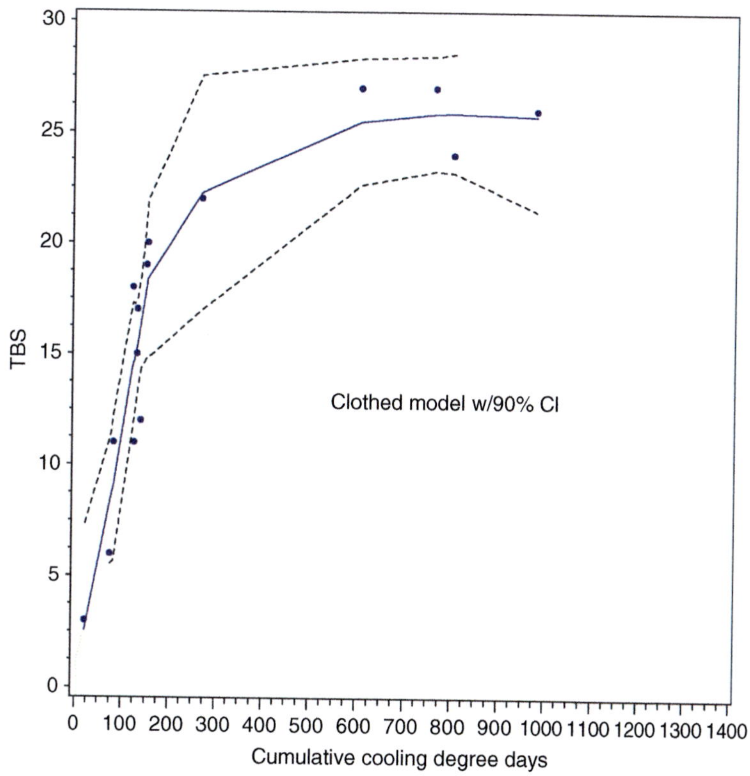

Figure 14.2 LOESS regression, with 90% CI, of observed TBS values versus their cumulative cooling degree days for outdoors, clothed contexts. The smoothing parameter was 0.6.

and their associated CDD ranges. Lacking larger TBS measures reduces the accuracy associated with higher CDD indices; this is displayed in the large CI beyond CDD sums of 200. As in any similar modeling exercise, more data points would enhance the model by reducing the breadth of the CI.

More not clothed contexts would help clarify the differences in the two models. This sample suggests clothed bodies decay slightly faster than not clothed when found in an outdoor setting (Figure 14.4). The nature of not clothed decay rates above CDD indexes of 400, as represented in Figure 14.4, may be an anomaly of the underrepresented sample and the possible outlier status of Case 11 (TBS = 29; CDD = 1116.05).

Figures 14.5 and 14.6 show the application of the models on the 12 excluded outdoor cases, where the max/min temperatures occasionally fell below 0 °C. Their case specifics can be found in Table 14.4. The predicted TBS values fell within the CI 7 of 12 times and were not accurate for the two not clothed cases. Clearly, more observations are needed to better represent these multi-seasonal situations.

Returning to the nature of decay as a nonlinear process, Figures 14.7 and 14.8 present two decay rate approximations derived from the model results. Figure 14.7

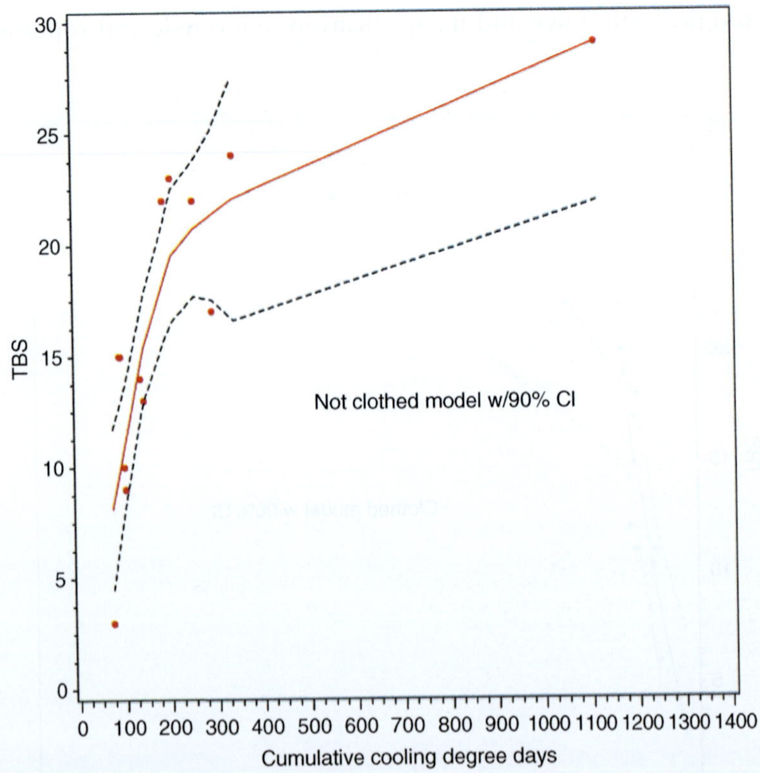

Figure 14.3 LOESS regression, with 90% CI, of observed TBS values versus their cumulative cooling degree days for outdoors, not clothed contexts. The smoothing parameter was 0.9.

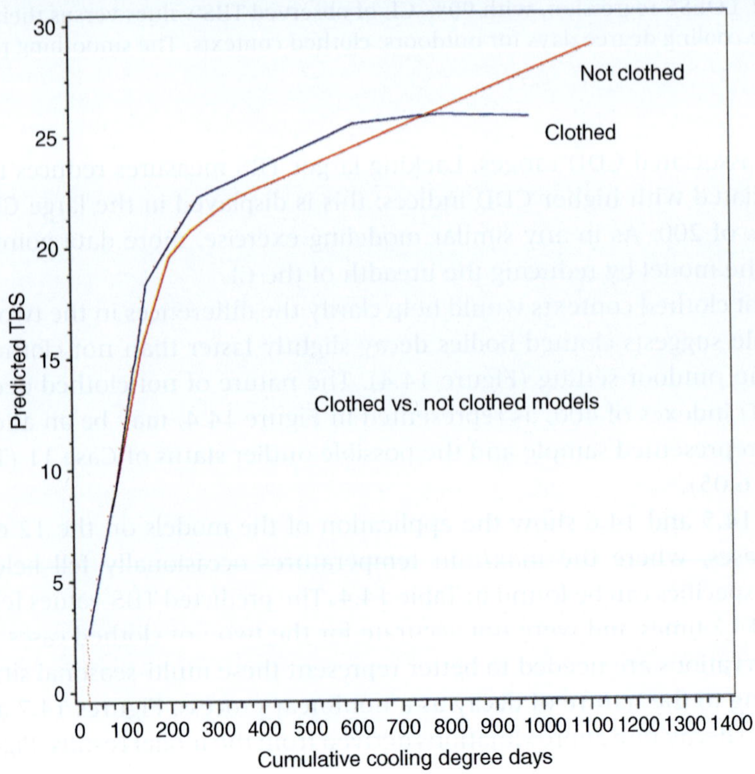

Figure 14.4 Comparative LOESS regressions of clothed versus not clothed contexts.

Table 14.2 Predicted TBS for model cases

Case no.	Clothed	Cumulative cooling degree days	TBS	Predicted TBS	Residual	Lower 90% CI	Upper 90% CI
4	No	252.55	22	20.73	1.27	17.7	23.76
11	No	1116.05	29	29.01	−0.01	21.92	35
37	No	92.75	15	10.17	4.83	7.24	13.11
44	No	141.95	13	15.39	−2.39	13.03	17.76
63	No	101.4	9	11.1	−2.1	8.4	13.79
65	No	205.3	23	19.54	3.46	16.57	22.51
78	No	291.8	17	21.34	−4.34	17.53	25.16
79	No	187.62	22	18.39	3.61	15.73	21.04
85	No	99.2	10	10.86	−0.86	8.11	13.62
92	No	338.05	24	22.07	1.93	16.61	27.52
93	No	73.6	3	8.13	−5.13	4.53	11.73
95	No	90.5	15	9.93	5.07	6.93	12.93
101	No	134.95	14	14.67	−0.67	12.35	17
5	Yes	764.5	27	25.84	1.16	23.25	28.44
39	Yes	605.55	27	25.48	1.52	22.63	28.33
43	Yes	125.8	11	14.73	−3.73	12.23	17.23
52	Yes	150.1	19	18.02	0.98	14.76	21.27
56	Yes	803.3	24	25.87	−1.87	23.18	28.55
57	Yes	979.3	26	25.76	0.24	21.49	30.04
58	Yes	75	6	8.4	−2.4	5.55	11.25
72	Yes	130.5	15	15.27	−0.27	13.11	17.43
80	Yes	81.95	11	9.02	1.98	5.69	12.35
82	Yes	121.5	18	14.43	3.57	11.58	17.28
87	Yes	131.1	17	15.35	1.65	13.22	17.48
89	Yes	152.3	20	18.35	1.65	14.78	21.91
94	Yes	139.2	12	16.45	−4.45	14.33	18.57
97	Yes	21.1	3	2.53	0.47	0	7.34
102	Yes	268	22	22.25	−0.25	16.95	27.54

is comparable with Figure 14.1's ratio of TBS values to CDD sums over time. The form of the curve for clothed contexts is similar to Figure 14.1's. Decay scores increase fastest through the first 200 degree days. The limited sample for not clothed cases suggests a similar process, but with less detail.

Figure 14.8 is a smoothed approximation of the localized rates of decay based on the graphically decomposed segments of the model produced in Figure 14.4. The rate of change in TBS is essentially the slope of the linear regression lines within each scatterplot neighborhood. Each horizontal section is associated with a CDD range where this rate applies. Again, the most rapid periods of decay occur through 200 CDDs followed by a rapid slowing of the process until 300–400 CDDs when

Table 14.3 Predicted TBS for cumulative cooling degree days

Clothed model				Not clothed model			
Cumulative cooling degree days	**Lower limit**	**Predicted TBS**	**Upper limit**	**Cumulative cooling degree days**	**Lower limit**	**Predicted TBS**	**Upper limit**
22	0	3	7	74	5	8	12
30	0	4	8	78	5	9	12
40	1	5	8	87	6	10	13
49	2	6	9	96	8	11	13
58	4	7	10	106	9	12	14
67	5	8	10	115	10	13	15
77	6	9	12	124	11	14	16
86	7	10	13	134	12	15	17
93	8	11	13	144	13	16	18
101	9	12	14	159	14	17	19
108	10	13	15	175	15	18	20
115	11	14	16	190	16	19	21
123	12	15	17	205	17	20	22
133	14	16	18	244	18	21	23
140	14	17	19	302	17	22	26
147	15	18	20	387	17	23	28
157	15	19	22	499	19	24	28
187	16	20	23	611	20	25	29
217	17	21	24	723	21	26	30
246	17	22	26	835	22	27	31
295	18	23	27	947	22	28	33
399	20	24	27	1059	22	29	35
503	22	25	27				
613	23	26	28				

the changes in TBS stabilize. If the decay process had been a linear one, these curves would have shown rates proportional to CDD along a continuous line.

Conceptually, the area under each curve in Figure 14.8 represents the total dissipated decay energy expended as CDDs increase. Any given corpse might be expected to have a specific maximum value for this decay energy related to the body's mass. Even though the body contexts differ and the rates of decay vary, the areas should be approximately equal. For clothed contexts, the rate of decay drops to zero after 803 CDD. The area under the clothed curve up to this point is 23.23. The area under the not clothed curve to 803 CDD is 18.05. Although these values are close, clothed bodies appear to dissipate more energy than not clothed—especially during the first few days of the PMI. As noted by Card *et al.* (2015:979), some studies observed accelerated rates of decomposition in clothed

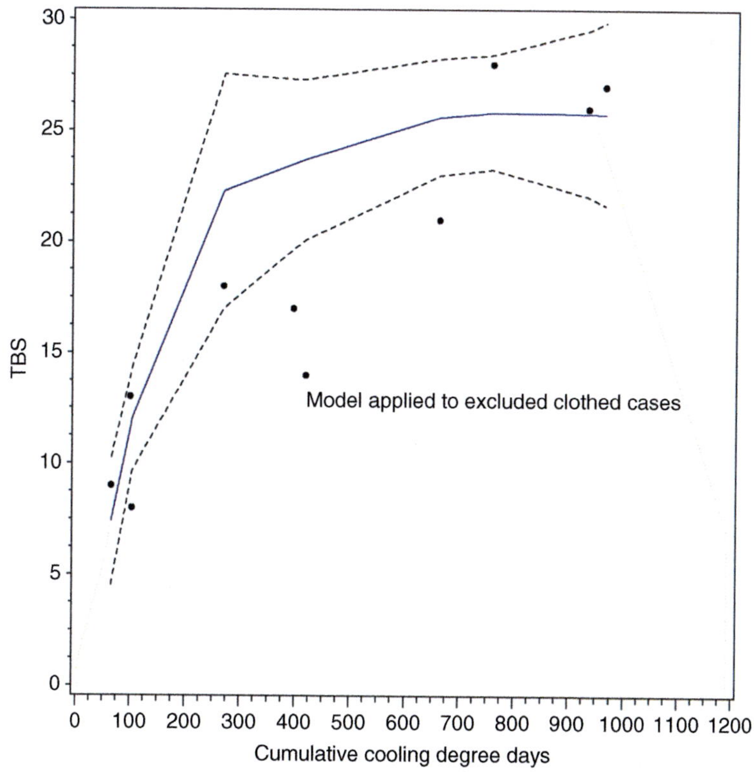

Figure 14.5 LOESS regression, with 90% CI, of observed TBS values versus their cumulative cooling degree days for outdoors, clothed contexts not included in the model-building sample.

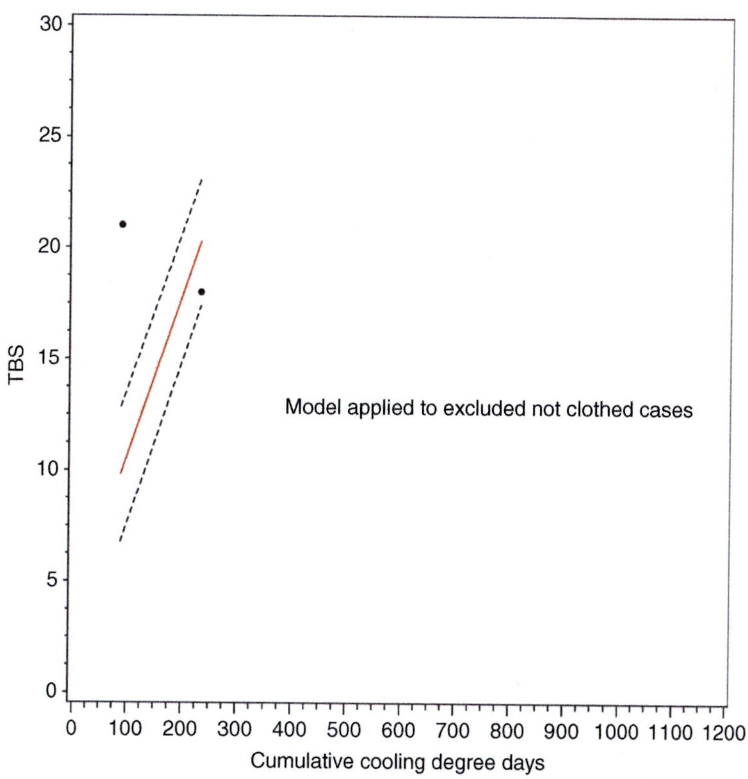

Figure 14.6 LOESS regression, with 90% CI, of observed TBS values versus their cumulative cooling degree days for outdoors, clothed contexts not included in the model-building sample.

Table 14.4 Models applied to excluded outdoor cases from Megyesi *et al.* (2005)

Case no.	County, state	Date died	Date found	PMI[a]	Clothed?	ADD	Cumulative cooling degree days	Observed TBS	Predicted TBS	Lower limit	Upper limit
53	Missoula, MT	10/17/1993	11/07/1993	21	No	91.5	89.35	21	9.8096	7	13
68	Spokane, WA	05/27/1996	06/14/1996	18	No	273	233.65	18	20.2548	17	23
27	Jackson, IN	02/24/1995	04/14/1995	49	Yes	406.9	419.35	14	23.6991	20	27
36	Fulton, IN	11/11/1994	05/06/1995	176	Yes	723.5	759.375	28	25.8332	23	28
45	Howard, IN	09/15/1995	11/19/1995	65	Yes	676.2	662.75	21	25.6133	23	28
47	Rock, WI	09/02/1996	03/20/1997	199	Yes	920	933.917	26	25.7889	22	30
62	Escambia, FL	02/27/1996	03/05/1996	7	Yes	91.4	103.75	8	12.0022	10	14
70	Allen, IN	01/03/1998	04/07/1998	94	Yes	360.6	396.6	17	23.4811	20	27
84	Marion, IN	02/15/1994	04/05/1994	49	Yes	279.4	269.3	18	22.2614	17	28
86	Jo Daviess, IL	03/28/1994	04/10/1994	13	Yes	62.8	65.7	9	7.3891	5	10
90	Jefferson, IL	07/22/1993	12/05/1993	136	Yes	2370.9	965.125	27	25.7706	22	30
99	Boundary, ID	08/03/1996	08/09/1996	6	Yes	118.2	99.95	13	11.4822	9	14

Source: Reproduced with permission of ASTM International.

[a] PMI is one day less than originally reported.

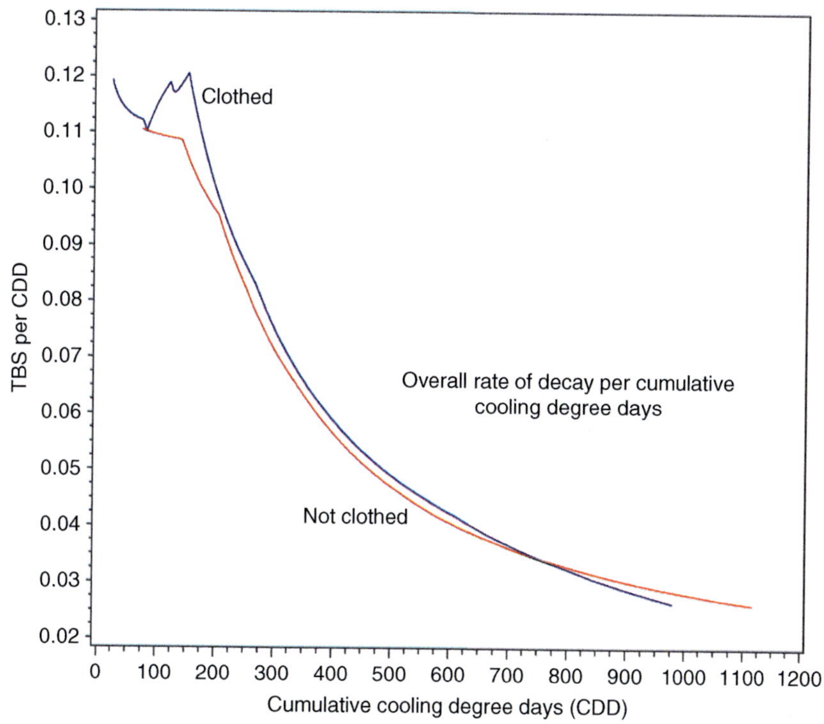

Figure 14.7 Modeled rates of decay expressed as expected TBS value per cumulative cooling degree days. Similar to Figure 14.1.

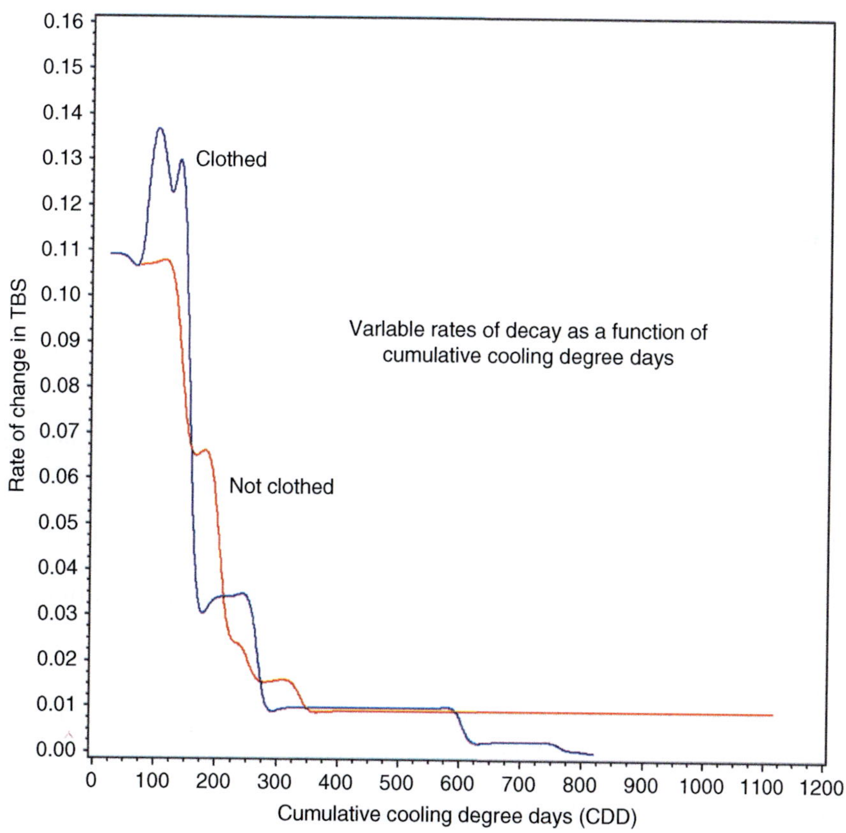

Figure 14.8 Approximation of the rate of change in TBS as cumulative cooling degree days increase.

specimens "because clothing creates new areas for insect oviposition and reduces tissue desiccation…" Dautartas (2009) also noted that covering bodies affected time since death estimations. Again, more complete observations under controlled conditions would enhance the value of these curves in understanding the decay process.

Finally, work needs to be undertaken to empirically determine the best base temperature value for forensic applications. Both 0 and 10 degrees are somewhat arbitrary and in need of verification with more complete data. It is possible, for example, that clothed contexts might use a different temperature than not clothed. This refinement is most applicable to time sequences that include periods where temperatures drop below the base temperature.

In conclusion, forensic anthropologists, as well as archaeologists, are notorious borrowers of theoretical and methodological concepts from other disciplines. But this should not be seen as a bad thing. Reconstructing the past (whether recent or prehistoric) is a complex, multivariate problem, requiring interdisciplinary data and coordination of research methods and goals. The complex process of change in material objects—both animate and inanimate—over time should not be modeled simplistically, but should be depicted in a more realistic manner, which mirrors the actual process and its sequence. Taphonomic experimental and actualistic research has provided us with data on change through direct observation. Using this knowledge, predictive models should be developed and used that represent this nonlinear reality. In light of the recently documented variation in the rates of decomposition of human remains (Dautartas *et al.*, 2016), such nonlinear models will be vital in developing more accurate estimations of PMI.

References

Baden, W.W. (2005) Modelling prehistoric maize agriculture as a dissipative process. In: *Nonlinear Models for Archaeology and Anthropology: Continuing the Revolution* (eds. C.S. Beekman and W.W. Baden). Ashgate Publishing Company, Burlington, VT, pp. 95–122.

Bass, W.M. (1984) Time interval since death: a difficult decision. In: *Human Identification* (eds. T.A. Rathbun and J.E. Buikstra). Charles C. Thomas, Springfield, IL, pp. 136–147.

Bass, W.M. (1997) Outdoor decomposition rates in Tennessee. In: *Forensic Taphonomy: the Postmortem Fate of Human Remains* (eds. W.D. Haglund and M.H. Sorg). CRC Press, Boca Raton, FL, pp. 181–186.

Beekman, C.S. (2005) Agency, collectives, and emergence: social theory and agent based simulations. In: *Nonlinear Models for Archaeology and Anthropology: Continuing the Revolution* (eds. C.S. Beekman and W.W. Baden). Ashgate Publishing Company, Burlington, VT, pp. 51–78.

Beekman, C.S. and Baden, W.W. (eds.) (2005a) *Nonlinear Models for Archaeology and Anthropology: Continuing the Revolution*. Ashgate Publishing Company, Burlington, VT.

Beekman, C.S. and Baden, W.W. (2005b) Continuing the revolution. In: *Nonlinear Models for Archaeology and Anthropology: Continuing the Revolution* (eds. C.S. Beekman and W.W. Baden). Ashgate Publishing Company, Burlington, VT, pp. 1–12.

Binford, L.R. (1972) *An Archaeological Perspective*. Seminar Press, New York.

Binford, L.R. (1983) *Working at Archaeology*. Academic Press, New York.

Binford, L.R. (1989) *Debating Archaeology*. Academic Press, New York.

Bourdieu, P. (1977) *Outline of a Theory of Practice*. Cambridge University Press, Cambridge.

Bourdieu, P. (1992) *The Logic of Practice*. Stanford University Press, Palo Alto, CA.

Boyd, C.C. and Boyd, D.C. (2011) Theory and the scientific basis for forensic anthropology. *Journal of Forensic Sciences*, **56**, 1407–1415.

Boyd, C.C., Baden, W.W., and Boyd, D.C. (2015) Nonlinear systems theory and its application to the determination of the postmortem interval. *Proceedings of the 67th American Academy of Forensic Sciences*, **XXI**, 206.

Card, A., Cross, P., Moffatt, C., and Simmons, T. (2015) The effect of clothing on the rate of decomposition and Diptera colonization on *Sus scrofa* carcasses. *Journal of Forensic Sciences*, **60**, 979–982.

Cleveland, W.S. (1979) Robust locally weighted regression and smoothing scatterplots. *Journal of the American Statistical Association*, **74**, 829–836.

Cleveland, W.S., Delvin, S.J., and Grosse, E. (1988) Regression by local fitting. *Journal of Econometrics*, **37**, 87–114.

Congram, D. (2014) Deposition and dispersal of human remains as a result of criminal acts: *Homo sapiens* as a taphonomic agent. In: *Manual of Forensic Taphonomy* (eds. J.T. Pokines and S.A. Symes). CRC Press, Boca Raton, FL, pp. 249–285.

Dautartas, A.M. (2009) *The Effect of Various Coverings on the Rate of Human Decomposition*. M.A. Thesis, Department of Anthropology, The University of Tennessee, Knoxville.

Dautartas, A.M., Steadman, D.W., Mundorff, A.Z., *et al.* (2016) A comparison of seasonal decomposition patterns between human and non-human animal models. *Proceedings of the 68th American Academy of Forensic Sciences*, **XXII**, 180.

Dobres, M.-A. (2010) Technology's links and *Chaines:* the processual unfolding of technique and technician. In: *Contemporary Archaeology in Theory: The New Pragmatism* (eds. R.W. Preucel and S.A. Mrozowski). Wiley-Blackwell, Chichester, UK, pp. 156–169.

Dobres, M.-A. and Robb, J.E. (2005) "Doing" agency: introductory remarks on methodology. *Journal of Archaeological Method and Theory*, **12**, 159–166.

Dunnell, R.C. (1978) Style and function: a fundamental dichotomy. *American Antiquity*, **43**, 192–202.

Dunnell, R.C. (1980) Evolutionary theory and archaeology. *Advances in Archaeological Method and Theory*, **3**, 35–99.

Dunnell, R.C. (1989) Aspects of the application of evolutionary theory in archaeology. In: *Archaeological Thought in America* (ed. C.C. Lamberg-Karlovsky). Cambridge University Press, Cambridge, pp. 35–49.

Foucault, M. (1984) *The Foucault Reader* (ed. P. Rabinow). Penguin, Harmondsworth, England.

Galloway, A., Birkby, W.H., Jones, A.M., *et al.* (1989) Decay rates of human remains in an arid environment. *Journal of Forensic Sciences*, **34**, 607–616.

Giddens, A. (1979) *Central Problems in Social Theory*. Macmillan, London.

Giddens, A. (1984) *The Constitution of Society: Outline of the Theory of Structuration*. University of California Press, Berkeley.

Groen, W.J.M., Marquez-Grant, N., and Janaway, R.C. (2015a) Concluding remarks. In: *Forensic Archaeology: A Global Perspective* (eds. W.J.M. Groen, N. Marquez-Grant, and R.C. Janaway). Wiley-Blackwell, Chichester, UK, pp. 517–536.

Groen, W.J.M., Marquez-Grant, N., and Janaway, R.C. (eds.) (2015b) *Forensic Archaeology: A Global Perspective*. Wiley-Blackwell, Chichester, UK.

Haglund, W.D. and Sorg, M.H. (eds.) (1997) *Forensic Taphonomy: The Postmortem Fate of Human Remains*. CRC Press, Boca Raton, FL.

Haglund, W.D. and Sorg, M.H. (eds.) (2002) *Advances in Forensic Taphonomy: Method, Theory, and Archaeological Perspectives*. CRC Press, Boca Raton, FL.

Jacoby, W.G. (2000) LOESS: a nonparametric, graphical tool for depicting relationships between variables. *Electoral Studies*, **19**, 577–613.

Joyce, R.A. and Lopiparo, J. (2005) Postscript: doing agency in archaeology. *Journal of Archaeological Method and Theory*, **12**, 365–374.

Keeley, L. (1980) *Experimental Determination of Stone Tool Uses: A Microwear Analysis*. University of Chicago Press, Chicago, IL.

Lyman, R.L. (1994) *Vertebrate Taphonomy*. Cambridge University Press, Cambridge, UK.

Lyman, R.L. and O'Brien, M.J. (1998) The goals of evolutionary archaeology: history and explanation. *Current Anthropology*, **39**, 615–652.

Mann, R., Bass, W.M., and Meadows, L. (1990) Time since death and decomposition of the human body: variables and observations in case and experimental field studies. *Journal of Forensic Sciences*, **35**, 103–111.

Megyesi, M.S. (2001) *The Effects of Temperature on the Decomposition Rate of Human Remains*. M.A. thesis, University of Indianapolis, Indianapolis, IN.

Megyesi, M.S., Narwocki, S.P., and Haskell, N.H. (2005) Using accumulated degree days to estimate the postmortem interval from decomposed human remains. *Journal of Forensic Sciences*, **50**, 618–626.

Micozzi, M. (1991) *Postmortem Change in Human and Animal Remains*. Charles C. Thomas, Springfield, IL.

Moffatt, C., Simmons, T., and Lynch-Aird, J. (2016) An improved equation for TBS and ADD: establishing a reliable postmortem interval framework for casework and experimental studies. *Journal of Forensic Sciences*, **61**, S201–S207.

Nicolis, G. and Prigogine, I. (1977) *Self-organization in Nonequilibrium Systems: From Dissipative Structures to Order Through Fluctuations*. Wiley, New York.

Nicolis, G. and Prigogine, I. (1989) *Exploring Complexity: An Introduction*. W. H. Freeman, New York.

Pauketat, T.R. (1994) *The Ascent of Chiefs: Cahokia and Mississippian Politics in Native North America*. The University of Alabama Press, Tuscaloosa.

Pauketat, T.R. (2010) Practice and history in archaeology: an emerging paradigm. In: *Contemporary Archaeology in Theory: The New Pragmatism* (eds. R.W. Preucel and S.A. Mrozowski). Wiley-Blackwell, Chichester, UK, pp. 137–155.

Pokines, J.T. and Symes, S.A. (2014) *Manual of Forensic Taphonomy*. CRC Press, Boca Raton, FL.

Preucel, R.W. (1991) *Processual and Postprocessual Archaeologies: Multiple Ways of Knowing the Past*. Center for Archaeological Investigations, Southern Illinois University at Carbondale, Occasional Paper No. 10.

Preucel, R.W. and Mrozowski, S.A. (eds.) (2010) *Contemporary Archaeological Theory: The New Pragmatism* (2nd ed.). Wiley-Blackwell, Chichester, UK.

Prigogine, I., Nicolis, G., and Babloyantz, A. (1972) Thermodynamics of evolution. *Physics Today*, November, 23–28.

Rodriguez, W.C. and Bass, W.M. (1983) Insect activity and its relationship to decay rates of human cadavers in East Tennessee. *Journal of Forensic Sciences*, **28**, 423–432.

SAS Institute, Inc. (2015a) *SAS/GRAPH 9.4 User's Guide: The GPLOT Procedure*. SAS Institute, Inc., Cary, NC.

SAS Institute, Inc. (2015b) *SAS/STAT 14.1 User's Guide: The LOESS Procedure*. SAS Institute, Inc. Cary, NC.

Schiffer, M.B. (1976) *Behavioral Archaeology*. Academic Press, New York.

Schiffer, M.B. and Skibo, J.M. (1997) The explanation of artifact variability. *American Antiquity*, **62**, 27–50.

Schmitt, S. (2002) Mass graves and the collection of forensic evidence: genocide, war crimes, and crimes against humanity. In: *Advances in Forensic Taphonomy: Method, Theory, and Archaeological Perspectives* (eds. W.D. Haglund and M.H. Sorg). CRC Press, Boca Raton, FL, pp. 277–292.

Schoenly, K., Griest, K., and Rhine, S. (1991) An experimental field protocol for investigating the postmortem interval using multidisciplinary indicators. *Journal of Forensic Sciences*, **36**, 1395–1415.

Shean, B.S., Messinger, L., and Papworth, M. (1993) Observations of differential decomposition on sun exposed v. shaded pig carrion in coastal Washington State. *Journal of Forensic Sciences*, **38**, 938–949.

Silliman, S. (2001) Agency, practical politics and the archaeology of culture contact. *Journal of Social Archaeology*, **1**, 190–209.

Sledzik, P.S. (1998) Forensic taphonomy: postmortem decomposition and decay. In: *Forensic Osteology: Advances in the Identification of Human Remains* (ed. K. Reichs). Charles C. Thomas, Springfield, IL, pp. 109–119.

South, S. (1977) *Method and Theory in Historical Archaeology*. Academic Press, New York.

Vass, A., Bass, W.M., Wolt, J.D., *et al.* (1992) Time since death of human cadavers using soil solution. *Journal of Forensic Sciences*, **37**, 1236–1253.

Vaughan, P.C. (1985) *Use-Wear Analysis of Flaked Stone Tools*. University of Arizona Press, Tucson.

Willey, P. and Heilman, A. (1987) Estimating time since death using plant roots and stems. *Journal of Forensic Sciences*, **32**, 1264–1270.

Yoshida, Z. (2010) *Nonlinear Science: The Challenge to Complex Systems*. Springer, Heidelberg.

CHAPTER 15

Arrows of influence: The give and take of theory between forensic anthropology, archaeology, and geophysics

John F. Schweikart[1] and Cheryl A. Johnston[2]
[1] *Search Recovery Consultants L.L.C., Columbus, OH, USA*
[2] *The Ohio State University, Columbus, OH, USA*

15.1 Introduction

Forensic anthropology has historically been derived, and heavily influenced, by other disciplines, notably anatomy and biological science. In recent years, forensic anthropology has undergone exponential change as the contextual framework, perception, and practice of the discipline have developed under the influence of theoretical and methodological constructs from other fields and subdisciplines of anthropology.

In this chapter, we will consider the give and take, or mutual influences, that have occurred between forensic anthropology and two fields that have contributed to, and benefited from, interactions with forensic anthropology: these fields are archaeology, a subdiscipline of anthropology, and geophysics, a subdiscipline of geology. Current as well as future aspects of informational, theoretical, and methodological "backflow" from contemporary forensic anthropology to archaeology and geophysics, from which it has borrowed and adapted theory or methodology, are considered. The authors argue that forensic anthropology has emerged from a formative period of borrowing from other fields into a new era of contribution to other fields. This may be accomplished by linking current to past behaviors via similarities in the signatures each leaves in the environment, the basis of many interpretive theories.

Unlike other forms of anthropological research, the variables for designing and implementing methods, approaches, data collection procedures, permitted analyses, and the dissemination of case or project information to peers may be

Forensic Anthropology: Theoretical Framework and Scientific Basis, First Edition.
Edited by C. Clifford Boyd Jr and Donna C. Boyd.

beyond the control of the forensic anthropologist(s) involved. All activities prior to, during, and after a medicolegal investigation under the force of law must be negotiated and set by the appropriate medicolegal authorities who are ultimately responsible for each investigation. By definition, the *forensic* anthropologist serves a prescribed role, which can be (and often is) a limited one within the total context of a much more comprehensive medicolegal investigation.

Because of these necessary prescriptions, there is a perception that the practice of forensic anthropology is inherently lesser and limited in its potential to contribute new approaches, methods, or theories of substantial consequence back to its parent disciplines. Nevertheless, Boyd and Boyd (2011) recently countered this criticism and (in this volume) have explored and illustrated foundational, interpretive, and methodological theory in forensic anthropology. We embrace the merits of this and, in particular, consider some current and future directions of interpretive theory. In support of this approach, we offer the following.

The history of forensic anthropology is replete with novel approaches and developments related to the estimation of a comprehensive biological profile for deceased individuals, as well as important aids to the interpretation of antemortem, perimortem, and postmortem influences on sets of remains and placement of remains within an interpretable locational context. While all of these developments have been of great value to medicolegal investigations, they predominantly represent "lower levels" of general inquiry designed to address straightforward questions through specific lines of empirical inquiry (Merton, 1949). For example, bones and teeth form at relatively regular rates during human development and certain discrete and metric skeletal and dental traits offer statistically significant distribution frequencies in their phenotypic expression between the sexes and in various human populations originating from different parts of the world.

In order to guide empirical inquiry to a higher level, we suggest that forensic anthropology has reached a point where practitioners need to bridge the gap between their observations and the interpretable behavior(s) that created the "anthropological stuff" of medicolegal interest (Praetzellis, 2000). Many researchers are, of course, already engaged in this type of analysis (see Chapter 13, this volume). This, in sum, is what interpretive theory is all about, as reflected in its origins in sociology (Merton, 1949), and the later "New Archeology" emphasis on middle-range research in the 1960s and 1970s (Binford, 1977).

To put this in perspective, consider Galileo's experiments in which he dropped small stones and cannon balls from a tall tower to answer simple questions about how gravity actually worked on earth (methodological theory). Galileo's results were essential foundations to the development of Newton's higher level or intermediate theories concerning gravity's nature at the universal scale, which are able to explain not only how objects on earth behaved but also how and why heavenly bodies such as planets and stars move the way that they do (i.e., interpretive theory). In spite of this important achievement, Newton's laws are intermediate themselves because they cannot explain why matter in our universe (especially at the subatomic level) behaves the way it does (i.e., this is a "higher" level foundational theory). Nevertheless, Newton's laws allowed us to predictably send objects to the far reaches of our solar system and to safely send human beings to the moon and back again, which is no small achievement.

Like archaeologists trying to infer behavior from artifacts (Whitley, 1998), forensic anthropologists have to contend with a limited ability to interpret forensic evidence and infer the past behavior that created it. Thus, for both disciplines, abductive reasoning (inference to the best explanation, given available data) (Walton, 2004) is the most common form of logic used.

Therefore, an "observational language" is needed for forensic anthropologists to interpret materials and contexts within the theoretical limitations of the discipline. Forensic anthropologists stand to benefit from the use of the Occam's razor concept: that the simplest explanation is the most likely to be true based on our ability to observe and interpret what is there (Whitley, 1998; Praetzellis, 2000). So, instead of disparaging the fact that forensic anthropology as it has developed to the present falls short of employing "high-order theories" due to it being an "applied science," hope springs eternal as we briefly consider how it is already having a "backflow" of influence on archaeology and geophysics through intermediate or interpretive theoretical developments that are opening up new avenues of future inquiry.

15.2 Influences of archaeology on forensic anthropology

While most would support the notion that modern forensic anthropology is primarily the offspring of physical (i.e., biological) anthropology, influence from archaeology has played an integral part in the development of forensic anthropology since its earliest beginnings and continues to do so as both fields have adapted and evolved over the past century. For example, archaeological collections have been (and in many cases continue to be) primary source material for comparative study of both metric and nonmetric hard tissue variation in human populations from around the world. In addition, methods of site identification and systematic recovery borrowed from archaeology reflect a growing emphasis in forensic anthropology on how to best document forensic contexts and maximize the interpretation of both biological and nonbiological materials of potential medicolegal interest (Dirkmaat *et al.*, 2008; Duhig and Turnbull, 2007). The key contribution of archaeology to forensic anthropology has been summarized by Dirkmaat *et al.* (2008:41): "The evidentiary value of any item at the scene will depend on its relative position and contextual relationships with other evidence and elements at the scene."

One of the fundamental differences between the application of archaeological methods to forensic anthropology and "typical" archaeological investigations is the desired level of analysis and interpretation. Most archaeological investigations work to interpret remains of past human behaviors in the collective and to interpret them in terms of what they say about a group of past people over an extended period of time—often spanning multiple generations. On the other hand, forensic anthropologists by necessity focus on interpreting a singular event or a series of closely related events involving the evidence of behaviors of specific perpetrators in relation to individual decedents within a limited temporal and geographic boundary.

The statement by Dirkmaat *et al.* (2008:41) that "...the main difference between conventional archaeology and forensic archaeology resides in the presence of soft tissues at forensic scenes..." is too narrow for what both fields have become. Beginning with discoveries associated with radiometric dating in the 1950s, the past half-century in modern archaeology has undergone a profound revolution of ever-increasing "new" approaches and applications being brought to bear on even the most conventional of investigations, leading to the identification of novel forms of "artifacts" (i.e., evidence) and new opportunities for interpretation and evaluation. These include new forms of data derived from trace elemental identification and analysis, identification of various geophysical signatures of archaeological phenomena, and the identification, collection, and analysis of preserved "soft tissue" and microbiological materials (e.g., DNA) from humans and other organisms that have been preserved in archaeological contexts. Therefore, to say that there is a major barrier between modern archaeology and forensic anthropology in terms of classes of materials worthy of study or investigation would be shortsighted. New approaches and new tools for analysis are likely to continue to develop for both fields in the future.

Concurrently, the past two decades have seen a great deal of interest in the application of taphonomic principles to the field of forensic anthropology, and while in the strictest sense, taphonomy developed first out of paleontology, it has had its most profound influence on forensic anthropology through developments borrowed from archaeological investigation—particularly zooarchaeology (Lyman, 1994). Taphonomic research in zooarchaeology led to a growing awareness on the part of forensic anthropologists that it is possible to contribute significantly to the reconstruction of past events, anthropogenic and otherwise, that surround an individual's death, including the interpretation of the means by which disposal of remains occurred, as well as other relevant site formation processes that may have contributed to the condition of a given scene at the time of its investigation and recovery (Haglund and Sorg, 1997, 2002; Pokines and Symes, 2014).This recognition of the importance of taphonomy of the site or scene and consideration of site formation processes has and will continue to profoundly affect the practice and direction of forensic anthropology for years to come. Clearly, the days of the forensic anthropologist not being compelled by professional obligation to contribute fully to scene documentation and systematic recovery are over, thanks to methods derived from archaeology.

What differs most between forensic anthropology and archaeology today is not the specific types of materials or evidence that are of exclusive interest to the archaeologist versus those of interest to the forensic anthropologist, but rather the differences in research design. Specifically, this relates to the questions each field needs to identify to get at the contextual relationships of importance for their specific types of investigation. Therefore, the long association between these two fields will surely continue albeit with different objectives and outcomes.

15.3 Influences of geophysics on forensic anthropology

Geophysics is the study of contrasting physical properties of the Earth, primarily developed out of geological applications for the prospection and identification of large-scale geological phenomena such as productive oil and gas fields and underground aquifers, characterization of bedrock strata, and applications for stability and engineering assessments prior to large-scale project construction. Initially, large-scale geological applications of geophysics had little influence on the development and application of forensic anthropology due to the vast difference in scale of interest; however, this changed with the development of near surface levels of investigation, which were instigated for other fields of inquiry (Bevan, 1991; Cheetham, 2005). Developments occurred as a result of a better understanding of various wave properties along much of the electromagnetic (EM) spectrum (Cheetham, 2005; Larson *et al.*, 2011). Following is a list of the most prominent methods that have found use in forensic anthropology:

1. *Photography* (particularly aerial) across the surface of the Earth captures variation within and outside of the visible spectrum (such as with the use of infrared imaging) and has been used as a means of identifying contrasting surface conditions that may be of interest in locating remains.
2. *Resistivity* measures the varying degree of electrical resistance of electrical current passing through the subsurface of the Earth.
3. *Magnetometry* measures anomalies in the Earth's magnetic field below the ground surface.
4. *EM systems* include metal detectors that generate EM fields that induce small electrical currents into conducting targets (i.e., metals) that are then detected by a receiving coil.
5. *Ground-penetrating radar (GPR)* or subsurface interface radar (SIR) transmits a pulse of microwaves into the ground, which then become reflected and refracted back to a receiver in different ways based on the physical properties of the subsurface materials encountered by those microwaves (Schultz, 2007).

Developments in applied engineering, environmental, and industrial geophysics led to technological developments allowing application of geophysics to smaller-scale near-surface contexts. This made them more useful for both archaeological and forensic anthropological prospection. While these developments can trace their origins back to the early 1970s, if not earlier, widespread use of geophysics in near-surface investigations was limited by the ability and speed by which geophysical data could be filtered and manipulated to reveal specific anomalies of potential interest at the level of individual "features" or "targets" produced by the actions of individuals at a given point in time (Bevan, 1991; Davenport, 2001; Cheetham, 2005). In spite of technological improvements, in many cases, data obtained were still somewhat difficult to interpret. This was due to unforeseen variables encountered in the field combined with a lack of familiarity by many early practitioners as to what sort of EM signatures were to be expected for the specific anomalies/targets of forensic interest.

However, the most significant factor leading to the routine incorporation of geophysical prospection into forensic anthropological investigations resulted from advancements in computing and microprocessing in the 1990s and 2000s. This effectively brought the computer into the field so that geophysical data could be filtered and processed on-site, thereby maximizing the ability to gather high quality data in real-time and making it possible to quickly compare and contrast different geophysical prospecting methods simultaneously. These microprocessors concurrently led to a revolution in the ability to collect and display distributional information and to produce accurate high quality maps in the field that can be overlaid on top of pertinent data, such as geo-referenced aerial photography, soils data, hydrology data, and other data sets collected and stored in geographic information system (GIS) databases. Therefore, there is now an expectation that forensic field data, including those collected by the forensic anthropologist on-site, will be gathered, compiled, and possibly interpreted while conducting forensic anthropological investigations in the field.

These technological changes were accompanied by the concurrent development of a generation of geophysical specialists who have gained expertise through experience as to what sort of signatures are to be expected from near-surface activities of forensic anthropological interest (Dupras *et al.*, 2012). Equally important is that this new generation of specialists in forensic anthropology, in order to remain relevant, need to be receptive to the adoption of new avenues of inquiry in order to interpret forensic anthropological remains in ever wider taphonomic and behavioral contexts, many of which were not considered just a few years before. Thus, continuing education from, and connection with, active practitioners in this evolving field is a vital part of good practice.

15.4 "Backflow" to other disciplines: Site formation processes in archaeology

As previously summarized, one of the most important additions to the field of forensic anthropology over the past two decades has been recognition of the importance of documenting relevant data that may have influenced physical, anthropogenic, and preservational conditions at a forensic scene. While much has been gained in forensic anthropology from contributions from paleontology and archaeology, there is much that forensic anthropology can (and already has) contribute back to these and other "parent" disciplines.

In particular, nearly all paleontological and archaeological investigations involve interpretation and recovery of biological materials that have either degraded to a point where they are at or very near complete organic disintegration. These materials of interest may still be recognizable because they have been interrupted on their path toward oblivion by some kind of decompositional stasis. These arresting factors may have resulted from some combination of desiccation, freezing, antimicrobial conditions, mineralization, and/or fossilization. While traditional paleontologists and archaeologists are well acquainted with the later stages of preservation or decomposition, they often have little firsthand experience interpreting the earliest and most dramatic stages of organic decomposition and are therefore poorly prepared to evaluate how and to what degree recent decomposition has impacted the surrounding flora, fauna, and chemical composition in the immediate area of a given scene. Importantly, they may be in doubt as to which (if any) of these factors is most important.

Furthermore, in contrast, the contemporary forensic anthropologist is motivated by self-preservation and legal requirements of what has been called the "trilogy" for admissibility of expert witness testimony (i.e., *Daubert, Kumho,* and *Joiner*) and is very much aware of the requirement to operate under a standardized protocol and in a multidisciplinary framework (Grivas and Komar, 2008; Christensen and Crowder, 2009). This has led to a new kind of forensic anthropology specialist—that is, one who is prepared and is comfortable working within a multidisciplinary team in developing new methodologies and protocols for the identification and interpretation of these earliest stages of biological decomposition or dissolution. These practitioners are adept at understanding what this means for evidence collection, as early-stage decomposition is likely to be encountered during field recovery (e.g., Blackledge, 2007; Harrison and Donnelly, 2009; Larson *et al.*, 2011; Dupras *et al.*, 2012).

Some forms of forensic analysis have already made their way back to influence these parent fields. These include use wear (i.e., tool mark), firearms, and blood residue analyses, methods, and strategies for the collection of DNA from decomposed or damaged contexts and a multitude of trace elemental, soil, and chemical analyses related to changes imparted to an individual set of remains or to the surrounding matrix of materials in proximity to them (Connor and Scott, 2001; Larson *et al.*, 2011).

15.5 Backflow: Interpretation/understanding of geophysical signatures

One of the most interesting and productive areas of "backflow" has been the development of a new class of forensic anthropologist well versed in the challenges and potential utility of geophysical applications to forensic anthropology.

In combination with forensic taphonomy and forensic archaeology, forensic geophysics has highlighted the fact that near-surface phenomena of forensic interest have their own distinct set of challenges for identification. Equally, phenomena of forensic interest will have their own particular "lexicon" or set of distinguishing "signatures" to be recognized and defined and will in many cases differ qualitatively and quantitatively from the contexts and "signatures" that paleontologists and archaeologists are used to identifying. Nevertheless, this altered focus earlier in the decomposition process rather than later can provide valuable data for a better understanding of the full spectrum of anthropogenic and natural formation processes related to deposition and material preservation of evidence and will in all likelihood lead to new insights that can be tested.

As discussed previously, technological innovations that have enabled computing capabilities to be brought into the field have also been a critically important development, along with the widespread application of various geophysical methods to forensic anthropology in the last two decades. In essence, the strict barrier between field collection and analysis in the laboratory has been broken, and as more and more testing can be done in real-time on-site, results will be used to better inform and direct ongoing multidisciplinary forensic investigations.

There have also been concurrent developments of increasing sophistication and interpretive potential rendered by combining multiple layers of geophysical and cartographic data with GIS to interpret and explain the interactions between human behaviors and natural processes across a given landscape. Manheim *et al.* (2006) demonstrated this for forensic anthropology in their application of GIS and spatial analysis to evaluate relationships between various areas of dumped and subsequently scattered human remains. These kinds of analyses open new doors for developing predictive models for locating sites of clandestine or criminal behaviors. Like any human activity, there are certain factors with differing levels of visibility that will affect where, when, and possibly even why certain activities happen more frequently in certain places rather than in others. Not only does this have great potential for interpreting individual cases of forensic interest, but it could also be very helpful in documenting what could be predictive evidence left by police, military, or paramilitary groups shown to be perpetrators of crimes against humanity or other large-scale human rights violations.

When most people think of forensic anthropology, they think of dealing with the (human) dead. Nevertheless, as the field has developed, so has its applicability to cases other than human death investigations. Examples include the application of forensic anthropological methods of investigation and analysis to animal cruelty, wildlife poaching, and cases of suspected trafficking in endangered species (Weidner *et al.*, 1997).

Another avenue of significant "backflow" has been the adoption of systematic recovery methods derived from forensic archaeology and applied to other kinds of criminal investigations such as fire scenes, cases involving the discharge of firearms, as well as sexual assault cases. These types of cases require careful recovery methods that can yield significant trace chemical, ballistic, and body fluid evidence that would have been missed or not subjected to specific analyses using standard law enforcement recovery techniques (Schweikart, 2000; Connor and Scott, 2001).

15.6 Conclusion

Within the last generation, forensic anthropology has undergone rapid expansion in terms of how it can contribute to an ever-growing list of types of medicolegal investigations. As has been advocated by Boyd and Boyd (2011; Chapter 1, this volume), forensic anthropology is now at the point where it is ready for explicit theoretical development and for consideration as a fully contributing subdiscipline to American anthropology in its own right. In addition, the dialectic between forensic anthropology and all subfields of anthropology, including physical anthropology, archaeology, and cultural anthropology, is already demonstrating methodological and theoretical "backflow" of ideas and methods, and the potential for more development exists.

The task ahead for forensic anthropologists is to codify the "observational language" so that the interrelationships and influence of biological, anthropogenic (i.e., behavioral), and physical characteristics are considered to enhance the overall interpretive value of a forensic investigation. In combination, all these phenomena need to be identified and interpreted in a consistent manner, following established protocols, to benefit the investigation as a whole. This will involve careful consideration and advocacy regarding the kinds of forensic anthropologists that are needed to adequately conduct a particular phase of an investigation. The field itself is developing technically and intellectually and demands the development of subfields of specific expertise. While all these new tasks or roles are still evolving, what is clear is that the forensic anthropologist of the near future will need, more than ever, to be involved from the earliest stages of field investigation. He or she will increasingly be required to work within and between complementary disciplines and with new and unique combinations of key players as the nature and range of situations for interdisciplinary collaboration continue to increase.

References

Bevan, B.W. (1991) The search for graves. *Geophysics*, **56**, 1310–1319.

Binford, L.R. (1977) *For Theory Building in Archaeology: Essays on Faunal Remains, Aquatic Resources, Spatial Analysis, and Systemic Modeling*. Academic Press, New York.

Blackledge, R.D. (ed.). (2007). *Forensic Analysis on the Cutting Edge: New Methods for Trace Evidence Analysis*. John Wiley & Sons, Inc., Hoboken, NJ.

Boyd, C.C. and Boyd, D.C. (2011) Theory and the scientific basis for forensic anthropology. *Journal of Forensic Sciences*, **56**(6), 1407–1415.

Cheetham, P. (2005) Forensic geophysical survey. In: *Forensic Archaeology: Advances in Theory and Practice* (eds. J. Hunter and M. Cox). Routledge, London, UK, pp. 62–95.

Christensen, A.M. and Crowder, C.M. (2009) Evidentiary standards for forensic anthropology. *Journal of Forensic Sciences*, **54**(6), 1211–1216.

Connor, M.A. and Scott, D.D. (2001) Archaeologists as forensic investigators: defining the role. *Historical Archaeology*, **35**(1), 1–6.

Davenport, C.G. (2001) Remote sensing applications in forensic investigations. *Historical Archaeology*, **35**(1), 87–100.

Dirkmaat, D.C., Cabo, L.L., Ousley, S.D., and Symes, S.A. (2008) New perspectives in forensic anthropology. *Yearbook of Physical Anthropology*, **51**, 33–52.

Duhig, C. and Turnbull, R. (2007) Crime scene management and forensic anthropology: observations and recommendations from the United Kingdom and international cases. In: *Forensic Archaeology and Human Rights Violations* (ed. R. Ferllini). Charles C. Thomas, Springfield, IL, pp. 76–100.

Dupras, T.L., Schultz, J.J., Wheeler, S.M., and Williams, L.J. (2012) *Forensic Recovery of Human Remains: Archaeological Approaches* (2nd edn.). CRC Press, Boca Raton, FL.

Grivas, C.R. and Komar, D.A. (2008) Kumho, Daubert, and the nature of scientific inquiry: implications for forensic anthropology. *Journal of Forensic Sciences*, **53**(4), 771–776.

Haglund, W.D. and Sorg, M.H. (eds.). (1997) *Forensic Taphonomy: The Postmortem Fate of Human Remains*. CRC Press, Boca Raton, FL.

Haglund, W.D. and Sorg, M.H. (eds.). (2002) *Advances in Forensic Taphonomy: Method, Theory, and Archaeological Perspectives*. CRC Press, Boca Raton, FL.

Harrison, M. and Donnelly, L.J. (2009) Locating concealed homicide victims: developing the role of geoforensics. In: *Criminal and Environmental Soil Forensics* (eds. K. Ritz, L. Dawson, and D. Miller). Springer, Dordrecht, The Netherlands, pp. 197–219.

Larson, D.O., Vass, A.P., and Wise, M. (2011) Advanced scientific methods and procedures in the forensic investigation of clandestine graves. *Journal of Contemporary Criminal Justice*, **27**(2), 149–182.

Lyman, R.L. (1994) *Vertebrate Taphonomy*. Cambridge University Press, Cambridge, UK.

Manheim, M.H., Listi, G.A., and Leitner, M. (2006) The application of geographic information systems and spatial analysis to assess dumped and subsequently scattered human remains. *Journal of Forensic Sciences*, **51**(3), 469–473.

Merton, R.K. (1949) *Social Theory and Social Structure*. Simon and Schuster, The Free Press, New York.

Pokines, J.T. and Symes, S.A. (2014) *Manual of Forensic Taphonomy*. CRC Press, Boca Raton, FL.

Praetzellis, A. (2000) *Death by Theory: A Tale of Mystery and Archaeological Theory*. AltaMira Press, Walnut Creek, CA.

Schultz, J.J. (2007) Using ground-penetrating radar to locate clandestine graves of homicide victims: forming forensic archaeology partnerships with law enforcement. *Homicide Studies*, **11**, 15–29.

Schweikart, J.F. (2000) The investigation of fire scenes. *Paper Presented at the 22nd Annual Spring Seminar of the Society for the Scientific Detection of Crime, Reynoldsburg*, Ohio.

Walton, D.N. (2004) *Abductive Reasoning*. The University of Alabama Press, Tuscaloosa.

Weidner, D., Johnston, C., and Lee, A. (1997) Elephant ears and orangutan skulls. *North East Forensic Anthropology Association meeting*, Erie, PA, October 3–4, 1997.

Whitley, D.S. (1998) New approaches to old problems: archaeology in search of an ever elusive past. In: *Reader in Archaeological Theory: Post-Processual and Cognitive Approaches* (ed. D.S. Whitley). Routledge, New York, pp. 1–30.

CHAPTER 16

Forensic anthropology, scientific evidence, and the law: Why theory matters

Donna C. Boyd[1,2] and C. Clifford Boyd Jr[1]
[1] *Department of Anthropological Sciences, Radford University Forensic Science Institute, Radford University, Radford, VA, USA*
[2] *Department of Biomedical Science, Virginia Tech Carilion School of Medicine, Roanoke, VA, USA*

16.1 Introduction: Theory in practice

This chapter discusses the importance of theory for legal applications of forensic anthropology. As such, it explores the difficulties associated with court testimony regarding admissibility and interpretation of forensic anthropology evidence. Many of these difficulties arise from the ambiguous and sometimes contentious relationship between science and the law, while others derive from an absence of a clear recognition and understanding of the scientific basis for the research forensic anthropologists conduct. It is argued here that a strong and explicit theoretical and scientific framework for forensic anthropology research is critical to ensuring admission and accurate evaluation of the scientific evidence it engenders. Theory is also useful for understanding and bridging the often tense divide between the scientific and legal arenas, as illustrated by the following case study.

16.1.1 *Commonwealth of Virginia v Lockett*: Why theory matters

In early 2010, investigators were called to the Virginia home of a 2-year-old boy by his stepfather, who claimed that intruders had broken into the home and abducted the child. After an unproductive AMBER Alert search, the stepfather admitted that the child was not kidnapped. He stated that the boy died accidentally due to choking on ingested food and provided information that ultimately led investigators to recover partially decomposed remains of the juvenile at the county landfill 2 weeks later. These remains had undergone significant postmortem (heavy equipment) damage and the medical examiner was not able to establish

Forensic Anthropology: Theoretical Framework and Scientific Basis, First Edition.
Edited by C. Clifford Boyd Jr and Donna C. Boyd.

cause of death; however, they were intact enough for an autopsy to show evidence of numerous past injuries (e.g., soft tissue scarring, burns) as well as evidence of malnutrition and neglect. Forensic anthropological analysis by the authors of this chapter documented the presence of a prior untreated complete spiral fracture of the right humerus with evidence of significant callus development and beginning bridging. Time since injury (TSI) was estimated as likely 10 days to 3 weeks.

The juvenile's stepfather was charged with first-degree murder but avoided trial by pleading no contest to second-degree murder and receiving a 50-year prison sentence. The mother was also charged with first-degree murder, but this charge was later reduced to second-degree murder, child abuse, and neglect. During the mother's trial, contention focused on the role of the forensic anthropologist (DB) as an expert witness and the admissibility of the antemortem fracture evidence. Defense attorneys questioned the board-certified forensic anthropologist's credentials to testify as an expert witness. The judge concurred, stating that only medical doctors could testify about the nature and cause of an injury. In addition, defense attorneys objected to admission of the forensic anthropology report that documented the fractured humerus and its estimated healing time. With the jury excused, debate ensued about the scientific validity of TSI estimation for antemortem fractures. The court considered TSI estimation as not yet recognized as a "generally accepted" scientifically-based analysis with known error rates or theoretical underpinning for the science. Questions were raised about the number of reference samples with identical variables (age of decedent, fracture type and location, known healing time) available for comparison. The expert witness was asked if she was "100% certain" that the TSI fell within this range, to which she replied "no." The end result was an exclusion of forensic anthropology testimony regarding all aspects of the fracture analysis except for the technical aspects of chain-of-custody receiving and processing of the humerus in the forensic anthropology laboratory.

This case study illustrates a number of important difficulties with regard to admissibility of expert forensic anthropology evidence and testimony and why the continued development of a sound scientific theoretical basis for forensic anthropology research is so important. These issues include ambiguities regarding the role of forensic anthropologists as expert witnesses and the nature of their evidence (both its reliability and validity) in the post-*Daubert* world. They also relate to inherent differences between science and the law in regard to their theoretical basis, methodological approaches, and expected outcomes. This has led to much tension between scientists and legal practitioners, rooted in the differential natures of their professions. These barriers between forensic anthropologists and the legal application of their evidence are discussed more fully in the succeeding sections.

16.2 Science and the law: The disconnect

As many forensic scientists will attest, testifying in court is often not a positive experience, regardless of the scientist's preparation and training. In fact, the interaction between forensic scientists and legal professionals has been described as being "fraught with much fear, loathing, pain and inefficiency" (Forrest and Kennedy, 2013:313), and many guidebooks (e.g., Feder and Houck, 2008; Wall, 2009) offer advice to forensic scientists about how to "survive" the court testimony experience. Concern about the relationship between science and the law is expressed not just by forensic scientists, but by legal professionals as well (e.g., Forrest and Kennedy, 2013; Smith, 2014; Vosk and Kennedy, 2014).

Forrest and Kennedy (2013) attribute much of the tension between science and the law to the explosion of new scientific advances and the court and its members' struggle to keep abreast of them. Most judges and, certainly, jurors are not trained in the sciences or statistical analysis, making it a challenge for scientific specialists to explain their observations and conclusions in court. This overall absence of understanding of science was emphasized as a problem in the National Academy of Sciences (NAS) (National Research Council, 2009) report:

> Lawyers and judges often have insufficient training and background in scientific methods, and they often fail to fully comprehend the approaches employed by different forensic science disciplines and the strengths and vulnerabilities of forensic science evidence offered during trials *(National Research Council, 2009:238).*

In many cases, attorneys' failures to comprehend scientific testimony and scientific validity may contribute to admissibility issues with regard to expert testimony (Lesciotto, 2015). Equally disconcerting is an inadequate understanding of the legal process on the part of many scientists, heralded by the numerous "how-to" manuals and courses available as court testimony survival guides (e.g., Feder and Houck, 2008; Wall, 2009; Mattson, 2012; Cohen, 2015).

The science/law disconnect also emanates from their inherent differences in foundational methods, objectives, and intended outcome. Science is a means for understanding and explaining observations at different levels of complexity by using different forms of logical reasoning and inference. As an open-ended method of investigation, it is an ongoing process—the continuous testing, evaluation, reevaluation, and interpretation of data ideally leads to better explanations of perceived patterns or regularities in the data.

The ultimate goal for science is to attain *truth*—an accurate, objective depiction of the subject of interest while recognizing and managing errors and biases. Thus, as Ousley and Hollinger (2012) note, scientific results (or conclusions) cannot stand alone—they must be interpreted and, even then, are not 100% certainties but are measures of *probabilities* awaiting further testing. In this sense, there is no such thing as "certainty" in science and forensic scientists in court cannot attest to it.

With regard to evidence, scientific evidence consists of the data collected through operationalizing the scientific method during the course of an investigation. Scientific evidence can support or refute, but not *prove* a hypothesis. This extends to negative evidence, which can be used to refute a hypothesis and is useful in science as a means to redirect experimentation and research toward a more positive direction (Walton, 2002).

In contrast, legal investigations are limited in time and scope. The law strives for finality (proof)—a clear end and decision to the legal process (Kennedy, 2014).

Legal evidence (specifically, evidence that is admitted in court) is information that can *prove* "a fact necessary to a legal decision" (Kennedy, 2014). It may be empirical, tangible, and physical or circumstantial, but not negative—negative evidence is an anathema in law (Walton, 2002). Successful attorneys have not only presented this evidence, but their interpretation of its meaning, in a form that is both persuasive and reasonable (in the perception of the jurors) and that provides a plausible explanation for the events in question (Walton, 2002; Gabbay and Woods, 2005). The jury reaches a determination of innocence or guilt based on the relevance and perceived credibility of this evidence.

In terms of overall objectives, the legal system has some built-in contradictions. In order for a case to come to trial, law enforcement and prosecuting attorneys have to build a probable case of guilt for the accused with the available evidence. However, during trial, the court's (and the trier's) primary goal is to avoid a wrongful conviction (Gabbay and Woods, 2005). Strict procedural rules and requirements (e.g., the Federal Rules of Evidence (FRE)) must be followed in order to ensure this. The accused is presumed to be innocent, with the burden of proof on the prosecution, and the standard of proof of guilt "beyond a reasonable doubt" (Walton, 2002:13). Thus, a primary goal of the legal system is to avoid judicial errors and biases in the courtroom, even at the expense of the truth, so that the chance of a wrongful conviction may be avoided. So, it can be said that "justice trumps truth" in a legal proceeding (Gabbay and Woods, 2005:256).

16.3 Science and the law: Commonalities

In spite of the differences discussed earlier, science and the law share a common dialogue, logical reasoning, and need for probabilistic evaluation of competing arguments/hypotheses to strengthen confidence in conclusions or findings. Understanding these commonalities offers the means to bridge the intellectual and methodological gap between the two arenas.

16.3.1 Legal and scientific dialogue

At first glance, forensic science and the law appear to engage in very different dialogues. In a legal proceeding, there is an argumentative discourse between the prosecution and defense. In the United States as well as Canada, Australia, and the

United Kingdom, legal proceedings are adversarial (Wall, 2009; Kennedy, 2014; Adam, 2016), with the prosecution and defense engaging in a dialogue regarding admitted evidence—"the most complete and deep information on the subject [of interest]…" (Walton, 2002:242). Walton (2002:335) calls this discourse "persuasion dialogue," where attorneys attack the arguments of the other side with the goal of persuading a third party (the trier—the judge or jury) the validity of *their* argument regarding the accused. Persuasion dialogue is the main type of dialogue in a trial and may induce anxiety in a forensic scientist at the receiving end of such dialogue.

Walton (2004) identifies four stages of dialogue that the law follows in some form: confrontation, opening, argumentation, and closing. Confrontation dialogue in a legal setting involves bringing charges against the accused, opening dialogue marks the beginning dialectic between the defense and prosecution, while argumentation dialogue continues it. Closing dialogue includes final arguments and the court's decision.

However, these types of dialogue are also seen in forensic science. Confrontation dialogue can be envisioned as the beginning of the scientific method, where hypothesis generation follows a new observation. Opening dialogue by the defense and prosecution mirrors the definition of if-then testable hypotheses by scientists using deductive reasoning. Argumentation dialogue in the scientist's lab involves evaluation of evidence, while closing dialogue relates to hypothesis support or rejection by the scientist. To succeed in the legal arena, forensic anthropologists need to not only recognize and understand the commonalities in these types of legal and scientific dialogue but also be able to conduct discourse in both.

16.3.2 Abductive reasoning

Recognition of similarities in logical reasoning in the legal and scientific arenas is equally important, for it is the logical basis for reasoning in evaluation of evidence that perhaps most closely links scientists (particularly forensic anthropologists) with the legal setting in which they operate; in both cases, it is abductive reasoning (Walton, 2001, 2008; Gabbay and Woods, 2005), as defined in Chapter 1. Since both forensic anthropology and criminal law are dealing with the reconstruction of past events and their interpretation, both rely on abductive argumentation or reasoning in the process of arriving at their conclusions. Both reason from the present to the past and reach conclusions based on available evidence. Most importantly, as Walton (2001:161) states, "the structure of the abductive argument form is more explicitly *dialectical*" (emphasis ours). As in a courtroom, "…each single abductive argument [to the best explanation] needs to be evaluated in a dialogue containing other abductive arguments as well" (Walton, 2001:162). So, the debate between the defense and prosecution, presenting their conflicting "best explanation" for the transpired events in question, is a model of abductive reasoning—a cornerstone of all logical reasoning in the historical sciences. In this sense, science and the law are theoretically united.

As noted in Chapter 1, abduction directs subsequent investigation and this is true both in science and the law. Scientific discoveries lead to inferences to the best explanation, which can ultimately be tested. Criminal investigations, by definition, are abductive in that they proceed from observed consequences to infer prior causes: "Causal reasoning, when analyzed abductively, provides a model that is useful for evaluating argumentation of the most common and important kind in legal evidence gathering" (Walton, 2004:174). The concept of causality is important, since addressing causal questions explains the process of creation of an object or event and helps answer the broader, epistemologically significant "how" and "why" questions about the subject of interest.

Causal arguments are based on the relationship (or correlation) between two variables (Walton, 2008). Variable B results from the influence of variable A (e.g., the gunshot wound on the victim (variable B) was caused by the firearm recovered from the scene (variable A)). When reconstructing historical events and processes, whether in the historical sciences or criminal investigations, causal arguments are those that are the most *plausible*, given the available evidence. Again, it is *presumed* that the most plausible arguments are the best explanations, but plausibility and presumption are not fixed—they are defeasible, based on new information. In a trial, however, only the admitted evidence (as identified by the judge) is under evaluation.

Abductive reasoning is most evident in the application of circumstantial evidence in legal cases: "Direct evidence proves a fact without inference... Circumstantial evidence is evidence from which a fact is reasonably inferred but not directly proven" (Klotter, 1992:67–68). Most trials involve the presentation of both direct and circumstantial evidence, on which the prosecution and defense elaborate in order to support their arguments for the guilt or innocence of the accused. The jury has to rely on abductive reasoning (inference) to evaluate the circumstantial evidence and its significance.

Once the jury reaches a consensus and is satisfied with the plausibility of opposing arguments, they render their decision (verdict). As Gabbay and Woods (2005:268) note, "A verdict in a criminal trial is not a conjecture. It is a finding; hence, something that is forwarded assertively. Even so, especially in cases built upon circumstantial evidence, verdicts are reached abductively. They are solutions to abductive problems." Gabbay and Woods (2005:273) go on to state in their Proposition 8.33 (beyond reasonable doubt): "The judicial question of proof beyond a reasonable doubt has a solution in the logic of abduction."

16.3.3 Probabilistic evaluation of the strength of evidence

Both scientific and legal evidence require probabilistic evaluation of their significance in a standardized manner. As has already been seen, definitions of legal and scientific "certainty" are often disparate, but both reflect the necessity to assess the strength of conclusions reached. As was seen in the case study at the introduction of this chapter, inadequate knowledge of evidence significance can contribute to its exclusion in court. Much inconsistency and lack of standardization in evaluation and presentation of the *weight* of scientific evidence has been noted across most forensic science disciplines, including forensic anthropology, to the point where Adam (2016:74) calls much of it "incoherent." Expressions of significance in the form of "match," "lack of exclusion," "is consistent with," "is probably or likely," "could have," or "unique" are vague, undefined, and sometimes used interchangeably. They also pretend to attach levels of significance to an opinion but may lead to unintended inferences by the court regarding an accurate judgment of the weight of the evidence. Equally problematic is that no consideration of the weight of *alternative* hypotheses is given. A more uniform and consistent approach has been called for (Steadman *et al.*, 2006; Adam, 2016).

Bayesian inference can form the basis for statistical models in both the scientific and legal arena, providing an important potential source of probabilistic strength for both scientific and legal evidence. Bayesian methods can lead to the creation and revision of statistical probabilities for hypotheses by incorporating both previous and newly-observed relevant evidence and can offer statements of probability regarding the "best overall explanation" derived from abductive reasoning (Gabbay and Woods, 2005; Taroni *et al.*, 2006). At its core are three concepts: prior probability, posterior probability, and likelihood (Prince and Konigsberg, 2008; Adam, 2016). Bayes' theorem is represented by the following formula (Taroni *et al.*, 2006; Emery, 2014; Taroni, 2014; Taroni and Biedermann, 2014):

$$P(H|E) = \frac{P(E|H) \times P(H)}{P(E)}$$

where

H, hypotheses whose probability is affected by data or evidence (E) (the proposed theory reconstructing how a forensic event occurred)

E, evidence, or data, not used in computing prior probability (P(H)) (the specific evidence forensically linked to the event described by H)

P(H), the *prior* probability of H before E is observed (the likelihood event H occurs without regard to any specific evidence)

P(H|E), the *posterior* probability of H, given E (the likelihood event H would occur given E's associated evidence)

P(E|H), the probability of E, given H, or the *likelihood* (or compatibility) of E given H (the likelihood the evidence (E) is associated with similar events)

P(E), the commonality of the evidence or data (the likelihood the evidence (E) occurs in any context)

The terms "relevance" and "plausibility" (probability) appear as components of Bayes' theorem and relate this theorem to both science and law. Bayesian inference can be used to assign probabilities to plausible hypotheses, or hypotheses about data that are believed, based on that available data. As Taroni *et al.* (2006:xiii) state, "...forensic scientists should consider probability theory as the fundamental concept to govern their reasoning." By turning hypothetical beliefs into numerical probabilities, we can provide statistical estimates for the validity of these beliefs, which, in turn, can satisfy the *Daubert* requirement of evidence having a known potential error rate (Konigsberg *et al.*, 1998; Steadman *et al.*, 2006; Grivas and Komar, 2008).

Probabilities calculated by Bayes' theorem can also be considered a vital component in the justification of what constitutes relevant evidence. For scientific evidence to be admissible in court, it must be relevant, meaning that it must contain knowledge that will increase or decrease the probability of the claim of either guilt or innocence. Factual evidence (e.g., regarding prior offenses of the accused) may not be admitted for presentation at trial by the judge if it is not deemed relevant to the specific case being tried. FRE 401 states: "'Relevant evidence' means evidence having any tendency to make the existence of any fact that is of consequence to the determination of the action *more probable* or *less probable* than it would be without the evidence" (Mueller and Kirkpatrick, 1988:33, emphasis ours). Thus, statistical information about probability may be used to justify the admittance of evidence as "relevant."

Bayes' theorem can be used to update probability estimates by incorporating new evidence (data) into the formula (Taroni *et al.*, 2006). The posterior probability now becomes the prior probability and a new posterior probability is calculated, with reference to the new data. So, as in science, the concept of probability estimation can be seen as a continuous process of alteration of previous hypotheses.

Bayes' theorem and likelihood ratios have been successfully applied to the evaluation of scientific evidence in the UK court system. Hypotheses, referred to as "propositions" (Adam, 2016), are accompanied by competing or alternative hypotheses, which are in need of logical evaluation. Each proposition (H0) is accompanied by an alternative proposition (H1), both of which undergo statistical evaluation through Bayesian methods to assess the strength of each. Bayes' theorem and likelihood ratios have also been successfully applied to the evaluation of scientific evidence (e.g., DNA) in the United States, albeit on a more limited scale.

In sum, while differing in their goals, science and the law do share some important, largely methodological practices. They both engage in dialogues and debates regarding explanations and reconstructions of past events (especially in the case of historical sciences). They both take pains to base their conclusions on relevant evidence that is obtained as objectively as possible. They both use similar logical processes (abduction) to arrive at their conclusions. They are both amenable to and, under legal and ethical stipulations, required to represent evidence and conclusions in a probabilistic form.

This background discussion examining scientific and legal commonalities and discordances has important repercussions for forensic anthropology both in terms of acceptance of forensic anthropologists as expert witnesses and admissibility of their evidence. These are discussed in the following text.

16.4 Forensic anthropologists as expert witnesses

Adam (2016:59) describes the goal of the scientist as an expert witness: "to provide a balanced and considered opinion on the evidence, thereby assisting the court in reaching a valid and sustainable verdict." An expert witness is defined as someone (a "scientist") who may provide specialized knowledge that falls outside or beyond the common knowledge of the court (Federal Rules of Evidence, 1975; Adam, 2016). In 2000, however, FRE 702 was amended to include expert testimony from those outside the traditional scientific realm (including those with "technical knowledge,") as long as they employed accepted scientific principles (Federal Rules of Evidence, 2000).

Qualifying as an expert witness can be considered an ethical obligation for forensic anthropologists—it is a forensic anthropologist's responsibility as an expert witness to be as knowledgeable as possible regarding the opinion that he or she is giving. The Board Certification process (through the American Board of Forensic Anthropology) provides diplomates the rigorous training, education, and experience required to meet that obligation and has constituted, for over 40 years, the "highest recognized level of professional qualification" in the discipline (www.theabfa.org). However, partly because it is not currently required to practice, a significant number of eligible forensic anthropologists have opted to not seek it (although this is beginning to change). Formal forensic anthropology certification will become increasingly important as forensic standards are developed under the auspices of the Organization of Scientific Area Committees (OSAC) and the American Academy of Forensic Sciences Academy Standards Board (AAFS ASB).

In the previously discussed case study, even though the testifying forensic anthropologist was board-certified, the court still questioned her credentials and her ability to make any statements regarding injury. This reflects a misunderstanding about what types of specialized training forensic anthropologists have and, in fact, the very core of what a forensic anthropologist does. Given the increasing emphasis in forensic anthropology on obtaining advanced (e.g., medical school) training in anatomy (see Langley and Dudzik, this volume) and experience working with soft tissue in a clinical (medical examiner) setting, a clarification and, arguably, redefinition and recognition of the specialized knowledge about which a forensic anthropologist can testify is needed. This is particularly true given that an increasing amount of forensic anthropology testimony is centered on trauma interpretation, often involving soft tissue (Boyd and Boyd, 2015; Lesciotto, 2015).

Adam (2016) discusses the roles and responsibilities of a qualifying expert witness who, by virtue of his or her status as an expert witness, can provide testimony not just about facts but also opinions. Since facts cannot speak for themselves, it is up to forensic anthropologists and other forensic scientists to speak for them in the form of an opinion. The court may have limited knowledge of their scientific area, creating a burden of responsibility on the part of forensic anthropologists to interpret and present evidence as clearly, logically, intelligently, objectively, honestly, and without bias as possible. This reflects, in fact, an ethical and professional obligation on the part of forensic scientists to serve the court, not the prosecution or defense. Other expert witness responsibilities include providing alternative opinions, hypotheses, and approaches that might assist in explaining the evidence, not speaking beyond one's expertise, and not omitting evidence that might not support an opinion (Adam, 2016).

16.5 Admissibility of forensic anthropology evidence in the post-*Daubert* world

Clarifying the relationship between science and the law is most critical at the juncture of admissibility of evidence and judgment regarding its accuracy and significance. Scientific evidence must be relevant, reliable, and valid to be admitted in court. Much has been written about the legal rulings that affect these requirements for acceptance of forensic anthropological evidence, beginning with *Frye v United States* (1923) and including *Daubert v Merrell Dow Pharmaceuticals, Inc.* (1993), *Kumho Tire Company, Ltd. v Carmichael* (1999), *Melendez-Diaz v Massachusetts* (2009), and others (Christensen, 2004; Grivas and Komar, 2008; Christensen and Crowder, 2009; Ousley and Hollinger, 2012; Christensen *et al.*, 2014; Lesciotto, 2015; Love and Fulginiti, 2017). In federal and many state courts, the *Daubert v Merrell Dow Pharmaceuticals, Inc.* (1993) ruling has been the most influential, requiring prior testing of a theory or technique following agreed-upon standards derived from the scientific method. Stipulations also include peer review through publication, known error rates, and the prior *Frye v United States* (1923) requirement for general acceptance by the wider scientific community (*Frye v United States*, 1923; *Daubert v Merrell Dow Pharmaceuticals, Inc.*, 1993; Lesciotto, 2015).

It has been anticipated that these more stringent *Daubert* standards for scientific evidence admissibility would lead to an increase in exclusion of evidence in courts following *Daubert* rules. Recent reviews of the impact of *Daubert* on anthropological evidence by Lesciotto (2015) and Love and Fulginiti (2017), however, suggest otherwise. According to these authors, there have been fewer than expected recorded *Daubert*-related exclusions of forensic anthropological expert testimony by the courts since 1993, even when the admissibility was challenged. Lesciotto records only 16 *Daubert* challenges to forensic anthropology testimony since 1993, with only one resulting in exclusion. However, she acknowledges that a larger number of forensic anthropology testimonies (with unknown outcomes) were likely not included in the search results—the case study at the beginning of this chapter being one. What is also apparent is an overall wide range of variability across federal and state courts in how *Daubert* is interpreted and enforced. Although the majority ($n = 34$) of states follow *Daubert* standards for admissibility of evidence, these guidelines are seen as a flexible framework for interpretation of evidence. The end result is that the outcome of admissibility determinations is, overall, widely variable and unpredictable (Lesciotto, 2015).

In spite of this variability, it is clear that acceptance of forensic anthropology evidence in court is ultimately dependent upon explicitly following the core tenets of the scientific method including explicit and valid hypothesis statements and predictions, statistical testing through comparison with appropriate reference samples, and quantitative assessment of error and strength of conclusions.

Boyd and Boyd's (2015 and Chapter 1, this volume) review of all forensic anthropology research articles from the *Journal of Forensic Sciences* (JFS) published over the past 25 years of *Daubert* shows that, overall, forensic anthropologists have met these requirements, but not consistently or overtly. Over this period, approximately 83% of JFS publications incorporated a research hypothesis into their study; however, only 29.3% of these articles did so explicitly, meaning that the authors specifically stated, usually in their introduction, their research question or hypothesis to be tested. More often than not, hypotheses (and the predictions derived from them) were implied, not stated. In terms of temporal trends, there has been a statistically significant increase in both the use of research hypotheses and their explicit statement across the two and a half decades. The vast majority of JFS authors have employed the scientific method in their research articles, and this is something that has remained consistent across the 25-year study review sample. However, up until recently, less than a third of authors explained their research methods explicitly, addressing testing, falsifiability, and probabilities of outcomes. Just in the past 5 years, this number has doubled and is undoubtedly related to the implications of living in a *Daubert*-era judicial system. In fact, many of the more recent research papers specifically cite the *Daubert* ruling as a justification for their research designs and analyses.

There has been a consistent use of statistical evaluation of data across this period, primarily in the form of univariate or multivariate assessments of hypothesis acceptance or rejection, and this has been a major impetus for recent research in forensic anthropology in the post-*Daubert* world (Boyd and Boyd, 2015). Application of statistical (probability) theory to evaluate these data was and still is a cornerstone of the majority of research in forensic anthropology.

Bayesian statistical methods have been regularly used in forensic anthropology hypothesis testing. Bayesian statistics have been used in forensic anthropology research to estimate age at death from the dentition (Lucy *et al.*, 1996; Prince *et al.*, 2008; Schmitt *et al.*, 2010), subadult cranium (Lottering *et al.*, 2016), clavicle (Langley-Shirley and Jantz, 2010), ribs (Kimmerle and Konigsberg, 2004—actually multi-trait ribs and teeth), shoulder (Brennaman *et al.*, 2017), and innominate (Kimmerle *et al.*, 2008; Hens and Godde, 2016; Miranker, 2016) (also see Aykroyd *et al.*, 1997, 1999; Konigsberg and Frankenberg, 2002; Lucy *et al.*, 2002; Schmitt *et al.*, 2002; Konigsberg *et al.*, 2008; Garvin and Passalacqua 2012). They have also been used in sex (Konigsberg and Hens, 1998), ancestry (Klales and Kenyhercz, 2015), stature estimation (Konigsberg *et al.*, 1998; Ross and Konigsberg, 2002), and pathology-based personal ID (e.g., Cawley and Steadman, 2017).

However, these methods have not been routinely applied by forensic anthropologists to evaluate the weight of their evidence in court. Probabilistic statements of the strength of forensic anthropology evidence and the generation of known error rates have not been routinely applied to forensic anthropology evidence—Steadman *et al.* (2006) points out that forensic anthropologists have, in the past, tended not to quantify the strength of their evidence. While assessments of personal ID and the "uniqueness" of a biological profile have undergone probabilistic evaluation (through Bayesian likelihood ratios) with regard to appropriate reference samples and "populations at large" (Steadman *et al.*, 2006), a significant number of research areas exist in forensic anthropology for which these *Daubert* requirements have not been met. This includes a significant amount of research on antemortem and perimortem trauma. The estimation of TSI illustrated in the previous case study serves as an important example. Without a knowledge of the known TSI of a comparative reference population for estimation of strength of evidence and associated error, this research must be viewed as deficient in scientific rigor. Development of an antemortem bone fracture archive (e.g., Boyd, Chapter 9, this volume; Boyd *et al.*, 2016) is a beginning step toward this goal. Further validation research and development of additional reference populations are needed in other areas of antemortem and perimortem trauma as well as postmortem processes to mitigate these deficiencies and increase our ability to meet *Daubert* requirements for evidence admissibility.

16.6 The legal application of forensic anthropology: Why theory matters

Although one of the primary conclusions of the 2009 NAS report was the need in numerous forensic science disciplines for "serious research about their underlying theories and the ability of their methods to support conclusions to which their experts testify" (Kennedy, 2014), the end result of these criticisms as well as court rulings like *Daubert* has been an increased focus on doing "good science," particularly in forensic anthropology (Ousley and Hollinger, 2012). Ultimately, Lesciotto (2015) notes that recent self-regulating efforts by many forensic anthropologists to refine methodological procedures and engage in testing and improved statistical analyses "…may have allowed the field to stay a few steps ahead of the legal requirements for the admissibility of expert testimony" (Lesciotto, 2015:554).

It has been argued here that continued and explicit development of a sound theoretical and scientific basis for forensic anthropology is the key to avoiding its misrepresentation and evidence exclusion in court. Addressing and strengthening the science within forensic anthropology can ameliorate many of the antagonisms between scientists and the judicial system and address the discipline's perceived shortcomings as it is applied in legal settings.

There are several points that, if addressed, can enhance the status and role of forensic anthropologists as forensic scientists in the view of the legal system and, importantly, among ourselves:

- Recognize the strong theoretical basis for the research and analysis that forensic anthropologists (and archaeologists) do (Boyd and Boyd, 2011; Chapter 1, this volume). Through educational and professional presentations, clarify this theoretical grounding in the perception of our non-forensic anthropological colleagues and other nonanthropological forensic scientists and legal experts.
- Expand our validation studies of time-honored traditional as well as more recent forensic anthropology methods to provide more explicit evaluation of their effectiveness that can be stated in court.
- Test the applicability and efficiency of new, innovative methods drawn from other fields in answering questions relevant to forensic anthropology. This concept is suggested and applied by several authors in this volume. Actively explore the interdisciplinary nature, both in theory and method, of the goals of forensic anthropologists.
- Stress the utilization of well-known, established statistical and probability determination methods in the evaluation and presentation of research results in forms that allow them to be widely understood by all forensic scientists and legal specialists. Expand known population reference frequencies for forensic anthropological data (e.g., fracture data) to enhance the validity of these statistical comparisons.
- Support and follow standards and best practice methods in forensic anthropology vetted by OSAC and the Anthropology Consensus Body of the AAFS ASB.
- Obtain the highest education and training possible as a forensic anthropologist, including board certification.
- When possible, engage with and educate law enforcement and legal professionals about the roles and capabilities of forensic anthropologists. This often occurs on a case-by-case basis, but we should explore more comprehensive methods, such as periodic workshops for law enforcement officers and other legal experts (based on available funding from legal or educational institutions).

This last suggestion is perhaps the most important in ensuring that the expertise of forensic anthropologists is realized and their research, analyses, and opinions as expert witnesses are admitted in court.

16.7 Final comments

There is a clear need for mutual understanding between science and the law that both sides must work hard to achieve. Smith notes, for example, "To avoid unnecessary acquittals of the guilty and wrongful convictions of the innocent due to faulty forensic science evidence, police and prosecutors must work harder to think and act more like scientists, constantly critiquing their theories and tentative conclusions, and learn how to detect and eliminate the implicit biases in themselves and in the forensic experts they must increasingly rely on" (Smith, 2014). Likewise, it is an obligation on the part of forensic anthropologists to achieve and maintain their highest expert credentials, engage in scientifically valid and theoretically sound evaluation of evidence, and present this evidence objectively and fairly, with quantitative assessments of its strength. Most important is for forensic anthropologists to engage in legal discourse and achieve and maintain cognizance of the legal process in which they actively participate.

Most forensic scientists and legal professionals realize they need to work together to successfully accomplish the goals of the legal process. By understanding the theoretical base and methodological processes of each other, successful collaboration and mutual respect can be enhanced.

Acknowledgments

The authors sincerely thank Bill Baden and Christian Crowder for reviewing and providing helpful comments on a previous draft of this chapter.

References

Adam, C. (2016) *Forensic Evidence in Court: Evaluation and Scientific Opinion*. Wiley, Chichester, UK.

Aykroyd, R. G., Lucy, D., Pollard, A. M., and Solheim, T. (1997) Regression analysis in adult age estimation. *American Journal of Physical Anthropology* **104**, 259–265.

Aykroyd, R. G., Lucy, D., Pollard, A. M., Roberts, C. A., and Roberts, A. (1999) Nasty, brutish, but not necessarily short: a reconstruction of the statistical methods used to calculate age-at-death from adult human skeletal and dental age indicators. *American Antiquity* **64**, 55–70.

Boyd, C. C. and Boyd, D. C. (2011) Theory and the scientific basis for forensic anthropology. *Journal of Forensic Sciences* **58**, 1407–1415.

Boyd, C. C. and Boyd, D. C. (2015) Theory in forensic anthropology: a retrospective and look forward. *Proceedings of the 67th American Academy of Forensic Sciences* **XXI**, 193–194.

Boyd, D., Boyd, C., and Roller, S. (2016) Pediatric antemortem healing standards based on microscopic analysis of fractures in known forensic child abuse cases. *Proceedings of the 68th Scientific Session of the American Academy of Forensic Sciences* **XXII**, 130.

Brennaman, A. L., Love, K. R., Brethard, J. D., and Pokines, J. T. (2017) A Bayesian approach to age-at-death estimation from osteoarthritis of the shoulder in modern Americans. *Journal of Forensic Sciences* **62**, 573–584.

Cawley W. D. and Steadman, D. W. (2017) Identity by the numbers: cancerous lesions and likelihood ratios. *Proceedings of the 69th American Academy of Forensic Sciences* **XXIII**, 140.

Christensen, A. M. (2004) The impact of Daubert: implications for testimony and research in forensic anthropology (and the use of frontal sinuses in personal identification). *Journal of Forensic Sciences* **49**, 427–430.

Christensen, A. M. and Crowder, C. M. (2009) Evidentiary standards for forensic anthropology. *Journal of Forensic Sciences* **54**, 1211–1216.

Christensen, A. M., Crowder, C. M., Ousley, S. D., and Houck, M. M. (2014) Error and its meaning in forensic science. *Journal of Forensic Sciences* **59**(1), 123–126.

Cohen, K. S. (2015) *Expert Witnessing and Scientific Testimony*, 2nd ed. CRC Press, Boca Raton, FL.

Daubert v. Merrell Dow Pharmaceuticals, Inc. (1993) 509 US 579. United States Supreme Court.

Emery, A. F. (2014) Epistemological robustness in quantitative results: measurement uncertainty. Paper presented in Workshop No. 16, 66th Annual Scientific Meeting, American Academy of Forensic Sciences, Seattle, Washington. *Proceedings of the American Academy of Forensic Sciences* **XX**, 21.

Feder, H. A. and Houck, M. M. (2008) *Feder's How to Succeed as an Expert Witness*, 4th ed. CRC Press, Boca Raton, FL.

Federal Rules of Evidence (FRE), 702 (1975) Publ. L No. 93-595, § 1, 88 Stat. 1926. Effective January 2, 1975.

Federal Rules of Evidence (FRE), 702 (2000) Publ. L. No. 93-595, § 1, 88 Stat. 1926. Amended April 17, 2000. Effective December 1, 2000.

Forrest, A. R. W. and Kennedy, R. T. (2013) Jurisprudence. In: *Forensic Science: Current Issues, Future Directions (ed. D. H. Ubelaker)*. Wiley-Blackwell, Chichester, UK. pp. 310–336.

Frye v. United States. (1923) 293F, 1013, 1014. District of Columbia Court of Appeals.

Gabbay, D. M. and Woods, J. (2005) *The Reach of Abduction: Insight and Trial, a Practical Logic of Cognitive Systems*, vol. 2. Elsevier, Amsterdam.

Garvin, H. M. and Passalacqua, N. V. (2012) Current practices by forensic anthropologists in adult skeletal age estimation. *Journal of Forensic Sciences* **57**(2), 427–433.

Grivas, C. R. and Komar, D. A. (2008) *Kumho, Daubert*, and the nature of scientific inquiry: implications for forensic anthropology. *Journal of Forensic Sciences* **53**, 771–776.

Hens, S. M. and Godde, K. (2016) Auricular surface aging: comparing two methods that assess morphological change in the ilium with Bayesian analyses. *Journal of Forensic Sciences* **61**(S1), S30–S38.

Kennedy, R. (2014) Jurisprudential goals and decision making. Paper presented in Workshop No. 16, 66th Annual Scientific Meeting, American Academy of Forensic Sciences, Seattle, Washington. *Proceedings of the American Academy of Forensic Sciences* **XX**, 21.

Kimmerle, E. H. and Konigsberg, L. W. (2004) Estimating individual age-at-death parameters through multi-trait Bayesian analysis. *Proceedings of the 73rd Annual Meeting of the American Association of Physical Anthropology*, April 14–17, 2004. American Association of Physical Anthropology, Tampa, FL, 45.

Kimmerle, E. H., Konigsberg, L. W., Jantz, R. L., and Barybar, J. P. (2008) Analysis of age-at-death estimation using pubic symphyseal data. *Journal of Forensic Sciences* **53**(3), 558–568.

Klales, A. R. and Kenyhercz, M. W. (2015) Morphological assessment of ancestry using cranial macromorphoscopics. *Journal of Forensic Sciences* **60**(1), 13–20.

Klotter, J. C. (1992) *Criminal Evidence*. 5th edn. Anderson Publishing, Cincinnati, OH.

Konigsberg, L. W. and Frankenberg, S. R. (2002) Deconstructing death in paleodemography. *American Journal of Physical Anthropology* **117**, 297–309.

Konigsberg, L. W. and Hens, S. M. (1998) Use of ordinal categorical variables in skeletal assessment of sex from the cranium. *American Journal of Physical Anthropology* **107**, 97–112.

Konigsberg, L. W., Hens, S. M., Jantz, L. M., and Jungers, W. L. (1998) Stature estimation and calibration: Bayesian and maximum likelihood perspectives in physical anthropology. *Yearbook of Physical Anthropology* **41**, 65–92.

Konigsberg, L., Herrmann, N., Wescott, D., and Kimmerle, E. (2008) Estimation and evidence in forensic anthropology: age-at-death. *Journal of Forensic Sciences* **53**(3), 541–557.

Kumho Tire Company, Ltd. v. Carmichael. (1999) 526 US 137. United States Supreme Court.

Langley-Shirley, N. and Jantz, R. L. (2010) A Bayesian approach to age estimation in modern Americans from the clavicle. *Journal of Forensic Sciences* **55**(3), 571–583.

Lesciotto, K. M. (2015) The impact of *Daubert* on the admissibility of forensic anthropology testimony. *Journal of Forensic Sciences* **60**, 549–555.

Lottering, N., MacGregor, D. M., Alston, C. L., Watson, D., and Gregory, L. S. (2016) Introducing computed tomography age standards for age estimation of modern Australian subadults using postnatal ossification timings of select cranial and cervical sites. *Journal of Forensic Sciences* **61**(S1), S39–S52.

Love J. and Fulginiti, L. C. (2017) Evolution of forensic anthropology: influences of court rulings, legislative actions and social trends. *Proceedings of the American Academy of Forensic Sciences* **XXIII**, 280–281.

Lucy, D., Aykroyd, R. G., Pollard, A. M., and Solheim, T. A. (1996) Bayesian approach to adult human age estimation from dental observations by Johanson's age changes. *Journal of Forensic Sciences* **41**, 189–194.

Lucy, D., Aykroyd, R. G., and Pollard, A. M. (2002) Nonparametric calibration for age estimation. *Journal of the Royal Statistical Society: Series C* **51**, 183–196.

Mattson, J. V. (2012) *Effective Expert Witnessing: Practices for the 21st Century*, 5th ed. CRC Press, Boca Raton, FL.

Melendez-Diaz v. Massachusetts. (2009) 129 S. Ct. 2527. U.S. Supreme Court No. 07-591.

Miranker, M. (2016) A comparison of different age estimation methods of the adult pelvis. *Journal of Forensic Sciences* **61**(5), 1173–1179.

Mueller, C. and Kirkpatrick, L. (1988) *Federal Rules of Evidence*. Little, Brown, and Company, Boston, MA.

National Research Council. (2009) *Strengthening Forensic Science in the United States: A Path Forward*. The National Academies Press, Washington, DC.

Ousley, S. D. and Hollinger, R. E. (2012) The pervasiveness of *Daubert*. In: *A Companion to Forensic Anthropology* (ed. D. C. Dirkmaat). Wiley-Blackwell, Chichester, UK, pp. 654–665.

Prince, D. A. and Konigsberg, L. W. (2008) New formulae for estimating age-at-death in the Balkans utilizing Lamendin's dental technique and Bayesian analysis. *Journal of Forensic Sciences* **53**(3), 578–587.

Prince, D. A., Kimmerle, E. H., and Konigsberg, L. A. (2008) Bayesian approach to estimate skeletal age-at-death utilizing dental wear. *Journal of Forensic Sciences* **53**, 588–593.

Ross, A. H. and Konigsberg, L. W. (2002) New formulae for estimating stature in the Balkans. *Journal of Forensic Sciences* **47**, 165–167.

Schmitt, A., Murail, P., Cunha, E., and Rougé, D. (2002) Variability of the pattern of aging on the human skeleton: evidence from bone indicators and implications on age at death estimation. *Journal of Forensic Sciences* **47**, 1203–1209.

Schmitt, A., Saliba-Serre, B., Tremblay, M., and Laurent, M. (2010) An evaluation of statistical methods for determination of age at death using dental root translucency and periodontosis. *Journal of Forensic Sciences* **55**(3), 590–596.

Smith, F. C. (2014) Scientific and legal inferences: complimentary or competing processes? Paper presented in Workshop No. 16, 66th Annual Scientific Meeting, American Academy of Forensic Sciences, Seattle, Washington. *Proceedings of the American Academy of Forensic Sciences* **XX**, 21.

Steadman, D., Adams, B., and Konigsberg, L. W. (2006) Statistical basis for positive identification in forensic anthropology. *American Journal of Physical Anthropology* **131**(1), 15–26.

Taroni, F. (2014) Bayesian networks as tools and models of forensic inference. Paper presented in Workshop No. 16, 66th Annual Scientific Meeting, American Academy of Forensic Sciences, Seattle, Washington. *Proceedings of the American Academy of Forensic Sciences* **XX**, 21.

Taroni, F. and Biedermann, A. (2014) Bayesian inference in forensic science. Paper presented in Workshop No. 16, 66th Annual Scientific Meeting, American Academy of Forensic Sciences, Seattle, Washington. *Proceedings of the American Academy of Forensic Sciences* **XX**, 21.

Taroni, F., Aitken, C., Garbolini, P., and Biedermann, A. (2006) *Bayesian Networks and Probabilistic Inference in Forensic Science*. Wiley, Chichester, England.

Vosk, T. W. and Kennedy, R. T. (2014) Science, law, and the inferential process—the epistemology of scientific conclusions and their role in the legal fact-finding process. Workshop No. 16, 66th Annual Scientific Meeting, American Academy of Forensic Sciences, Seattle, Washington. *Proceedings of the American Academy of Forensic Sciences* **XX**, 21.

Wall, W. (2009) *Forensic Science in Court: The Role of the Expert Witness*. Wiley-Blackwell, Chichester, UK.

Walton, D. N. (2001) Abductive, presumptive, and plausible arguments. *Informal Logic* **21**, 141–169.

Walton, D. N. (2002) *Legal Argumentation and Evidence*. The Pennsylvania State University Press, University Park.

Walton, D. N. (2004) *Abductive Reasoning*. The University of Alabama Press, Tuscaloosa.

Walton, D. N. (2008) *Informal Logic: A Pragmatic Approach*, 2nd edn. Cambridge University Press, New York.

www.theabfa.org.

CHAPTER 17

Epilogue: Theory and science in forensic anthropology: Avenues for further research and development

C. Clifford Boyd Jr[1] and Donna C. Boyd[1,2]
[1] *Department of Anthropological Sciences, Radford University Forensic Science Institute, Radford University, Radford, VA, USA*
[2] *Department of Biomedical Science, Virginia Tech Carilion School of Medicine, Roanoke, VA, USA*

17.1 The science of forensic anthropology

When perceived as simply an applied aspect of biological anthropology, forensic anthropology has often been characterized as a technical field devoid of theory and, therefore, lacking a solid scientific foundation (Adovasio, 2012) or, at least, so methodologically complex that theoretical models for what forensic anthropologists do might not be possible (Nordby, 2002). However, as forensic anthropology becomes more recognized as a distinct discipline, there is a critical need for its strong but often unstated theoretical framework and scientific basis to be acknowledged and further developed—this is what this volume is all about.

Scientifically-based disciplines are those that have at their foundation empirically testable theories. Ideas and organizational concepts (theories) form the basis of all epistemological and empirical examinations of the material, physical world. Scientific theories are basic premises or postulates that can be used to explain and predict empirical phenomena—we have to *think* about what we observe and propose hypotheses explaining it before we can understand it. Thus, theory drives our collection, evaluation, and interpretation of physical data, the analysis of which is the basis of science.

As we have shown in this volume, theory is alive and well in our discipline—directing and influencing forensic anthropological data collection and analysis and stimulating further research in virtually every specialty within it. Foundational, interpretive, and methodological forms of theory comprise the basis of forensic anthropology, interacting with each other in an informed dynamic. The methods we use as forensic anthropologists in the field and laboratory influence our interpretations of the data we analyze. These interpretations, in turn, can strengthen

Forensic Anthropology: Theoretical Framework and Scientific Basis, First Edition.
Edited by C. Clifford Boyd Jr and Donna C. Boyd.

and build a more robust foundational theory. These theoretical approaches, when joined with abductive, inductive, and deductive logical reasoning, form integral parts of the theory building process.

The chapters in this volume have illustrated the vibrant but at times unrecognized theoretical underpinnings initiated by our mentors and undergoing further development by professional forensic anthropologists today. As a discipline originating from (and still closely related to) not only biological anthropology but also clinical medicine and anatomy (Langley and Dudzik, Chapter 6), forensic anthropology is grounded in the overarching foundational theory of biological evolution and resultant human variation (Darwin, 1859; Mayr, 2001). Much of the basis for our estimation of the biological profile (e.g., age, sex, and ancestry) derives from this theoretical underpinning. Ousley *et al.*, for example, illustrate how morphoscopic and morphometric population variability underpin and influence concepts of social *and* biological race. Langley and Dudzik as well as Crowder *et al.* show how foundational principles of bone development and growth provide a scientific basis for age estimation, while Chesson *et al.* rely on principles of individual and population variation to assist with identifications of geographic origin. Interpretive and methodological theories often form the core of forensic anthropological research, as it is applied in the investigation of cases. This is best exemplified by Berryman *et* al.'s theoretical modeling of perimortem fractures from a knowledge of both extrinsic and intrinsic variables. Likewise, Love and Soto Martinez's and Boyd's interpretations of non-accidental pediatric deaths depend upon on interpretive theories (and their resultant predictions) surrounding bone fracture, whether antemortem or perimortem. Taphonomic observations, as Wescott and Boyd and Baden indicate, are heavily reliant on interpretive theories explaining postmortem processes, including those relating to decomposition and determination of PMI. Finally, advances in the often overlooked area of methodological theory are well-illustrated by many chapters in this volume, most notably Williams and Davis' application of GIS to sharp force trauma analysis and Chesson *et al.*'s extensive detailing of stable isotope methodology for isoscape estimation.

As seen in many of the chapters of this volume, borrowing methods and theories from other disciplines is a long-standing characteristic of forensic anthropology and is one that should not be criticized or dismissed but supported and encouraged. Much has been learned, for example, about fracture healing and dating through biomedical theories of bone biology. Perimortem trauma (blunt force, sharp force, gunshot) is informed by biomechanical theories from physics and engineering, while theories derived from archaeology, geology, geography, soil science, and others can be quite useful in providing a more accurate and fuller interpretation of decompositional and other postmortem events.

Acknowledgement and development of the theories underlying our methods and analyses not only drive research but also lead to a sounder scientific foundation in our discipline. As Boyd and Boyd emphasize in Chapter 16, this ultimately provides us with more solid credibility as expert witnesses and a greater likelihood of admissibility of our evidence in court. And as we saw in the preliminary chapters of this volume (Winburn, Warren *et al.*, Blau), recognizing bias associated with our methods is an integral part of this theory building that provides us with an even stronger legal and scientific footing. Thus, theory is critical to the success of everything that we, as forensic anthropologists, do.

17.2 Looking forward

While current research is based on a rich repertoire of both a borrowed and unique theoretical framework, some additional avenues for forensic anthropology theory development are suggested here. For example, with DNA more commonly being applied to issues of identification, an anthropological focus on research in antemortem, perimortem, and postmortem processes and how better to define, describe, and explain them is heralded. Accurate interpretation of the signatures of these processes (particularly antemortem bone repair, perimortem fracture dynamics, and taphonomy) is strengthened through theoretical and methodological development based on a solid foundation of empirical research.

The traditional emphasis in forensic anthropology on estimating aspects of the biological profile requires further open exploration and acknowledgment of the theoretical basis underlying the methods and analyses used for age, sex, ancestry, and stature estimation. Cognitive bias should be recognized and mitigated (as much as is feasible) openly and objectively along this process—confronting past and present bias is especially critical in conducting meaningful research on patterned human variation associated with biological race and furthering our understanding of its relationship to social race in the context of modern world problems. Validation studies of our major identification methods necessitate quantitative assessments of error and bias and the statistical strength of these assessments for court testimony. Newly proposed methods of identification should also have their theoretical basis explicitly outlined and their probabilities defined through testing.

Finally, we encourage forensic anthropologists not only to engage in careful consideration and realistic assessments of the methods and theories they use in their research but also to thoughtfully consider the broader and more philosophical aspects of their research as an expression and exemplification of the epistemology of science. As a lens through which we evaluate and come to understand the complexities of our world, science is predicated on both ignorance and curiosity—ignorance about what we don't know and curiosity about how we can mitigate these unknowns. The "why" questions about the research we do and how we conduct it are just as important as the questions embedded within the research itself. Ultimately, this continual reflection on the nature of science and how our research embodies it provides our discipline with the solid scientific foundation and framework to carry it forward. As the main goal of this volume, we have endeavored to provide the impetus for a continuation of this conversation about the evolving scientific and theoretical basis for forensic anthropology and look forward to the maturation and strengthening of our discipline through this important dialogue.

References

Adovasio, J.M. (2012) An "outsider" look at forensic anthropology. In: *A Companion to Forensic Anthropology* (ed. D.C. Dirkmaat). Wiley-Blackwell, Chichester, UK, pp. 683–689.

Darwin, C. (1859) *The Origin of Species (reprinted 1998)*. The Modern Library, New York.

Mayr, E. (2001) *What Evolution Is*. Basic Books, New York.

Nordby, J.J. (2002) Is forensic taphonomy scientific? In: *Advances in Forensic Taphonomy: Method, Theory and Archaeological Perspectives* (eds. W.D. Haglund and M.H. Sorg). CRC Press, Boca Raton, FL, pp. 31–42.

Index

Forensic Anthropology: Theoretical Framework and Scientific Basis, First Edition.
Edited by C. Clifford Boyd Jr and Donna C. Boyd.

Printed and bound by CPI Group (UK) Ltd, Croydon, CR0 4YY
17/09/2026
14964269-0008